Prevention's

THE
SUGAR
SOLUTION

YOUR SYMPTOMS ARE REAL—
AND YOUR SOLUTION IS HERE

By the Editors of **Prevention.** magazine with Ann Fittante, MS, RD

RODALE

©2007 by Rodale Inc.

All rights reserved. No part of this publication may be reproduced or transmitted in any form or by any means, electronic or mechanical, including photocopying, recording, or any other information storage and retrieval system, without the written permission of the publisher.

Prevention is a registered trademark of Rodale Inc.

Printed in the United States of America
Rodale Inc. makes every effort to use acid-free ♾, recycled paper ♻.

Writer: Sarí Harrar
Exercise photographs by Hilmar
Book design by Christina Gaugler

ISBN-13 978–1–59486–693–7
ISBN-10 1–59486–693–7

4   6   8   10   9   7   5   3   hardcover

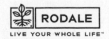

We inspire and enable people to improve their lives and the world around them

For more of our products visit **rodalestore.com** or call 800-848-4735

CONTENTS

INTRODUCTION

I f one simple thing could energize you within hours, soothe cranki-
ness and fatigue within a day, allow you to (finally!) shed extra pounds,
and dramatically reduce your lifetime risk of heart attack, stroke, and
dementia—you'd say it's magic. Or a wonder drug.

The good news is, this wonderful "something" is real—and it can
change your life without drugs or magic. All you need to do is *take
charge of your blood sugar.*

Controlling blood sugar isn't just for people with diabetes. It's for
everybody—women, men, and even kids who want to stay fit, healthy,
and happy. Luckily, getting there is a delicious, fun, and fascinating
journey with Prevention's *The Sugar Solution.*

This book is for you if:

- You rely on goodies and sweet beverages to get you through the
  dreaded 3:00 p.m. slump, yet you feel groggier and even more tired
  by 4:45.
- Your attempts to lose weight end in late-night refrigerator raids.
- You want to do all you can to lower your risk for heart attack, stroke,
  and dementia.
- You're a woman with fertility problems or a history of pregnancy
  diabetes.
- You are slightly overweight, have slightly high blood sugar, and have
  slightly elevated cholesterol or triglycerides—a deadly combination
  overlooked by most family doctors.
- You're looking for an eating plan for life that balances protein, "good"
  fats, and carbohydrates so that you can still enjoy the foods you like
  and even eat out without guilt.

Inside this book, you'll find cutting-edge medical research on blood
sugar, insulin resistance, and diabetes and related conditions. Top

medical researchers are discovering that well before blood sugar reaches levels most doctors consider dangerous, your risk of heart attack and stroke—two of America's top three killers—may be many times higher than normal. Even newer evidence links out-of-whack blood sugar and the condition behind it—insulin resistance—to loss of mental functioning and perhaps even cancer.

You'll also find a satisfying eating plan based on low-glycemic-index foods, plus an exercise program that fits your fitness level and schedule and stress-relief tips to further control blood sugar. Try it! You can lose weight, safeguard your future health, and sail through your busiest day with energy to spare.

1

WHY BLOOD SUGAR MATTERS

CHAPTER 1

THE "SWEET" CRISIS

Imagine pouring a 5-pound bag of sugar down your throat. Absurd, right? Wrong. New research shows that this is how much sugar each American man, woman, and child gets each month—and most of it doesn't come from the sugar bowl. Sweeteners go by more than 50 names and hide out in virtually all processed foods, from your morning doughnut to those lunchtime baked beans, from fruit-flavored yogurt to the ketchup on your burger.

Added sugars in the American diet have grown exponentially since the early 1900s—by more than 2,100 percent—adding calories and edging out more nutritious fare. Researchers say it's no coincidence that as the food we eat grows sweeter, rates of overweight and blood sugar problems—including insulin resistance, metabolic syndrome, prediabetes, full-blown type 2 diabetes, and even pregnancy diabetes—have soared.

Sugar entwines us in a love-hate relationship. Your body needs a steady supply of blood sugar, the primary fuel burned by your cells. It plays a central role in physical and mental well-being. Your brain, for example, runs almost entirely on blood sugar. Your muscles can burn fat in a pinch, but they prefer blood sugar (glucose) for zip. A baby growing in a mother's womb relies on it, too.

But the carbohydrates we eat and drink—the source of virtually all blood sugar—are more treacherous than ever before. Refined carbs (white bread, cakes, and snack foods) can make blood sugar skyrocket

RISK CHECK: DOC, HOW'S MY BLOOD SUGAR?

We encourage you to call your doctor soon to schedule a fasting blood sugar test, one of the easiest in-office screenings (and one that's covered by most insurance plans). Far too many Americans live with undiagnosed type 2 diabetes and unrecognized prediabetes—uncontrolled high blood sugar that accelerates your chances of serious, life-threatening complications. Here's what you need to know.

Test as Soon as Possible If You Have Any of These Risk Factors for Type 2 Diabetes

- Family history of type 2 diabetes
- Overweight
- History of diabetes during pregnancy (gestational diabetes) or having a baby weighing 9 pounds or more at birth
- Low HDL cholesterol level (under 50 for women, below 40 for men), high total cholesterol (above 200), or triglycerides above 150
- High blood pressure (over 130/85)
- Age over 45
- Inactive lifestyle
- African American, Latino, Asian, Native American, or Pacific Island ethnicity

Choose the Best Test for You

The Sugar Solution recommends a fasting plasma glucose test for most people. For this check, you will first fast for 8 to 12 hours, then visit the doctor's office or a lab to have your blood drawn. Your blood sugar is normal if the result is 99 milligrams of glucose per deciliter of blood (mg/dl) or lower; prediabetic if your sugar level is between 100 and 125 mg/dl; or potentially diabetic if it's over 125 mg/dl (your doctor will retest, on another day, before diagnosing type 2 diabetes).

If you are pregnant, experiencing infertility or miscarriage problems, or concerned about prediabetes despite a normal fasting check, your doctor will perform an oral glucose tolerance test. You'll fast, then drink a sugary concoction of 75 grams of glucose (100 grams for a pregnant woman). Blood is drawn before you drink and up to four times afterward. Prediabetes is indicated when readings after 2 hours are between 140 and 199 mg/dl. Readings of 200 mg/dl or higher are considered indicative of full-blown diabetes. You've got gestational diabetes if you have any two of these results: fasting blood sugar over 95 mg/dl; blood sugar of 180 mg/dl 1 hour after drinking the sugary beverage; 155 mg/dl after 2 hours; 140 mg/dl after 3 hours.

If you couldn't fast or weren't expecting a blood sugar check at your doctor's appointment, your doctor may perform a random plasma glucose test. This nonfasting check is the least sensitive blood-sugar check; it can miss slightly elevated sugar levels, making it a poor choice for people concerned about prediabetes. Your blood sugar is considered normal if the result is 140 mg/dl or lower and diabetic at 200 mg/dl or higher. If you opt for this test, ask for a follow-up fasting check to confirm your results.

Test in the Morning

You're apt to get a truer picture of where your blood sugar stands if you get tested in the morning as opposed to the afternoon. This realization emerged when scientists from the National Institute of Diabetes and Digestive and Kidney Diseases compared results of fasting plasma glucose tests given to 12,800 people. Only half the people with morning levels high enough to qualify as diabetic would have been detected if their tests had been done in the afternoon.

And Test Again

If your blood sugar is normal, your doctor will probably recommend rechecking it in 1 to 3 years. If you are at risk for diabetes, however, ask for annual rechecks to catch creeping sugar levels early, when lifestyle changes can do the most to control them. If you have prediabetes or diabetes, follow the steps in Chapters 21 and 22 to track and lower your levels.

to dangerous levels. And there's growing evidence that high-fructose corn syrup (HFCS), now the most ubiquitous sweetener in the American food supply, is directly linked to the nation's twin epidemics of overweight and diabetes. HFCS's role? This sweetener seems to bypass the body's "I feel full" mechanisms. In a study of 93,000 women, Harvard School of Public Health researchers recently linked a 10-pound weight gain and 83 percent higher diabetes risk directly to the consumption of HFCS.

Add other 21st-century factors that also pack on pounds and disrupt blood sugar levels—including big portions, fatty fast foods, and inactivity—and you've got a blood sugar crisis. Up to half of Americans have a prediabetic condition called insulin resistance—a serious, early stage blood sugar control problem that won't even show up on a blood sugar test. As many as 41 million have prediabetes (above-normal blood sugar levels), and 21 million have full-blown type 2 diabetes. Meanwhile, the number of children and teens with type 2 diabetes has increased six- to tenfold since 1994, mirroring the childhood obesity epidemic.

The bottom line for you: Blood sugar problems can zap your energy levels, make weight loss difficult or nearly impossible, and put you at risk for an astonishing variety of serious health problems, including heart attack, stroke, Alzheimer's disease, some cancers, infertility, blindness, kidney failure, amputation, and sexual difficulties. And that's not sweet.

PREHISTORIC BODIES, DRIVE-THRU LIFESTYLES

"Our bodies are essentially the same as they were 40,000 years ago, but our eating and exercise habits have changed tremendously," says Bryant Stamford, PhD, director of the Health Promotion and Wellness Center at the University of Louisville in Kentucky. "The same number of calories it might have taken our prehistoric ancestors an entire day to hunt and gather we can now have brought to our door with a phone call. We simply eat too much and exercise too little."

The Sugar Solution can help you bring your lifestyle back into harmony with your body's true needs. It's a simple, delicious, and drug-free approach that supports your blood sugar control system, reducing your blood sugar and dampening elevated levels of insulin, a key blood sugar control hormone. The advantage: You can step off the sugar "spike and dip" roller coaster that contributes to stubborn weight gain, fatigue, moodiness, and cravings. You'll protect yourself against the profoundly damaging effects of high insulin and high blood sugar. You'll feel more energetic.

The Sugar Solution's foundation is a smart, "good carb" eating plan recommended by top nutrition experts and *Prevention* magazine. It features whole grains, fresh fruits and vegetables, good fats, and sensible portions so that you can lose weight without feeling hungry. (And there's still room for pasta, cheese, even chocolate!) You'll also find a physical-activity routine customized to your fitness personality and schedule, as well as spa-quality pampering to soothe stress and help you sleep better. Each of these components can tame out-of-control blood sugar, research shows. By combining them, you get a powerful plan with enormous benefits—now and for years to come.

7 BENEFITS OF BALANCE

The quiz in Chapter 2 can help you size up your risk. But first, check out these compelling benefits of lowering and balancing your blood sugar.

1. **Easier weight loss—without food cravings.** If your blood sugar control system is out of whack, high levels of insulin may slow your body's fat-burning ability even on a low-calorie diet. And low blood sugar levels—the result of insulin doing its job *too* well—can trigger food cravings. You're stuck in a cycle of overeating and weight gain.

   Bringing blood sugar and insulin down to healthier levels can stop cravings that prompt you to reach for another cookie at 3:00 p.m. or another handful of chips while you watch Jay or Conan or Dave late at night. And as Tufts University researchers discovered in a recent study, it helps overweight people with high insulin levels lose more weight—perhaps by allowing fat cells to release their stores so that the body can burn them at last. (For more details about this exciting study, turn to Chapter 3.)

2. **Energy to burn.** What you eat affects your energy levels as well as your weight. Overeating high-glycemic carbs such as white bread, sweet snacks, and sugary drinks floods your bloodstream with sugar, triggering a corresponding flood of insulin to move it out of the blood. The result: low blood sugar, which causes fatigue. Switching to better-quality body fuel like fiber-rich fruits and vegetables and healthy fats will keep you alert and energized for hours.

3. **Improved fertility.** Polycystic ovary syndrome (PCOS)—the leading cause of infertility among women—is a serious blood sugar control problem that involves insulin resistance (when cells ignore insulin's signals to absorb blood sugar) and high insulin levels, experts now know. (Research also shows that PCOS can occur with or without ovarian cysts.) High insulin prompts your ovaries to churn out male hormones that disrupt ovulation, wreak havoc with your skin and hair, lock stubborn fat at your waistline, and raise your risk for diabetes, heart disease, and some cancers. Keeping your blood sugar steady and improving your insulin sensitivity can help right the balance.

4. **A healthier pregnancy and baby.** Balancing your blood sugar with a healthy diet and regular physical activity can help you avoid pregnancy diabetes, thus lowering your risk for full-blown type 2 diabetes later in life. You'll also protect your baby from injury during delivery and from blood sugar problems of her own after birth. Following this plan before pregnancy will cut your risk for this condition.

5. **Slimmer, healthier kids.** Inactivity, fast food, and a sugar- and fat-laden diet are big reasons that the number of overweight kids in America has doubled since 1980—and the number with type 2 diabetes has skyrocketed. The Sugar Solution eating plan belongs on your family table. In Chapter 25, we'll show you how to incorporate more activity into your child's day to further cut her risks for overweight and blood sugar problems.

6. **Lower risk for devastating health problems.** High levels of circulating blood sugar and insulin can damage virtually every cell and organ in the body, significantly raising your odds for heart

attack, stroke, high blood pressure, type 2 diabetes, cancer, blindness, kidney failure, amputation, and more. Controlling your blood sugar with the lifestyle strategies described in this book can reduce your risk for these potential killers and complications.

7. **A sharper memory.** People who don't process blood sugar normally are likely to have memory problems and even shrinkage of the brain region crucial for recall. However, a healthy Sugar Solution lifestyle can help shield your brain from age-related memory loss and perhaps protect against Alzheimer's disease.

LOSE WEIGHT, FEEL GREAT—IN 30 DAYS OR LESS

Designed by a nutritionist from the prestigious Joslin Diabetes Center in Seattle with expertise in blood sugar management strategies, *The Sugar Solution* 28-Day Lifestyle Makeover is based on three key principles: good nutrition, regular physical activity, and stress management.

Healthy eating is one of the cornerstones of blood sugar control. Our meal plan uses the glycemic index (GI), which ranks foods based on how swiftly and how much they raise blood sugar. The GI is one of the most significant dietary findings of the past 25 years. In Chapter 7, you'll learn how using the GI system can crush cravings, curb overeating, and jump-start weight loss.

You'll find that healthy eating can be tasty and satisfying. Our menu plan features lower-GI foods and five delicious—and filling—meals and snacks a day, so you'll never feel deprived. Many of the menus feature the mouthwatering recipes that begin on page 313.

Physical activity is also a critical factor in blood sugar balance. For example, building muscle helps the body use insulin more efficiently, which lowers your blood sugar and insulin levels, encourages weight loss, and cuts health risks. The plan suggests easy ways to incorporate more movement into your daily life. If you're a dedicated walker or would like to start, see Chapter 14 for a customized walking plan developed by *Prevention* magazine. And check out our resistance-training program designed by *Prevention*'s fitness director, Michele Stanten. Lifting weights has been proven to help lower blood sugar.

The third "leg" of blood sugar balance is adequate, restful sleep and stress reduction. Too little sleep and too much stress both raise levels of stress hormones that in turn raise blood sugar levels. Each day of our plan features one easy way to short-circuit stress and boost your well-being. A balanced life also requires the active pursuit of pleasure, not merely the avoidance of stress, so see Chapter 16 for ways to add more healthy joy to your life.

As you start your journey toward better health, keep in mind all the benefits of managing your blood sugar. You'll have more energy. Lose a few pounds. Prevent the symptoms of elevated blood sugar that erode your quality of life, such as fatigue, lethargy, and mood swings. And that's just for now. In the long run, you'll lower your chances of diseases that can rob you of precious years, and you'll ensure that you always live at peak energy and health.

CHAPTER 2

THE *SUGAR SOLUTION* QUIZ: WHAT'S YOUR RISK?

Living with high blood sugar or a related blood sugar control problem is a lot like having termites in your home: Serious damage can happen well before you notice something's wrong. But caught in time, most high blood sugar can be corrected before lasting damage occurs.

While it's not always possible to prevent high blood sugar, there's a lot you can do to lower your risk. And if your blood sugar is already above normal or you have a prediabetic condition called metabolic syndrome, you can start taking steps to reduce your chances of suffering its serious and even life-threatening consequences, including full-blown diabetes, heart attack, stroke, infertility, blindness, kidney failure, amputation, and even dementia and cancer.

"No question: Our research shows that many blood sugar problems can be controlled through lifestyle factors such as diet and exercise, especially if people act early," says David M. Nathan, MD, director of the diabetes center at Massachusetts General Hospital in Boston and chairman of the National Institutes of Health Diabetes Prevention Program (DPP). The DPP—a landmark study that looked at the effects of diet and exercise, medication, or a placebo in 3,234 people with high-normal blood sugar—demonstrated just how powerful even small lifestyle changes can be. People in the study who lost just 7 percent of their body weight and exercised just half an hour most days of the week cut their risk for developing diabetes by an amazing 58 percent. In contrast, study volunteers who took medication cut their risk by a lower 31 percent.

Take this quiz and find out if your lifestyle protects you from high blood sugar—or raises your risk. When you're done, read the brief explanation accompanying each correct answer. You're on your way to living the *Sugar Solution* way—with lower blood sugar, a trimmer figure, and a healthier future.

1. What do you usually eat for breakfast?
   a. High-fiber, whole grain cereal or oatmeal with fresh fruit and fat-free milk
   b. Scrambled eggs and buttered toast
   c. Pastry and a cup of coffee

2. You watch TV this often:
   a. 1 hour a day
   b. 2 hours a day
   c. 2+ hours a day

3. What type of milk do you use most often?
   a. Fat-free
   b. 2% fat
   c. Regular

4. You need to get to the third floor of a high-rise. Will you:
   a. Take the stairs and consider it a mini workout
   b. Take the stairs but huff and puff a bit
   c. Take the elevator

5. How much time do you spend each week on a physical activity that makes you sweat, such as walking or strenuous physical work?
   a. At least 2½ hours a week
   b. About 1½ hours a week
   c. Usually zero minutes a week

6. When you make toast or a sandwich, you use:
   a. Whole grain or multigrain bread
   b. Rye bread
   c. White bread

7. You sauté veggies in:
   a. Olive oil
   b. Vegetable oil
   c. Butter

8. You lift weights or do some other type of resistance training (resistance bands, weight machines):
   a. At least twice a week
   b. Less than twice a week
   c. Never

9. Which best describes your ability to handle stress?
   a. Most of the time, I can stay calm and productive despite stress
   b. I lose my cool once in a while
   c. I become tense and anxious the minute things don't go as expected

10. How often do you eat beans?
    a. Frequently—at least five times a week
    b. Fairly often—once or twice a week
    c. Rarely, if ever

11. Do you smoke cigarettes?
    a. No
    b. A few a day
    c. 10 or more a day

12. How often do you eat each day (including snacks), and how large are those meals?
    a. Three moderate meals and several small snacks
    b. Three square meals a day
    c. I skip meals and usually have one or two big meals only

13. What's your alcoholic beverage of choice?
    a. Don't drink
    b. Wine
    c. A mixed drink or beer

14. How many hours of sleep do you usually get at night?
    a. 7½ hours or more
    b. Between 6 and 7½ hours
    c. Fewer than 6 hours

15. If you've had a fasting blood sugar test in the past year, the test result was:
    a. Under 100 milligrams/deciliter (mg/dl)
    b. 100 to 125 mg/dl
    c. 126 mg/dl or higher

16. My cholesterol, triglycerides, and/or blood pressure are:
    a. At healthy levels
    b. Just a little out of whack—my blood pressure is slightly higher than 130/85, my triglycerides are a bit over 150 mg/dl, and/or my "good" HDL is below 50 mg/dl (for women) or below 40 mg/dl (for men)
    c. In the danger zone—my doctor has told me that my total cholesterol is over 200, my LDL is above 130 (or above 100 for people with diabetes or heart disease), my HDL is below 50 (for women) or 40 (for men), and/or my blood pressure is above 130/85

17. Grab a tape measure and measure your waist. The result is:
    a. Less than 35 inches if you're a woman or 40 inches if you're a man
    b. 35 inches or more if you're a woman
    c. 40 inches or more if you're a man

SCORING

Give yourself 3 points for every a, 2 for every b, and 1 for each c.

From 45 to 41 points: Way to go! You're doing a great job to help your body process its blood sugar properly.

From 40 to 36 points: Nice work! You'll need to make just a few changes, especially if you're overweight or have other risk factors for high blood sugar.

From 35 to 31 points: Careful! This score puts you close to the danger zone, particularly if you have any of the risk factors for high blood sugar.

If you scored 30 points or lower: Uh-oh! Call your doctor, who can test your blood sugar and recommend lifestyle changes.

HOW DID YOU DO?

The best answer to every question is "a." Here's why.

1. **Reach for fiber.** Research shows that foods high in fiber, especially the soluble fiber in oatmeal, slows the absorption of glucose—the sugar molecules that fuel every cell in your body—into the bloodstream, which helps control blood sugar levels. For more information about fiber and tips for fitting more of it into your day, see Chapters 7, 8 and 9.

2. **Move to lower blood sugar.** Moderate exercise keeps muscle cells sensitive to insulin, the hormone that helps usher blood sugar into cells. Being an inactive couch potato makes your cells resist insulin, so blood sugar has trouble getting inside them, raising your risk for diabetes, cardiovascular disease, and stubborn overweight. The best fitness plan? A combination of walking or another calorie-burning aerobic exercise such as swimming or an exercise class, easy strength training, and plenty of everyday activity. Turn to Part 4 for all the details.

3. **Sip diabetes-protecting milk.** Even if you're overweight, consuming more low-fat dairy products, like fat-free milk, could help reduce your risk of insulin resistance. In a 10-year study of 3,000 people, those who were overweight but got lots of dairy foods were 70 percent less likely to develop insulin resistance than those who avoided dairy. Milk sugar (lactose) is converted to blood sugar relatively slowly, which is good for blood sugar control and reducing insulin levels. Nutrients in dairy products (choose low-fat or

fat-free varieties), including calcium, magnesium, and potassium, also help. Our eating plan shows you how to get the calcium and other nutrients you need.

4. **Find fitness opportunities everywhere.** Climbing stairs burns extra calories and gives the heart a workout. It's one small way to help head off blood sugar problems due to inactivity and over-weight. Need more "fit in fitness" ideas? See Chapter 13.

5. **Activate the 30-minute exercise solution.** Exercising at a moder-ate intensity (walking briskly, for example) for just 30 minutes a day, 5 days a week, can reduce the risk of developing type 2 dia-betes by 58 to 80 percent. Exercise is most protective if you also adopt a healthy diet. People who don't exercise at all increase their risk by 25 percent.

6. **Choose low-glycemic grains.** Whole grain bread is higher in fiber, which helps slow the rate at which sugar enters the blood-stream. Fiber also helps you maintain a healthy weight. To make sure you're getting whole grain wheat, for example, look for the words "100 percent stone-ground whole wheat" on the ingredients list and for at least 3 grams of fiber per slice. We'll show you which other grains are low-glycemic in Chapters 7 and 9.

7. **Say yes to good fats.** Olive oil and other good sources of mono-unsaturated fat, like flaxseed oil, avocados, and nuts, may help lower your risk for blood sugar problems and related cardiovascu-lar conditions. Turn to Chapter 9 for more details about these healthy fats—and check out Chapter 19, our 4-week lifestyle makeover, for delicious meals that contain these everyday luxu-ries.

8. **Build sleek, sexy muscle.** Resistance training builds muscle den-sity—stronger muscles that use more glucose. Along with aerobic exercise, it also aids weight loss. In Chapter 15, you'll find out how to build toned muscle in just 10 minutes a day, even if you've never strength-trained before.

9. **Ease anxiety.** Chronic stress increases the risk for high blood sugar several ways: Stress hormones trigger the release of extra blood sugar and also direct the body to store more fat in the abdo-

men, which raises your risk for insulin resistance and, ultimately, diabetes. Find out how to release chronic stress in Part 5—with strategies ranging from yoga and deep breathing to knitting.

10. **Open a can of beans.** Whether they're kidney, pinto, black, or white, beans are packed with soluble fiber, which blunts the entry of glucose into the bloodstream. Soluble fiber also helps lower bad-guy LDL as well as homocysteine, a compound in the blood associated with heart disease. Our eating plan (see Chapters 7 and 19 for mouthwatering menus) features beans in delicious new ways.

11. **Make your life a no-smoking zone.** Smoking increases your risk for prediabetic conditions and more. Compared with nonsmoking folks who have type 2 diabetes, smokers with type 2 are three times more likely to die of cardiovascular disease.

12. **Eat more often.** Eating small meals frequently is better for blood sugar control than sitting down to occasional feasts. Large meals cause more glucose to enter the bloodstream quickly, taxing the ability of the pancreas to produce sufficient insulin. Studies show that people who eat smaller meals throughout the day tend to take in fewer calories and make healthier food choices. Our eating plan (see Chapters 7 and 19) combines moderately sized meals and generous snacks to keep your blood sugar on an even keel.

13. **Choose (a little) wine.** In one study of nearly 80,000 people, women who drank beer or hard liquor one to four times a week were more likely to carry extra weight in the abdomen than women who didn't drink at all. However, wine was not associated with waist size in the study—significant because large waistlines increase diabetes risk—and may, in moderation, offer heart-protective effects that other alcoholic beverages do not.

14. **Sleep for better insulin sensitivity.** Recent research found that people who averaged less than 6½ hours of sleep a night were 40 percent more insulin resistant—a major risk for developing diabetes—than people who slept 7½ hours or more. The insulin insensitivity of the short sleepers was typical of senior citizens over age 60, yet their real ages were between 23 and 42. Need some sleep tips? See Chapter 18.

15. **Schedule a blood sugar test.** Haven't been tested? *Prevention* magazine urges all adults to have their blood sugar checked and, if it's above normal, take steps to lower it. A blood sugar test is an absolute must if you're 45 or older and overweight or if you have any other risk factors for diabetes. In Chapter 1, we provide all the details on getting the best test. But don't stop there. You can have a serious prediabetic condition called metabolic syndrome and still have normal-looking blood sugar levels. Your answers to the next two questions will help assess your risk for this condition.

16. **Look for little signs of trouble.** If you have at least two of these risks—even if they seem small—plus a large waistline, odds are high that you've got metabolic syndrome. Your cells resist insulin's signal to absorb blood sugar, so your body pumps out extra blood sugar. This condition puts you at high risk for heart disease, stroke, diabetes, and other health dangers. Experts estimate that one in four, perhaps even one in two, Americans has metabolic syndrome. Get the lowdown in Chapter 20.

17. **Listen to your tape measure.** Research suggests that belly fat may be an even more potent risk factor for diabetes than weight alone. While experts aren't yet sure why, one theory is that insulin-resistant people store excess dietary fat in inappropriate places, such as in muscle cells and the liver, which makes it harder for their bodies to use sugar as fuel. Can't quite button your favorite jeans? Never tuck in your blouse anymore? All three components of the *Sugar Solution* plan—our eating program, exercise routines, and stress-reduction tips—work together to help you blast belly fat. You'll look great—and feel even better.

CHAPTER 3

LOSE WEIGHT AT LAST!

Skip the low-fat cookies and grab the walnuts, raspberries, and (*oh, yes!*) pasta: New research from the nation's top weight-loss labs shows that a simple secret—keeping blood sugar lower and steadier—can overcome even the toughest roadblocks to pounds-off success.

The *Sugar Solution* eating strategy is delicious enough for your whole family to enjoy. It uses easy-to-find, nutritious, well-loved foods and ingredients from your local supermarket and packs the fiber, good fats, antioxidants, and other nutrients that protect against heart disease, stroke, diabetes, cancer, and more. The key? Low-glycemic-index (GI) eating that stops blood sugar swings. Add our customized fitness plan and daily tips for better sleep and less stress, and you've got a plan that will make you feel great right away—and keep you feeling great as the weight falls away.

Better yet, this strategy is backed by a growing stack of research showing that a weight-loss diet based on low-GI foods (fruits, veggies, and whole grains that won't make blood sugar spike) may work better than low-carb and low-fat diets for many overweight Americans. The benefits:

Drop more pounds. If you have insulin resistance or metabolic syndrome—a prediabetic condition affecting up to half of all American adults—you could lose 60 percent *more* weight on a moderate-fat, low-GI diet than on a low-fat diet containing more refined carbohydrates, suggests a recent Tufts University–New England Medical Center study of 39 overweight women and men. Study volunteers with high insulin levels lost an average of 22 pounds in 6 months on the low-GI plan, but just 13 on a high-GI diet.

And keep 'em off. You want to lose weight once and for all—and choosing low-GI foods could help you achieve your goal. In a revealing study that tracked 572 nondieters for a year, University of Massachusetts Medical School researchers found that body weight was 9.6 pounds lighter for every 10-point decrease in the total glycemic load of a person's diet. That could be the difference between choosing a baked sweet potato (a GI of 54) instead of a baked white potato (85). "Nearly 10 pounds is a significant difference," says researcher Barbara Olendzki, RD, MPH, a registered dietitian and instructor at the medical school. "If people can lower the GI of their diet by choosing the best carbohydrates to eat, they should be able to lose some weight. Those lower-GI foods can also be helpful for appetite control."

Sidestep a metabolic downshift. The first law of weight loss is, you must burn more calories than you take in. But cutting calories usually triggers a significant metabolic slowdown as your body loses lean muscle mass and tries to hold on to fat reserves. The result: Weight loss stalls. Now, a study from Children's Hospital Boston and Brigham and Women's Hospital suggests that a reduced-calorie eating plan packed with good fats and smart carbohydrates could outsmart this frustrating obstacle. When 39 overweight and obese dieters followed either a low-fat or a low-GI diet for 10 weeks, the low-GI group's resting metabolic rate stayed higher. Their bodies burned an extra 80 calories per day. Translation: You could lose an extra 8 pounds per year. That's nearly a dress size!

Melt the most stubborn pounds of all. Insulin resistance—a widespread problem among overweight Americans—raises your insulin levels two to 10 times higher than normal and thwarts weight-loss efforts by prompting the body to store fat instead of burning it, say researchers from the University of California, San Diego, School of Medicine. (They discovered that too much insulin blocks catecholamine, a key fat-burning hormone.) The solution: Fill your plate with low-GI carbohydrates. This strategy cut insulin levels in half for 12 overweight people in a Tufts University study comparing the effects of high- and low-GI breakfasts.

Turn off crazy fat-and-sugar cravings. Refined carbs make blood sugar spike, then plummet. Suddenly, you're ravenous—and primed to overeat high-fat, high-sugar goodies. The fix: Junk-food-proof your weight-loss plan with low-GI choices. The Tufts researchers found that study volunteers snacked on 81 percent fewer calories after a low-GI breakfast than after the high-GI version.

Feel energetic, not cranky. Dieting can make you feel irritable, tired, and ready to quit. In the same Children's Hospital Boston study detailed above, study volunteers on the low-GI eating plan reported feeling more energetic. "If your metabolic rate doesn't fall as much, your body may not be as stressed by the weight loss," notes lead study author David Ludwig, MD, PhD, director of the obesity program at Children's Hospital Boston. "You may feel stronger and more energetic and have a better sense of well-being—and that could keep you on your diet and even get you off the couch and out the door to exercise."

WEIGHT LOSS THE *SUGAR SOLUTION* WAY

Our breakthrough 28-day lifestyle makeover tackles the underlying cause of America's obesity epidemic—your body's out-of-whack blood sugar control system—on many levels. Designed by a nutritionist with expertise in blood sugar control, the eating plan begins on page 53. Here's the art and the science behind it.

STRATEGY #1: EAT SMART CARBS, NOT FLABBY CARBS

Say no to the glazed doughnut, yes to strawberries and yogurt. Ignore the chips; crunch a handful of almonds. Reach for sweet potatoes instead of white in the produce aisle. Subtracting high-GI foods while you add low-GI alternatives to your plate multiplies your chances for weight-loss success. You banish the foods that crank up your blood sugar and your insulin levels—and that lead to cravings, binges, fatigue, and weight that won't budge. You eat more of the good stuff that keeps

THE SUGAR SURVIVORS: Jacqueline Daniels

Something felt terribly wrong when Jacqueline Daniels, then in her early forties, returned to her job as a nursing-home aide after recovering from a surgical procedure. "After 2 days back at work, I felt so weak that I asked one of the nurses to check my blood sugar," recalls Daniels, a Cincinnati resident. "It was 380." A normal, nonfasting level is 125 or lower.

She was determined not to end up like the diabetic patients she cares for. "I've seen them lose limbs, lose their eyesight, and pass away," she explains. "I never thought it could happen to me."

Everything Daniels ate seemed to raise her blood sugar. The turning point: Once she returned to work, she looked for help. "One of the nurses said, 'Eat less. Check your sugar more often. Instead of a whole apple, eat one-fourth and see what happens.'"

She also prayed with the nursing-home chaplain. "I remembered that little verse, 'God grant me the serenity . . .' That helped me a lot," she says.

Daniels also met with a diabetes educator to get a practical eating and activity plan. She left ready to change not just her own life but also her family's.

"I used to eat a lot of meat—I love pig's feet—and bread," Daniels says. "Instead, I started having more salad, chicken, fish, and veggie burgers. We always had sugary soda pop and chips in the house. That all changed. The kids didn't like it at first. They kicked and screamed. But now they beat me to the refrigerator. They like these healthy foods." Now she stocks her kitchen with diet drinks, fruits and veggies, lean meats, baked chips, and low-fat popcorn.

"I try to walk for at least 30 minutes a day and make the kids come, too," she adds. "On Saturdays, we walk to my brother's produce stand to get fruits and vegetables."

Daniels eats seven small meals and snacks per day. She's lost 42 pounds. She tracks her carbohydrate intake and measures healthy portions by comparing serving sizes to her hand. "A 5-ounce serving of protein is equal to my palm; a cup of pasta is the size of my fist."

The results? "Now I can laugh at diabetes. At work, they call me Miss Diabetical," says Daniels, who also stopped smoking.

you feeling full and satisfied, which helps you lose weight.

Researchers like Dr. Ludwig suspect that America's obesity epidemic is tied in part to our 30-year romance with low-fat diets high in refined carbohydrates—the high-GI stuff. Eating too many refined carbs (like low-fat diet cookies and cakes) overwhelms your body's ancient blood sugar control system—and can set off a cascade of hormones that pad fat cells.

Here's how it happens: A high-GI meal (say, a doughnut, coffee, and apple juice for breakfast) can drive blood sugar up twice as high as a low-GI alternative (such as steel-cut oatmeal with chopped apples and cinnamon). Insulin levels soar, pushing the sugar into your muscle and liver cells. That leaves your blood sugar lower than before you ate! You're famished and may reach for more high-GI foods. Meanwhile, high insulin levels deliver a one-two punch that makes your body gain stubborn weight: They send more excess calories into fat cells, and they prevent fat cells from releasing this stored energy when your body needs it. (Insulin suppresses the biochemical system that pulls fat from cells and burns it for energy.)

In contrast, a low-GI meal raises blood sugar slowly and steadily. Insulin levels rise only high enough to gently push glucose into waiting cells, where it is burned for energy. Your blood sugar stays low and steady for hours.

"The idea with low-GI eating is that we recruit fundamental biological mechanisms in the body so that blood sugar stays lower, you feel full faster, and the body doesn't seem to react to the diet with as much stress," Dr. Ludwig says. "Eating this way will help people stay on a weight-loss diet longer, without as much of a struggle. They'll be less hungry, their metabolic rate will stay a little higher, and they'll feel better."

You'll also eat more often. To lose weight, the *Sugar Solution* plan clocks in at 1,500 to 1,600 calories distributed in this manner: 225 at breakfast, 425 at lunch, and 550 at dinner. The rest? You'll eat three snacks daily—two at 80 calories apiece and one at 150 calories.

If you're a longtime meal skipper, this can seem like a lot of food. ("I can't eat this much!" is one of the first comments we get from new members of our *Sugar Solution* Web site, www.sugarsolutiononline.)

Start by scheduling time for breakfast or planning ahead to pack a portable meal, such as our Blueberry-Yogurt Muffins, to enjoy at your desk or our Berry-Good Smoothie, which you can sip on your commute. Then sit down to lunch, and you're on your way. Within a week or so, fit in snacks.

STRATEGY #2: SEIZE—AND SCHEDULE—FUN FITNESS OPPORTUNITIES

If you're among the 60 percent of Americans who've given up on regular physical activity because you don't have time; you think it's boring; or you think that you're too old, too tired, or too sick or that you just don't need it, welcome to the *Sugar Solution* plan. Here, fitness has nothing to do with monotonous, painful, tricky gym workouts and aerobics routines. You never have to squeeze into unflattering Spandex shorts or face a cold, uncomfortable locker room.

We've got a better idea. The *Sugar Solution* plan will help you identify the activities that fit your schedule, your fitness level, and even your personality. Our goal? To help you move for at least 30 minutes, at least 5 days a week. You might take a stroll around the mall; play tag with the kids in the backyard; pop in an energetically paced yoga video; or realize a dream and sign up for a dance class, horseback riding lessons, or karate. "Exercise doesn't have to be grueling," notes Michele Olson, PhD, professor of health and human performance at Auburn University in Alabama. "It's the accumulation of movement that counts."

Afraid that enjoying yourself at your own pace just won't cut it? Truth is, moderation can burn more calories than bursts of supervigorous exercise, say researchers at Maastricht University in the Netherlands. When they compared the fitness levels of 30 people who performed either moderate physical activity (such as walking and biking) or vigorous exercise, they discovered that the gung-ho athletic types compensated by being *less* active the rest of the day. In truth, the moderate exercisers tended to be more active overall.

You'll also find a gentle muscle-strengthening plan that will help you build a leaner body as you create denser muscles—the calorie-burning "engine" of your metabolism. In one University of Alabama study, women and men who worked out with weights three times a week for 6 months increased their metabolism by a respectable 12 percent. Thanks to the extra muscle, their bodies burned an extra 230 calories per day, every day. This change alone could help you drop 24 pounds in 1 year.

As you reexperience the joy of movement that we all possessed as children, you'll battle one cause of America's obesity epidemic: our push-button 21st-century life. Fifty years ago, Americans burned about 700 more calories per day than we do today—not by jogging but in performing daily activities from washing dishes by hand to typing on a manual typewriter to cranking the laundry through the wringer on the washing machine. Each time you take the steps instead of the elevator, join your kids on the playground, or park in the farthest spot from the office door, you invite more everyday, calorie-burning activity back into your life. We'll show you how.

THE STRESS-FAT CONNECTION

If your life could easily be subtitled *The High-Anxiety Story*, you're setting yourself up for a tummy pooch that's more deadly than cute—even if you're not overeating. Researchers at the University of California, San Francisco, have found that chronic stress jacks up levels of cortisol, the stress hormone that sends extra fat to your midsection.

Cortisol also persuades you to eat more high-fat, high-carb foods when you're feeling stressed, says physiologist Norman Pecoraro, PhD, a stress–belly flab researcher.

Magic calm trip: Develop an inner sense of control that allows you to nip stress in the bud so you don't snack your way out of it. "There are some very pragmatic ways to reduce persistent stress that don't involve eating," Dr. Pecoraro says. "Start with active coping—pay the bills!—rather than passive avoidance, such as refusing to open envelopes from your credit-card company." You also could try 5 minutes of calm, deep breathing or a quick walk around the block.

STRATEGY #3: STRESS LESS, SLEEP BETTER

The stresses of everyday life can affect how much and how well you sleep. And when emotional stress makes you lose sleep, it puts physical stress on your body—leading to overeating.

But lack of sleep doesn't just leave you vulnerable to cravings. Research shows that sleep deprivation also disrupts the body's normal ability to process and control blood sugar and weight-related hormones like cortisol and epinephrine. This imbalance leads to insulin resistance and to the elevated insulin levels that encourage cells to store excess fat instead of burning it.

Perhaps that's why women and men (ages 32 to 59) who snoozed 4 hours or less per night had a whopping 73 percent higher risk of obesity than their better-rested counterparts in a recent study from Columbia University's Mailman School of Public Health and the Obesity Research Center. Getting just 5 hours upped obesity risk 50 percent; 6 hours raised it 23 percent. You need at least 7½ hours per night to reduce this added risk to zero.

Quality counts, too. If you're among the 18 million Americans with sleep apnea, your sleep is disrupted dozens or even hundreds of times each night because you've stopped breathing for a moment. This condition, which may require medical intervention to fix, can raise your odds for insulin resistance by 50 percent.

The fix: It takes just three consecutive nights of 9 hours' sleep to correct the blood sugar and hormone imbalances sleep deprivation can cause. You'll find dozens of ways to catch up on your sleep in Chapter 18, plus advice on resolving sleep apnea. You'll feel better, and you may discover that weight loss is easier when you wake up refreshed each morning.

In addition, we'll show you how to take small stress-relieving breaks every day. These can help break the high-stress, high blood sugar cycle that can raise your risk for prediabetes and diabetes and may get in the way of effective weight loss.

2

THE BENEFITS
OF BALANCE

CHAPTER 4

YOUR BLOOD SUGAR CONTROL SYSTEM: AN OWNER'S MANUAL

Blood sugar is *not* a bad guy. This sweet stuff is your body's best friend—rocket fuel for hardworking muscles and brain cells, energy that (like extra flashlight batteries or the nation's strategic oil reserves) can be stored and then released at precisely the moment you need it most.

It's only when levels rise too high—or sink too low—that blood sugar has serious, negative consequences for your mood, your weight, your energy level, your health, and even your life. The trick to staying on blood sugar's good side is simple: Work with—not against—the intricate and intelligent biochemical system that keeps levels within a healthy range. Your first step? Understand how your blood sugar control system works by reading this brief owner's manual.

THE RIGHT FUEL

Nearly all of the blood sugar that powers your cells comes from the carbs on your plate—the fruits, veggies, grains, and sugar that your digestive system converts into the tiniest of sugar molecules: glucose.

In a sense, carbs are like candy. Whether you're eating corn chips, chocolate mousse, or broccoli spears, carbohydrate foods all contain chains of sugar molecules. Some chains are short. Others are long. Some, like the sugars glucose and fructose, need almost no digestion before they can be absorbed into your bloodstream. Others, like the fiber in oatmeal, are so tough that your body cannot break them down.

The moment you slide a forkful of apple pie or mashed potatoes into your mouth, a series of enzymes begins breaking apart these chains. Ultimately, all carbs are converted into glucose, fructose, or galactose—tiny sugar molecules that slide easily through your intestinal wall and into the bloodstream. There's one more stop before this new supply of blood sugar can reach hungry cells: the liver. Here, cells hold on to some glucose for later use (it's stored in a form called glycogen). And fructose and galactose are converted to glucose. Like gasoline pumped into the tank of your car at the start of a summer road trip, the glucose that circulates in your bloodstream is now ready to power your mind, muscles, and metabolism.

THE SIMPLE-CARB MYTH

Until recently, nutrition experts thought complex carbs—starches comprised of long chains of sugar molecules—were the "good" carbs that kept blood sugar low and steady. "Bad" carbs were simple sugars, with short chains that were absorbed quickly. But that's old think. Experts now know that some simple carbs are absorbed slowly, while some complex carbs convert swiftly into blood sugar.

A better ranking system: the glycemic index, which rates a food's effect on your blood sugar based on lab tests, not conjecture. This system is one of the foundations of the *Sugar Solution* plan, and you'll be hearing about it throughout this book.

SUGAR LESSON #1: GO FOR LOW-GLYCEMIC CARBS

Not all carbs are created equal. Some reach the finish line faster than others—and when it comes to healthy blood sugar, bet on the tortoise, not the hare.

THE SUGAR SURVIVORS: Alice McColgin

Alice McColgin controls her blood sugar the natural way: with diet and exercise.

A few years ago, McColgin, a 53-year-old account manager in Indianapolis, didn't feel well. She was extremely tired and thirsty, her vision was blurry, and she had to take frequent bathroom breaks. She got cold sweats, too. When she came down with a severe urinary tract infection, she went to her doctor, who tested her blood sugar. "Turned out my blood sugar was over 400," says McColgin. "I had become heavier and more inactive than ever and was paying the price."

To reduce her blood sugar quickly, her doctor prescribed a pill that makes cells more sensitive to insulin. But McColgin was determined not to become dependent on the medication and took matters into her own hands. She began walking for 10 to 15 minutes, four or five times a week. "My doctor was impressed with how much I had reduced my blood sugar in 6 weeks," she says. "From then on, with the encouragement of my family and friends, exercise became a part of my routine."

McColgin is careful to steer clear of refined sugars, and she watches her calorie and fat intake. To avoid temptation, she says, "I tell myself there are so many things I want to do, and eating the sugar will probably shorten my life."

Today, McColgin has built up to 50 to 55 minutes of aerobic exercise—walking, stationary cycling, or using a NordicTrack—4 or 5 days per week, and she's lost more than 30 pounds. She was weaned down and finally taken off the medication completely. "I have more energy, I sleep better, and I think more clearly," she says.

Eventually, almost everyone with type 2 diabetes needs medication to help control blood sugar. But losing weight, exercising, and eating well can help delay that inevitability, safeguard your health, and yield benefits no drug can achieve: You'll feel great, look great, and have the satisfaction of knowing you're in control of your health.

High-glycemic carbs, such as white rice and white bread, are broken down and absorbed swiftly, raising blood sugar fast. Low-glycemic carbs move through your digestive system slowly and release sugar into your bloodstream slowly. Many factors influence how rapidly or slowly a carb becomes blood sugar. Among them: whether you've also consumed something acidic (like vinaigrette dressing) or fatty (like butter on bread), both of which slow absorption; whether the starch in the food has been thoroughly cooked (the longer you cook a starch, the faster it's absorbed by your body); whether the carb is surrounded by a tough coating such as the covering on beans and seeds, which slows absorption; how finely a carb such as flour has been ground (finer grains absorb faster); and whether a carb comes with digestion-slowing viscous fiber (as do oatmeal and lentils).

SUGAR LESSON #2: BURN IT—OR WEAR IT ON YOUR HIPS

Muscle cells and the tissues of organs throughout your body rely on glucose for energy to function. Walking, breathing, sweating, digesting, producing new cells, growing a baby during pregnancy, and thousands of tiny intercellular functions are all driven by this teeny-tiny sugar.

Your body's top glucose hogs are your brain and nervous system, which collectively consume about half the glucose that circulates in your bloodstream. Even at rest, the brain devours a greater percentage of your glucose supply than your body uses while active.

It takes just 7 ounces of pure glucose—less than 1 cup—to fuel the daily work and play of your cells. Like a thrifty Boy Scout, your body's glucose abides by the motto "Be prepared." About 40 percent of the glucose released after a meal is stored in the liver and muscles in a form called glycogen. When blood sugar falls between meals or food isn't available, the liver releases its supply into the bloodstream as glucose. Muscle cells also hoard glycogen for their own private use. (And when your body runs out of glycogen, fat cells release fatty acids for use by skeletal muscles, your heart, and other tissues.)

Your glucose reserves must be replenished daily. Your body keeps only about 1,900 calories' worth of glycogen in its larder—enough to sustain you for about 16 hours. When that runs low, it burns fat and even uses protein to create more glucose. Most Americans have more than enough, however, thanks to overeating, inactivity, and a taste for refined carbohydrates. When there's an overload of glucose, your liver and muscle cells can run out of storage space. The excess sugar is stored—as fat.

But if you exercise (the *Sugar Solution* plan recommends at least 30 minutes at least five times a week), you not only burn more glucose, you also activate a mechanism that pulls blood sugar into cells that's independent of insulin. You get a double benefit: no excess insulin, lower glucose.

SUGAR LESSON #3: PROTECT YOUR INSULIN-PRODUCTION AND INSULIN-SENSING SYSTEMS

Normal blood sugar stays within a range of 60 to 90 milligrams of glucose per deciliter of blood (mg/dl) before a meal and rises to between 120 and 160 mg/dl after eating. Experts admire the body's ability to maintain this precise, narrow range around the clock and suspect its main purpose is to keep sugar supplies to the brain steady. (Brain cells can store only the smallest amount of extra glucose and cannot use fatty acids for power; they must constantly "sip" from the bloodstream.)

If blood sugar control is a balancing act, hormones act as the tightrope walker's pole. "Blood sugar regulation involves a balance between hormones that raise blood glucose and those that lower it," says Robert Cohen, MD, professor of medicine in the division of endocrinology and metabolism in the department of medicine at the University of Cincinnati and director of the diabetes clinic at University Hospital in Cincinnati. The key players: insulin, which lowers blood sugar by persuading cells to absorb it; and glucagon, which tells the liver to release stored glucose.

Insulin is produced by beta cells in the pancreas. Under healthy conditions, these clever cells sense glucose levels in the bloodstream and adjust their insulin output accordingly. After you eat, insulin levels rise. Once released, insulin ushers glucose out of the bloodstream and into waiting cells throughout the body. When sugar levels fall, so does insulin production.

But if you're overweight and inactive, receptors on muscle, liver, and organ cells throughout your body may grow deaf to insulin's signals. Then, your beta cells pump out extra insulin, raising your risk for stubborn overweight as well as health problems. Over time, overeating fatty and sugary foods may prompt your beta cells to lose their smart ability to sense changes in blood sugar levels. They stop producing the right amount at the right time. Blood sugar levels rise dangerously.

SUGAR LESSON #4: TAKE CARE OF YOUR BACKUP POWER SUPPLIES

If you haven't eaten in a while, alpha cells in the pancreas send glucagon into the blood. This hormone raises blood sugar by signaling the liver to give up its glycogen stores. Glycogen becomes blood sugar, ready to feed your body's fuel-hungry cells. If you overeat foods that raise blood sugar dramatically, this system can stay turned on and prevent your body from burning a secondary fuel: fatty acids stored in fat cells. This is a problem if you're trying to lose weight.

Meanwhile, chronic stress can keep another blood sugar backup plan switched on for too long. If you need a sudden burst of energy—to outrun a charging saber-toothed tiger, for example—your adrenal glands churn out stress hormones including epinephrine and cortisol, which tell your body to release and burn stored glucose. That worked well for cavemen and cavewomen, who faced short-term stresses like marauding cats. As you'll discover later in this book, 21st-century chronic stress can keep these hormones raging, leaving you with higher blood sugar around the clock. Chronic stress can also prompt you to overeat and store extra fat in your belly . . . which leads to more insulin resistance. Stress reduction isn't a luxury; it's a necessity for maintaining a healthy weight!

CHAPTER 5

ANCIENT BODY, MODERN LIFE: THE BLOOD SUGAR MISMATCH

Like a jewel-encrusted Fabergé egg or a vintage 1953 Studebaker, your body's system for managing blood sugar is a beautiful anachronism. Built to withstand the frequent famines, scarce feasts, and heavy physical demands of Stone Age life, it's out of place in a 21st-century landscape of Cinnabons, stuffed-crust pizza, and pay-per-view. Your body lives by prehistoric rules designed to keep mind and body running oh-so-frugally on a sometimes meager supply of glucose. It extracts every molecule of sugar from the foods you eat, then conserves precious glucose—hoarding the energy in muscle and liver cells for the times you need it most.

Yet Twinkies have replaced wild raspberries; grain-fed beef and supersize fries have replaced freshly dug roots and lean wild game rich in good fat. Calorie consumption has soared, and daily exercise means walking from the front door to the car—not a 15-mile trek to the next watering hole.

The world has changed; our bodies have not. And a growing stack of research links that fundamental mismatch to an amazing variety of modern-day, blood sugar–related health problems including heart attack, stroke, high blood pressure, diabetes, cancer, infertility, and even Alzheimer's disease, as well as birth defects, sexual dysfunction, blindness, kidney failure, and amputation. Even more alarming: The workings of this ancient sugar control system can put you at high risk for serious conditions *even if your blood sugar levels look normal*. Of course, risk rises higher if sugar levels soar into the prediabetic range, and higher still if you develop full-blown type 2 diabetes.

FROM INSULIN RESISTANCE TO DIABETES

The problem isn't just sugar. Insulin—the hormone that tells cells to absorb blood sugar—plays a major role, too. In tiny amounts, this powerful protein is healthy and essential. But if inactivity, belly fat, and a high-fat, high-sugar diet have made your cells insulin resistant—a condition affecting as many as one in two American adults—your body pumps out two to three times more insulin than normal in order to force sugar into cells. The ploy works. Your cells receive the sugar they need (and your blood sugar levels will look normal on a fasting blood sugar test). But the excess insulin can raise your blood pressure, clog your arteries, overtax your pancreas (raising diabetes risk), promote the growth of cancer cells, stop ovulation, and dim memory.

Once this hidden high blood sugar begins to do its damage, you develop a condition called metabolic syndrome, in which biochemical changes triggered by insulin resistance begin to alter systems throughout your body. Metabolic syndrome can simmer undetected for decades. (Turn to Chapter 20 for a list of the warning signals.) Blood sugar levels will rise into prediabetic and then diabetic zones if your pancreas can no longer produce enough insulin to overcome insulin resistance.

Diabetes adds new health risks, including vision problems, kidney failure, and bodywide nerve damage. A sobering new finding: These complications may begin to develop when your blood sugar is still in the prediabetic range (100 to 125 milligrams of glucose per deciliter of blood, or mg/dl, on a fasting blood sugar test). "The complications of diabetes may begin years before diagnosis and much earlier than we thought," said Richard Kahn, PhD, chief scientific and medical officer for the American Diabetes Association. "That is really the big news, because we have not known when the changes start to occur."

Here's more of the latest research on the profound links between blood sugar control and your health.

HEART DISEASE AND STROKE

In a new Swedish study that tracked 1,826 people for 20 years, researchers found that those with metabolic syndrome had a 69 percent higher risk for heart attack than those without it. Others estimate that metabolic syndrome could sometimes triple heart risk. Diabetes magnifies the problem, as high glucose levels further assault arteries. People with diabetes are four times more likely to have a heart attack or stroke and are more likely to die than people who don't have diabetes, say Harvard Medical School researchers. Atherosclerosis accounts for virtually 80 percent of all deaths among diabetes patients.

High insulin levels turn your blood into a superhighway for bad fats—raising triglycerides; lowering good HDL cholesterol, the kind that mops up artery-choking LDL cholesterol; and making nasty LDL extra small and better able to invade artery walls. They raise levels of fibrinogen, which makes blood clot, and up your risk for high blood pressure by altering the way your kidneys process sodium. People with metabolic syndrome also have signs of more chronic, low-level inflammation—as if their immune systems are constantly on alert. This churns out compounds such as C-reactive protein that help pack extra fatty gunk into artery walls and raise the risk for heart-stopping blood clots.

TYPE 2 DIABETES

One in three people with metabolic syndrome will go on to develop type 2 diabetes. The turning point may be encoded in your DNA.

Researchers from Iceland's Decode Genetics, a gene research company, recently announced the discovery of a "diabetes gene" carried by an astonishing 45 percent of humans around the world. The gene alone can't doom you to a diabetic future; experts say lifestyle pulls the trigger. A genetic "weakness" can prompt overtaxed insulin-producing cells

YOUR BLOOD SUGAR TIMELINE

The life cycle can profoundly affect blood sugar. Here's what happens.

Puberty

This life stage results in insulin resistance that has nothing to do with weight or fat, says Michael Goran, PhD, professor of preventive medicine at the Keck School of Medicine at the University of Southern California in Los Angeles. The cause? Probably a combination of the body's need for extra energy to fuel rapid growth, along with the sudden flood of sex hormones.

"Kids who go through puberty get very insulin resistant—regardless of how fat, thin, big, or small," Dr. Goran explains. If they're lean, their bodies can handle it with no long-term effects. But if they're overweight, the stress of puberty on the pancreas may push the entire system over the edge, resulting in longer-lasting insulin insensitivity or full-blown diabetes.

Pregnancy

Nearly all pregnant women develop some insulin resistance—that is, their cells don't readily obey insulin's signal to absorb blood sugar, says Thomas A. Buchanan, MD, professor of medicine, obstetrics and gynecology, and physiology and biophysics at the Keck School of Medicine. "As you become more and more resistant to insulin, your glucose and other nutrients stay in circulation a bit longer after you eat than if your insulin reactivity were normal," Dr. Buchanan explains. "That may be a way to get some of the maternal nutrients to the fetus." In other words: more for baby.

Menstruation and Menopause

Gabriele E. Sonnenberg, MD, professor of medicine at the Medical College of Wisconsin in Milwaukee, says many of her patients with type 1 diabetes (when the immune system destroys insulin-producing cells, so you must receive daily insulin injections) find it harder to control their blood sugar right before their periods. Some report problems at midcycle (during ovulation), while others say the changes come during menstruation itself. In fact, several of her patients change their insulin dose to coincide with their changing needs during the menstrual cycle.

Studies confirm this mysterious correlation. In one survey of 406 women with type 1, 67 percent said they had changes in blood glucose control just before their periods, and 70 percent reported changes during menstruation. Other studies find that even women without diabetes have higher blood sugar after meals during the 2 weeks between ovulation and menstruation.

Insulin may not dock as effectively with receptors on cell surfaces in the second half of the menstrual cycle. Or, estrogen may interact with insulin to raise or lower blood sugar.

Those cyclical/hormonal changes of menstruation should stop with menopause. But a new factor arises: weight gain, which can increase insulin resistance and ultimately raise sugar levels.

With age, the body's ability to produce insulin and absorb blood sugar declines. Blame it on wear-and-tear, genetics, and a tendency to eat more and sit more. Also, part of the reason may lie within tiny structures inside cells called mitochondria—the little power plants that turn glucose into energy. Mitochondria work less efficiently as we grow older, burning less blood sugar. The result: Risk for diabetes rises over age 40 and rises even faster after age 60.

The Rx: exercise. Muscle is one of the major users of glucose, Dr. Sonnenberg notes. If you maintain it—with resistance training and aerobic activity—you can improve your blood sugar status at any age.

in your pancreas to burn out, allowing blood sugar to rise. (Want to know if you're headed for type 2 diabetes? Ask your doctor for a fasting blood sugar check, as recommended in Chapter 1.)

CANCER

The link between insulin and cancer keeps getting stronger. High insulin levels tripled risk for breast cancer in a surprising University of Toronto study of 198 women. And among women with breast cancer, those with the highest levels were three times more likely to see cancer recur.

Researchers are also finding links between high insulin and prostate and colon cancer. National Cancer Institute scientists recently documented a doubled risk for pancreatic cancer among smokers with type 2 diabetes who had the highest levels of insulin and the most insulin resistance.

Insulin acts as a growth factor, making cancer cells grow quickly and divide wildly, says breast cancer researcher Pamela Goodwin, MD, of Toronto's Mount Sinai Hospital. Some cancer cells have more insulin receptors than normal cells do, allowing the hormone to dock easily.

INFERTILITY AND BIRTH DEFECTS

Women with a common infertility problem called polycystic ovary syndrome (PCOS) have insulin resistance and higher-than-normal insulin levels. While high insulin isn't the only cause of PCOS, it's a major factor—and helps explain why half of all women with PCOS develop diabetes by age 40 and 40 percent have signs of seriously clogged arteries by age 45.

In PCOS, high insulin may disrupt ovulation and prompt miscarriages by signaling a woman's ovaries to produce extra male hormones, says infertility specialist Sandra Carson, MD, a reproductive endocrinologist at Baylor College of Medicine in Houston. Signs of PCOS include menstrual periods that are more than 6 weeks apart, stubborn weight gain, acne, and abnormal facial or body hair.

Meanwhile, having diabetes before pregnancy can raise your baby's risk of birth defects—especially of the heart and spinal cord—two to five times higher than normal. Developing diabetes during pregnancy, a condition called gestational diabetes, raises your odds of delivering a high-birth-weight baby and developing preeclampsia, a dangerous pregnancy-related elevation in blood pressure.

DEMENTIA AND ALZHEIMER'S DISEASE

Both overweight and diabetes increase the odds for dementia. Now researchers think insulin resistance in brain cells is one reason why.

In lab studies at the Joslin Diabetes Center in Boston, researchers found that the brain cells of insulin-resistant mice produced a protein also found in the brain lesions of people with Alzheimer's disease. As you'll read in Chapter 6, diabetes and insulin resistance may also short-change a brain region responsible for memory—in some cases shrinking it significantly, new research shows.

VISION PROBLEMS AND BLINDNESS

If you have diabetes or even prediabetes, high blood sugar levels can damage and destroy tiny capillaries in the eyes. The capillaries swell and weaken, clog, and burst—a condition called diabetic retinopathy that blurs vision and often leads to blindness. Diabetes is the leading cause of blindness in adults age 20 on up.

Also, chronically high blood sugar levels activate a substance called protein kinase C, which causes abnormal production of new blood vessels in the eye. The problem is, you don't need these new vessels—and they're more prone to leaking and bursting.

NERVE DAMAGE AND AMPUTATION

About 70 percent of lower-leg amputations performed in 2003 were on people with diabetes, says the federal Agency for Healthcare Research and Quality. The cause: high blood glucose that damages nerves and reduces circulation, making even the smallest cut or blister potentially a wound that won't heal.

Nerve damage can also cause impotence, arousal and orgasm difficulty for women, out-of-rhythm heartbeats, slowed digestion, and urinary problems.

TEETH

High blood sugar presents a triple threat to good oral health. First, it compromises your ability to fight infection, so even a small cold sore or tiny pocket of bacteria below the gum line could lead to serious trouble. Second, it raises the level of glucose in saliva, says Sol Silverman Jr., DDS, professor of oral medicine at the University of California, San Francisco, School of Dentistry and a spokesman for the American Dental Association. This "sweeter" saliva supports the growth of fungal (thrush) and bacterial infections. Third, high blood sugar can dry up saliva, leaving you with less of this vital infection-fighting moisture when you need it most.

COMIC RELIEF: A REAL BLOOD SUGAR BUSTER

Laugh if you will, but a recent study conducted in Japan found that a chuckle a day just might keep high blood sugar at bay.

Researchers at the University of Tsukuba tested the guffaw/glucose connection by measuring the blood sugar levels of 19 men and women with high blood sugar. On one day, the participants listened to a 40-minute lecture, which the researchers described as "monotonous" and "without humorous content." On the second day, they were included in an audience of 1,000 people who laughed loud and long during a performance of manzai, the Japanese version of stand-up comedy.

Before both performances, volunteers ate a 500-calorie meal. Afterward, their blood sugar was tested. Sugar levels were significantly lower after the comedy.

Laughing makes us move, and as a result, muscle cells may absorb more blood sugar, speculates researcher Keiko Hayashi, PhD. It's also possible that mirth affects hormones that help regulate blood sugar.

The damage? In a new Italian study of 212 patients at the Dental Institute of the University of Sassari, researchers found three times more gum-disease bacteria in the mouths of people with diabetes than in those without diabetes. People with diabetes also had more dental plaque, more bleeding gums, and deeper openings at the gumline around each tooth, a sign of gum disease.

KIDNEY FAILURE

At least 41,000 Americans with diabetes live with kidney failure and need regular dialysis to filter waste products from their blood. Some even receive transplanted kidneys. Even more shocking: New research from the International Diabetes Institute in Caulfield, Australia, finds that 10 percent of people with prediabetes have higher-than-normal levels of a protein called albumin in their urine, a telltale sign of early kidney disease.

In a healthy kidney, millions of tiny blood vessels called glomeruli act as strainers, trapping waste that's eventually flushed from your body in urine. But high blood sugar can damage the glomeruli. They leak, then fail. Eventually, the damage can lead to kidney failure.

CHAPTER 6

FOOD FOR THOUGHT— OR MEMORY ROBBER?

Your brain is a sugar thief.

Whether you're solving a tricky math problem, engrossed in a hobby, daydreaming, or fast asleep, 200 billion neurons—brain cells responsible for thought and for communication with nerves throughout your body—are firing away. Neurons produce electrical signals and send them along miles of nerve pathways throughout your body; they also assemble and release neurotransmitters to communicate with each other. Some 10,000 different types of neurons are hard at work between your ears right now, processing information that makes every aspect of human life possible, from composing music to breathing, from holding a conversation to walking down the street.

All this brain work requires lots of fuel. Brain cells gobble nearly twice as much blood sugar as any other type of cell in your body—using about 80 milligrams of sugar per minute, compared with about 50 milligrams per minute for the rest of your body at rest. And brain cells are greedy: Neurons and the helper cells that feed them, called glial cells, store only a tiny percentage of the sugar the brain needs. Without a constant supply from your digestive system and liver, delivered via your bloodstream, your brain would run short in about 10 minutes.

Keeping hungry neurons fed and energized is one of your body's top priorities. You play an important role, too. Your little gray cells will work better—or worse—depending on the quality and quantity of carbohydrates you eat. If you've had any of these experiences, you've learned firsthand how the fuel you take in can profoundly affect your ability to think well.

- You wake up so groggy that making coffee feels like a final exam in advanced particle physics. Somehow, you assemble breakfast: cereal, milk, juice, java. *Ahhh!* Twenty minutes later, the mental fog lifts. Your thinking is sharp and clear.
- You're halfway through a complicated work project, and your mind just won't budge. Your body isn't tired, but your brain—at least the part you need right now—is wrung out.
- You skipped lunch and wish you hadn't. You feel shaky and can't think straight. You grab a cola and a candy bar and . . . *whoosh!* Clarity returns (for a little while).

Blood sugar fluctuations profoundly influence your thinking over the short term and can alter the health of your brain and its ability to process and recall information over the long term. Low blood sugar can dull your mental edge if an important prelunch meeting drags on for too long. Over time, high blood sugar and related sugar-control problems can change the brain itself—raising the risk for memory lapses, dementia, and even Alzheimer's disease.

Read on for the latest research breakthroughs on the brain/blood sugar interface. This food for thought could help you think more clearly today and for decades to come.

"I JUST CAN'T THINK ABOUT IT ANYMORE"

If you've ever wondered why you can hit a wall when you think about something for too long, neuroscience may finally have the answer. Landmark research has found that the hippocampus—a region of the brain crucial for processing short-term memory—may use up its glucose supply faster than other regions during intense problem solving, says neuroscientist Paul Gold, PhD, a professor at the University of Illinois in Champaign. In lab studies, Dr. Gold found that rats given glu-

THE DEPRESSION/BLOOD SUGAR LINK

Could it be that depression triggers or contributes to the development of diabetes?

Researchers at Kaiser Permanente Center for Health Research in Portland, Oregon, compared 1,680 HMO members newly diagnosed with diabetes and 1,680 members of the same age and sex without the condition. They found that people with diabetes were more likely than those who were diabetes-free to have been treated for or diagnosed with depression before they were diagnosed with diabetes. Moreover, when depression coexisted with diabetes, depression was diagnosed first 73 percent of the time, says Greg Nichols, PhD, senior research associate at Kaiser.

While experts aren't sure what to make of the link, they do have theories, says Dr. Nichols. There may be a relationship between the regulation of glucose and levels of various hormones responsible for depression, like catecholamine and serotonin. "In other words, both depression and diabetes share a common antecedent," says Dr. Nichols. "Obesity, a sedentary lifestyle, and poor diet—plus some genetic predisposition—lead to depression and diabetes, at least in some people. The big unanswered question is whether diabetes can be prevented by treating depression or even whether treating diabetes eases depression."

---

cose shots actually showed low glucose levels in this important region after navigating a new maze. He also discovered that the brains of older rats needed more time to recover after sugar supplies dropped.

Sugar *is* brain food. In another study by Dr. Gold, women and men in their sixties received either a sugar-sweetened or saccharin-sweetened drink after fasting overnight. After each drink, they were given an hour-long series of standardized memory tests while their blood glucose levels were monitored. "On the day our subjects got the sweetened drink, they performed 20 to 30 percent better on the memory tests," Dr. Gold says.

These findings shouldn't send you to the nearest Krispy Kreme shop, however. Yes, the simple sugars in a doughnut or a candy bar can spike your blood sugar—and perhaps your mental acuity—for a short time. Dr. Gold says that while certain doses of glucose improve memory and learning ability, higher doses actually impair memory. The optimal

RX FOR LOW BLOOD SUGAR

Beyond hungry, you're cranky, barely able to think clearly, and nearly on the verge of fainting. Your best bet? A glass of orange juice to raise your blood sugar swiftly and a peanut-butter-on-whole-wheat sandwich to keep levels steady 'til lunch.

Low blood sugar—doctors call it hypoglycemia—can leave you jittery, nauseous, shaky, and even sweaty and confused. If you have diabetes and use blood sugar–lowering medications, your dose may be off, or you may not have eaten enough at your last meal. If you don't have diabetes, you may have reactive hypoglycemia (when blood sugar levels plummet an hour or two after a meal) or fasting hypoglycemia (when levels fall steadily for hours after eating).

Reactive hypoglycemia may be a sign that your blood sugar control system overreacts to the stress hormone epinephrine or that your body doesn't release enough stored blood sugar between meals. Gastric bypass surgery and a rare enzyme deficiency, hereditary fructose intolerance, may also be behind it.

If you have fasting hypoglycemia, the cause could be a medicine you take (such as sulfa antibiotics and large, regular doses of aspirin) or the wine you had at your last meal. Your doctor may also check for a variety of kidney, heart, and liver conditions that can lower blood sugar.

The best Rx for garden-variety low blood sugar: Don't go more than 3 hours during the day without eating—include small snacks between meals. Go for high-fiber foods like whole fruit instead of fruit juice (except when you need to raise your blood sugar quickly), whole wheat instead of white bread, nuts instead of a snack cake. Avoid sugary goodies, especially on an empty stomach.

dose for improving memory probably varies from person to person, with other foods you've eaten recently, and even with your stress level at the moment.

The best fuel mix: good carbs—whole grains, fruits, and veggies. When University of Toronto researchers checked the memories of volunteers who breakfasted on plain water or on cereal, milk, and grape juice, they found that the cereal eaters remembered 25 percent more facts. And when breakfasters had either a sugary lemon drink or a bowl of barley, the barley eaters outperformed the sweet-drinks group on tests of long- and short-term memory.

HIGH BLOOD SUGAR NOW, MEMORY TROUBLE LATER

A small but well-designed study from New York University recently made headlines (and may have changed what a lot of middle-aged folks ordered for lunch that day) with the news that middle-aged and elderly people with blood sugar trouble actually had more memory problems and a smaller hippocampus.

First, the researchers gave 30 study volunteers, ages 53 to 89, a memory test. They were told a story and, after a short period of distraction, asked to retell the story with as many details as possible. The next day, after a good night's sleep but before breakfast, they received about two doughnuts' worth of glucose intravenously. Then researchers evaluated how quickly their bodies used the glucose and later imaged their brains with an MRI.

The result: People with insulin resistance, who had a tougher time absorbing sugar into cells, had smaller hippocampuses. This suggests that insulin resistance not only affects the way the brain processes information but also can change the physical structure of the brain itself. The researchers said that they detected insulin resistance in the hippocampus about a decade before this memory-processing center showed signs of shrinking.

The researchers have even developed a brain-scanning computer program that can predict Alzheimer's risk nearly a decade in advance. The system uses measurements of glucose uptake in the hippocampus. In a long-term study that followed 53 volunteers for 9 to 23 years, the

THE SUGAR SURVIVORS: Pamela Oldham

Freelance writer Pamela Oldham of Ashburn, Virginia, writes about health for a living, yet it took an ambulance ride to recognize her blood sugar problem.

Oldham often felt sluggish in the morning, but one day in fall 2002, she dialed 911. "I began to feel as though I was about to lose consciousness," she recalls. "My daughter was at school, and my husband had just left for work. My symptoms were strokelike, and that worried me, especially because I was alone in the house."

By the time the ambulance arrived, Oldham's speech was slurred and she couldn't think clearly. En route to the hospital, an emergency medical technician thought to test her blood sugar level. It was dangerously low. He immediately began a solution of intravenous glucose. By the time they reached the medical center a few minutes later, her symptoms had all but vanished.

Although she'd never been diagnosed with hypoglycemia (low blood sugar) before, she'd had the symptoms, including dizziness, nausea, and sluggishness,

for years. The morning she dialed 911, she hadn't eaten breakfast. "I felt awful from the moment I woke up," she says. "I was dizzy, as if I had a hangover or hadn't had enough sleep, yet I also felt shaky and nervous. It was weird."

The previous night, she'd eaten a candy bar before bed, which caused her blood sugar to rise, plummet as she slept, and bottom out just before she woke up.

To regulate her hypoglycemia, Oldham now eats several small meals throughout the day and tries to avoid simple sugars like candy and chocolate, especially on an empty stomach or late at night. In the morning, she eats mostly carbohydrates, such as high-fiber cereal and whole grain toast, to help steadily raise her blood sugar levels. If she starts to feel shaky, she downs a glass of orange or apple juice to balance her blood sugar.

"I'm much more aware of what I eat and drink and when," says Oldham. "I have to admit that even with the scare I had, it was tough to change my habits—like fitting breakfast into my day. But now I know a good breakfast is a must."

researchers found that those whose brains used 15 to 40 percent less glucose went on to develop memory problems ranging from mild impairment to Alzheimer's disease.

The research may have special significance for people with diabetes, who have a twofold higher risk for Alzheimer's disease and are at higher risk for age-related memory loss. When Harvard Medical School researchers tested the memory and mental function of 2,300 women in their seventies, those with diabetes were twice as likely to have low scores. Investigators estimate that diabetes adds at least 4 years to the age of the brain. Taking steps to lower blood sugar in middle age—via diet and exercise—could preserve your brain.

3

THE *SUGAR SOLUTION* EATING PLAN

CHAPTER 7

EAT WELL FOR LIFE: BETTER THAN A DIET!

Start with smart carbs that keep your blood sugar low and steady. Add good fats that taste good, too—nuts (even peanut butter!) and fish. Put lean, satisfying protein on your plate and have some bone-building, fat-burning milk, yogurt, and cheese. (And don't forget the chocolate brownies, wine, chips with salsa, and buffalo wings!)

This is the *Sugar Solution* eating plan—a diet that can help you lose weight now, keep it off forever, and protect you from a wide array of serious health problems, from heart attack and stroke to diabetes, cancer, and memory problems. Our daily menus don't look like health food or a skimpy low-calorie regimen; they do look (and taste) simply delicious! How about an omelet filled with asparagus and goat cheese for breakfast, a roast beef sandwich for lunch, and cheesy eggplant Parmesan with polenta for dinner—plus a chocolate chip cookie at snack time? Behind these satisfying meals is the latest nutrition and weight-loss research, harnessed to create an everyday eating plan in which virtually every food is a star, proven to help you lose weight and guard—or improve—your health.

Our menus and 100-plus recipes were developed by dietitian Ann Fittante, MS, RD, a certified diabetes educator, nutrition educator, and exercise physiologist at the renowned Joslin Diabetes Center at Swedish

Medical Center in Seattle. Her goal? To tickle your tastebuds, turn off between-meal cravings, optimize the way your body burns fat, and nurture your blood sugar control system. In the chapters ahead, you'll learn how to stock your kitchen to make *Sugar Solution* meals a snap,

5 WAYS TO BLUNT BLOOD SUGAR

These strategies can lower the overall effect of a meal on your blood sugar.

1. **Add beans.** Only have time to make instant rice? Just add some beans. Throwing in a low-glycemic-index food brings down the GI rating of the entire meal.

2. **Deploy good fat.** Bagels for breakfast? Slather with a tablespoon of peanut butter. Fat slows absorption of sugar into the bloodstream.

3. **Grab a cheese stick or precooked chicken strips.** For less than 100 calories, a stick of string cheese or a few pieces of chicken can transform a potentially blood sugar–raising snack (such as crackers or a piece of toast) into an oasis of satisfaction that will last for hours. Like fat, protein slows digestion and absorption of sugars.

4. **Have a salad with vinaigrette.** Start lunch or dinner with any vinaigrette-dressed veggie medley—field greens; chilled green beans; even a half cup of steamed, cooled red Bliss potatoes. Arizona State University nutritionists discovered that vinegar prevented blood sugar spikes after eating. They suspect that acetic acid (the compound that makes vinegar so, so sour) interferes with enzymes that break down carbs. Just 2 teaspoons per meal could help tame glucose.

5. **Sprinkle on some cinnamon.** Just half a teaspoon of cinnamon each day—dust a little on your morning toast, add a bit to your afternoon skim latte or your dinnertime sweet potato—improves your body's ability to obey insulin and take up glucose, report researchers at the USDA's Beltsville Human Nutrition Research Center in Maryland. Cinnamon contains a compound called methylhydroxy chalcone polymer that makes cells absorb glucose faster and convert it more easily into energy—so your blood sugar stays lower.

stick with the plan when you're eating in a restaurant, and fit in sweets and other treats, plus you'll get a month's worth of clever strategies that will help keep your body and mind on track for weight-loss success and better health.

This chapter outlines the five major components of the plan—we call them the *Sugar Solution* Food Groups—and shows you the research each one is based on. Let's get started!

SMART COMPONENT #1: A WEALTH OF FRUITS, VEGETABLES, AND WHOLE GRAINS

Serving Guide

You'll eat two to four servings of fruit, four to six servings of vegetables, and four to six servings of grains every day, for a total of 50 to 60 percent of your daily calories.

On the Menu

- A rainbow of fresh produce for crunching, including apples, apricots, pears, asparagus, red peppers, salads, sugar snap peas, and fresh soybeans (edamame)—plus dips for raw veggies
- Fruit showcased in berry smoothies, a raspberry tart, strawberries in phyllo dough, and more
- Delicious vegetable dishes such as broccoli with garlic and onions, mashed and baked potatoes, oven fries, and even eggplant Parmesan with melted cheese and an asparagus quiche
- Satisfying and sophisticated grain dishes such as polenta, quinoa (a mild, quick-cooking grain) with peppers, pasta, and barley with spring greens—plus breakfast favorites like waffles, crepes, toast, English muffins, and hearty hot cereals

The Blood Sugar Benefit

Low-glycemic-index (GI) carbohydrates—fresh fruits, vegetables, and whole grains—digest more slowly and release glucose to the bloodstream a little bit at a time over the course of hours. The benefit: Blood sugar and insulin (the hormone that tells cells to absorb blood sugar) stay lower. In contrast, high-GI foods like white bread, cake, and doughnuts make blood sugar spike, prompting your body to secrete a flood of insulin.

Recent research has linked lower insulin levels to a lower risk of type 2 diabetes, heart disease, and even memory loss. In one study of 23 young adults from Children's Hospital Boston—where some of the nation's most cutting-edge studies on the glycemic index, health, and weight in adults and children are under way—scientists found significant health benefits for volunteers following a low-GI eating plan, compared

SECRETS OF THE GLYCEMIC INDEX

Invented in the early 1980s by University of Toronto researchers as a tool for controlling high blood sugar, the glycemic index (GI) ranks carbohydrate foods according to their effect on blood sugar levels. High-GI carbs make blood sugar and insulin levels soar; low-GI carbs are slow-burning fuel that keeps your blood sugar low and steady—and as a result, keeps insulin levels lower. You feel full longer; have fewer food cravings; and reduce your risk for health problems, including type 2 diabetes, heart disease, stroke, cancer, and memory loss.

The GI assigns carbohydrate-containing foods a number based on their impact on your blood sugar. Foods with a GI below 55 cause only a little blip; those in the 55-to-70 range raise blood sugar a little higher;

and carbs with GIs over 70 send it soaring.

Why would different carbs have such radically divergent effects on blood sugar? No matter what form the carb initially takes—the lactose in milk, the starch in a bagel, the sucrose in table sugar—eventually, your body breaks it down to glucose. The longer your digestive system has to wrestle with the carb to break it down, the slower the rise in blood sugar and the lower the GI number assigned to the food.

Among the factors that make a carb low-GI: the presence of viscous fiber (such as in oatmeal and beans); the size of starch particles (finely milled flours have a higher GI than coarse flours); how thoroughly a starch is cooked (al dente pasta has a lower GI than soft, overcooked

with those eating a high-GI diet. Specifically, the low-GI group raised their heart-protecting HDL cholesterol further (by 12 points, versus one point for the high-GI group), cut harmful LDL cholesterol by an extra 20 percent, lowered heart-threatening triglycerides twice as much, and raised insulin sensitivity 20 percent more. Low-GI eating can also reduce levels of C-reactive protein, a compound associated with bodywide chronic inflammation, a risk factor for heart disease and diabetes.

"The beauty of the glycemic index for people with diabetes is that it not only helps control blood sugar and insulin but its appetite-sup-

---

noodles); and the presence of acids (like a vinaigrette dressing) or fat (such as margarine), which slows absorption of blood sugar.

Remember, the glycemic index describes the quality of a carbohydrate but not the quantity that exists within a food. Our plan takes into consideration a food's glycemic load—its true impact on blood sugar based on the carb's type *and* amount. Why does this matter?

Some healthy foods that have little effect on blood sugar, such as carrots and watermelon, contain carbs with a high GI. But they actually have very little of it—they're packed with water and fiber. It would be a mistake to miss out on them.

For a quick start with the glycemic index, try these simple food switches.

High-GI Favorite	Lower-GI Choice
French bread, 95	100 percent stone-ground whole wheat bread, 53
Jelly beans, 80	Dried apricots, 31
Mashed or baked potato, 73 or 85	Roasted sweet potato, 54
Pretzels, 83	Popcorn, 55
Side of bread stuffing mix, 74	Side of canned baked beans, 48
Vanilla wafers, 77	Oatmeal cookies, 55

pressing effects help them lose weight. And weight loss alone can reverse type 2," says Marc Rendell, MD, director of the Creighton Diabetes Center at Creighton University in Omaha, Nebraska, and medical director of the Rose Salter Medical Research Foundation in Baltimore.

Fruits, vegetables, and whole grains are also packed with cholesterol-lowering, digestion-improving fiber and a rainbow of powerful, natural antioxidants that protect your cells from damaging free radicals—rogue oxygen molecules produced naturally in the body that heighten your vulnerability to heart disease and cancer.

The Weight-Loss Bonus

If you're insulin resistant—and you probably are, since this condition affects as many as one in two American adults and nearly everyone who's overweight—your cells "ignore" signals from the hormone insulin to absorb blood sugar. Your body pumps out extra insulin to force sugar into cells. The excess may make weight loss a special challenge for insulin-resistant people. The hormone encourages cells to store more of your extra calories as fat and blocks your body's attempts to burn stored fat.

The answer? A low-glycemic, reduced-calorie eating plan like the *Sugar Solution*. In a recent Tufts University–New England Medical Center study of 39 overweight women and men, participants with high insulin levels lost an average of 22 pounds in 6 months on a low-GI plan, compared with 13 pounds on a higher-GI diet. Lower insulin levels seem to "unlock" fat cells so that extra body fat is finally burned off!

Other research suggests that a low-GI diet keeps your metabolism from downshifting dramatically, as happens on most weight-loss diets. Truth is, any low-calorie diet will slow your metabolic rate—the number of calories your body burns each day at rest. But researchers from Children's Hospital Boston found that adult dieters who ate low-GI foods burned 80 more calories per day than those on a higher-GI, lower-fat diet. They also felt more energetic and had a greater sense of well-being—feelings that can help you stick with a diet and feel more motivated to get up and exercise.

Low-GI diets can also stop food cravings. "GI is not the complete

(continued on page 63)

THE *SUGAR SOLUTION* GLYCEMIC INDEX TABLE

You don't really have to consult a glycemic index list before choosing foods. While the science behind this exciting nutrition and weight-loss breakthrough is complex, the basic on-your-plate strategy is simple: All you need to do to get the benefits is choose vegetables, whole fruits, and moderate portions of whole grains in place of a steady diet of white potatoes, fruit juices or sweetened fruit (such as canned in heavy syrup), and refined-grain products.

Foods listed in italic type are high-GI foods that you need not avoid. These foods, such as carrots and watermelon, contain very little carbohydrate (they're mostly water and fiber), so the actual impact on your blood sugar is small. Foods listed with an asterisk are low-GI foods that are best eaten sparingly. These foods, such as potato chips, are high in fat or calories—and don't offer much else nutritionally.

FOOD	GI	FOOD	GI	FOOD	GI
Baked Goods		*100 percent whole*		*Old-fashioned oats*	59
French bread	95	*rye bread*	65	Oat bran	55
Waffle	76	*Rye crispbread*	65	All-Bran	42
Graham cracker	74	Bran muffin	60	**Grains**	
Kaiser roll	73	Whole wheat pita	57	Instant rice	91
Bagel	72	Oatmeal cookie	55	*Millet*	71
Corn tortilla	70	Pumpernickel bread	4	Cornmeal	68
Melba toast	70	**Cereals**		White rice	68
White bread	70	Puffed rice	88	Couscous	65
Whole wheat bread	69	Cornflakes	84	Brown rice	55
Taco shell	68	Puffed wheat	74	Buckwheat	54
Angel food cake	67	Cream of Wheat	70	Bulgur	48
Croissant	67	*Shredded wheat*	69	Parboiled rice	47
Stoned wheat thins	67	Quick-cooking oats	66	Pearled barley	26

continued

FOOD	GI
Pasta	
Brown rice pasta	92
Gnocchi	68
Boxed macaroni and cheese	64
Rice vermicelli	58
Durum spaghetti	55
Cheese tortellini*	50
Linguine*	46
White spaghetti*	41
Meat-filled ravioli*	39
Whole grain spaghetti	37
Vermicelli	35
Fettuccine	32
Bean threads	26
Legumes	
Fava beans	79
Canned kidney beans	52
Canned baked beans	48
Canned pinto beans	45
Black-eyed peas	42
Canned chickpeas	42
Chickpeas	33
Lima beans	32
Yellow split peas	32
Butter beans	31
Green lentils	30
Kidney beans	27
Red lentils	26
Soybeans	18

FOOD	GI
Dairy and Ice Cream	
Tofu frozen dessert	115
Ice cream	61
Sweetened fruit yogurt	33
Fat-free milk	32
Whole milk	27
Artificially sweetened yogurt	14
Fruits	
Watermelon	72
Pineapple	66
Cantaloupe	65
Raisins	64
Orange juice	57
Mango	55
Banana	53
Kiwifruit	52
Grapefruit juice	48
Pineapple juice	46
Orange	43
Grapes	43
Apple juice	41
Apple	36
Pear	36
Strawberries	32
Dried apricots	31
Peach	28
Grapefruit	25
Plum	24
Cherries	22

FOOD	GI
Vegetables	
Parsnip	97
Baked potato	85
Instant mashed potato	83
French-fried potato	75
Pumpkin	75
Carrot	71
Fresh mashed potato	70
Beet	64
Boiled new potato	62
Fresh corn	59
Sweet potato	54
Yam	51
Green peas	48
Tomato	38
Snacks and Miscellaneous	
Pretzel	83
Rice cake	82
Vanilla wafers	77
Tortilla chips	74
Corn chips	72
Table sugar (sucrose)	65
Popcorn	55
Potato chips*	54
Chocolate	49
Chocolate-covered peanuts	32
Soy milk	31
Peanuts	14

answer to everyone's weight problem," says researcher Susan Roberts, PhD, professor of nutrition at Tufts University in Boston. "But aside from the research, I am personally convinced that low-GI diets help people lose weight, myself included. My husband and I were eating a relatively high-GI instant oatmeal for breakfast, but we both kept getting so hungry 2 hours after eating. [They switched to a low-GI Irish oatmeal and felt better.] I keep in mind the GI of what I eat and quite consistently find myself hungrier after very high-GI foods such as bagels and mashed potatoes."

SMART COMPONENT #2: LEAN, SATISFYING PROTEIN

Serving Guide

You'll eat some protein at each meal, for a total of 15 to 25 percent of your daily calories.

On the Menu

- Eggs in omelets and frittatas
- Beans in chili, lentil soup, Tuscan bean stew, and even baked beans
- Roll-ups and wrap sandwiches featuring tuna, chicken, turkey, and grilled veggies with melted lower-fat cheese
- Family favorites such as oven-fried chicken, grilled steak, barbecued spareribs, breaded cod with tartar sauce, clam chowder, chicken Parmesan, and shrimp and crab cakes
- Casseroles including eggplant stuffed with beef, Mexican lasagna, and chicken and mushrooms with rigatoni
- Meatless protein in whole wheat pasta, yogurt, whole grain cereal with nuts, snacks featuring nuts, and peanut butter

The Blood Sugar Benefit

Bringing their protein levels up to the amount recommended in the *Sugar Solution* plan (up to 25 percent of daily calories) allowed 25 Danish women and men to shed 10 percent more belly fat—the dangerous intra-abdominal fat that raises risk for diabetes and heart disease—than dieters whose plates held more carbs, say researchers from the

Royal Veterinary and Agricultural University in Copenhagen.

No one's sure why eating more protein would selectively target belly fat. One possible explanation: A higher protein intake may somehow trigger smaller releases of the anxiety hormone cortisol. Cortisol directs the body to store more fat in the abdomen—less cortisol, less belly fat.

The Weight-Loss Bonus

Protein switches on that "I'm full" feeling after you eat—and keeps you from feeling so hungry between meals. The effect can be powerful and long lasting. Thirty women who started their day with two eggs and toast felt so full and satisfied that they ate 274 fewer calories the rest of the day than those who had bagels and cream cheese, finds a new study from the Rochester Center for Obesity Research in Michigan. The egg eaters even ate fewer calories the following day. Eggs, note the researchers, are simply more satisfying than breads and bagels.

Protein—whether from meat, eggs, dairy foods, or nuts—boosts metabolism for up to 3 hours after a meal and to higher levels than carbs or fats do, so you burn more calories.

SMART COMPONENT #3: DAIRY FOR YOUR BONES— AND YOUR HEART

Serving Guide

You'll eat two servings of dairy products on most days. Dairy calories count toward your daily quota of protein, fat, and even carbs, because milk contains all of these components.

On the Menu

- Yogurt-berry smoothies and snacks that combine the cool, smooth texture of yogurt with the sweetness of fruit
- 1 percent milk
- Cheese. Surprised? You'll find generous amounts of melted cheese in our recipes for chicken and eggplant Parmesan and on our wrap sandwich with grilled veggies, plus a tasty helping of Parmesan on

pasta dishes and a satisfying layer of goat cheese or Jarlsberg on our chicken-pesto pizza.

The Blood Sugar Benefit

Dairy foods may protect against metabolic syndrome, a prediabetic condition that raises your risk of heart attack, stroke, high blood pressure, type 2 diabetes, cancer, and memory loss. In one landmark, multicenter study that followed 3,157 young women and men for a decade, insulin resistance risk dropped 21 percent for each daily serving of dairy products. Calcium and other nutrients in dairy foods can also help protect against high blood pressure.

Of course, calcium is also essential for maintaining bone density. That's why the *Sugar Solution* plan recommends that you take a daily calcium supplement of at least 500 milligrams, so that your body gets all it needs to protect your bones. Our eating plan provides about 850 milligrams per day, the amount in two regular dairy servings plus small amounts from the other foods you eat. You need 1,000 milligrams per day if you're between ages 19 and 50 and 1,200 milligrams per day if you're over 50.

One caveat: Be sure to spread your calcium supplements over the course of the day. Your body can absorb only about 500 milligrams at a time.

The Weight-Loss Bonus

On a reduced-calorie diet, the calcium in dairy products (and, to a lesser extent, in supplements) can turbocharge your weight-loss efforts. Despite recent controversies over whether milk can help shed pounds, two research studies from the University of Tennessee's Nutrition Institute are clear: If you haven't been getting enough calcium in your diet, adding more (up to safe, normal limits) can help you lose weight more easily. In one of the studies, 32 obese women and men who cut 500 calories a day from their meal plans lost more weight when they added 800 milligrams of supplemental calcium daily, and they shed even more weight and fat when they took supplements containing 1,200 to 1,300 milligrams of calcium. In the other study, 34 obese people on weight-loss diets lost more pounds and more fat if they had three daily servings of yogurt than if they had one.

SMART COMPONENT #4: GOOD FATS FOR YOUR HEART, MIND, AND TASTEBUDS

Serving Guide

You'll get 25 to 30 percent of your daily calories from fat, including daily servings of the good fats your body needs most.

On the Menu

- Omega-3 fatty acids in grilled salmon, ground flaxseed in our multigrain cereal and smoothies, and walnuts for snacking—and in our rich chocolate brownies
- Healthy monounsaturated fat in peanut butter and almond butter on your breakfast toast, olive and canola oils for sautéing and baking, the peanuts in our peanut butter cookies, avocado slices for salads, hummus dip for raw veggies, and cashews (and other nuts) for snacking
- No trans fats and just a smidgen of saturated fat

The Blood Sugar Benefit

Early research suggests that getting plenty of omega-3s may cool off chronic inflammation, a risk factor for metabolic syndrome and diabetes. Meanwhile, good fats have a proven track record as protectors against health problems brought on by metabolic syndrome.

Just one weekly serving of fish rich in omega-3s (such as salmon, sardines, or mackerel) can cut the risk of a fatal heart attack by 40 percent. The American Heart Association advises us to eat two servings a week. A 12-year Brigham and Women's Hospital study of 4,800 people found that those who ate any fish one to four times a week had a 28 percent lower risk of atrial fibrillation (AF) than those who avoided fish. AF disrupts the heart's rhythm, causing fatigue and shortness of breath.

Northwestern University scientists who had analyzed eight studies involving 200,575 people concluded that eating fatty fish (such as salmon, mackerel, and herring) just once a week cut the risk of ischemic stroke—the most common kind, caused by blood clots—by 13 percent. And a Harvard study of 727 women found that those who ate fatty fish almost every day—compared with those who ate it only three times a month—had 7 to 10 percent lower blood levels of molecules that bind plaque-building cells to artery walls.

Eating fish once a week could lower your risk of developing Alzheimer's disease, according to a study at Rush Presbyterian–St. Luke's Medical Center in Chicago. Researchers collected dietary information from 815 people ages 65 to 94 who were free from Alzheimer's at the start of the study. After an average follow-up of about 4 years, 131 of the participants developed Alzheimer's. Compared with those who rarely or never ate fish, those who ate it once a week had a 60 percent risk reduction.

Plant-based omega-3s are heart-healthy, too. Vigorous arteries pump fluid through smooth, untarnished "pipes." Eating walnuts may help them stay that way, suggest Spanish researchers. They gave two groups of people heart-healthy diets that differed in just one respect: One diet included eight to 13 walnuts a day. After 4 weeks, the walnut eaters had 64 percent stronger artery-pumping action and 20 percent less gunk-sticky molecules that initiate atherosclerotic plaque. Among nuts, walnuts alone are high in heart-healthy omega-3 fatty acids.

Meanwhile, almonds—a rich source of fiber, monounsaturated fats, and the antioxidant vitamin E—can cut heart disease risk 12.5 percent. After tracking more than 83,000 women with no history of diabetes, cardiovascular disease, or cancer for 16 years, Harvard researchers found that those who ate nuts at least five times per week reduced their risk of type 2 diabetes by almost 30 percent, compared with those who rarely or never noshed on these tasty nuggets. Those who ate peanut butter at least five times a week reduced their risk for type 2 diabetes by almost 20 percent, compared with women who rarely ate peanut butter.

The Weight-Loss Bonus

When 65 overweight women and men followed a 1,000-calorie-a-day diet for 24 weeks, those who ate almonds at snack time lost 18 percent of their body weight, while those whose treats were carbohydrate-based (such as crackers, baked potatoes, and popcorn) lost just 11 percent. The nut eaters whittled their waists 14 percent; the carb snackers, 9 percent. Researchers from the City of Hope National Medical Center in Duarte, California, suspect that the protein, fat, and fiber in almonds keep you feeling full longer—and that not all the calories in almonds are absorbed, thanks to the tough cell walls of these nuts.

SMART COMPONENT #5: ROOM FOR TREATS!

Serving Guide

You'll enjoy at least one treat every day.

On the Menu

- Wine—some menus include a glass of red or white wine—plus, advice on how to swap calories to fit in a drink on other days
- Real desserts that are fun to bake and guilt-free to eat, including chocolate chip cookies, raspberry tart, brownies, zucchini–chocolate chip bread, and rice pudding
- Tortilla chips at snack time, dips for veggies, a nacho plate for lunch, appetizers like shrimp in mustard-horseradish sauce and buffalo wings
- Easy treats like low-fat ice cream or sorbet, string cheese, and air-popped popcorn

The Blood-Sugar Benefit

Often, we've paired sweeter treats with fats, fiber, and proteins—a strategy that blunts the effect of sweets on your blood sugar—and trimmed the calories so these goodies won't add inches to your waistline (a risk factor for insulin resistance). We've also taken advantage of an underappreciated fact about sugar (yes, nearly all of our desserts use the real thing): Gram for gram, the carbs in *table* sugar have less effect on your blood sugar than do the starchy carbs in foods like white bread, some pastas and noodles, and many breakfast cereals. A moderately sized homemade treat or a sprinkle of sugar on oatmeal or strawberries won't make you fat. (Portions count, though; overdoing it will increase calories.)

We do urge you to avoid drinks sweetened with high fructose corn syrup. These high-calorie drinks seem to trigger a desire to drink even more—raising your risk for overweight and problems like diabetes.

The Weight-Loss Bonus

We firmly believe that regular treats will help you stay on track with your weight-loss plans. And to keep the luscious desserts in this book within your fat and calorie budget, we've made strategic and sparing use of low-fat baking ingredients (such as reduced-fat cream cheese) and, occasionally, the artificial sweetener Splenda. This allows us to keep in delicious, authentic ingredients such as real chocolate chips, butter, and sugar (in moderate quantities) so that *Sugar Solution* desserts taste like the real thing. You'll feel pampered—and satisfied. We used the same strategy in developing appetizer recipes that are delicious enough to serve company but won't throw you off your weight-loss plan.

CHAPTER 8

30 SMART FOOD AND WEIGHT-LOSS STRATEGIES

Oatmeal or toast and jelly? Pasta or broiled chicken and field greens? Fresh berries or a brownie sundae?

Ultimately, what you choose to eat—the little decisions you make in the kitchen, in the cafeteria line, or out to dinner—plays a major role in whether or not your blood sugar stays on an even keel, raising or lowering your risk for overweight, fatigue, and a host of major health problems.

Think of this chapter as a nutritional cheat sheet, with practical food wisdom that can help put you on the road to blood sugar control. Here, you'll find 30 nutritional tips that reflect the current thinking on the relationship between diet and blood sugar, including high-protein diets, "good" and "bad" carbs, the glycemic index, fitting sweets into your diet, and much more.

You'll even find quick and easy minirecipes to help you put these tips into action. And remember: The more often you practice these recommendations, the more your blood sugar numbers stand to benefit.

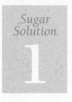

Sugar Solution

1

GO ON A FIBER HUNT

We'll skip the sermon about the health benefits of fruits and vegetables. But we'd like to remind you that if you're trying to lose weight or control your blood sugar, fiber is your friend. A recent study showed that people with diabetes who ate 50 grams of fiber a day—particularly the soluble kind, found in foods like apples and oatmeal—were able to control their blood sugar better than those who ate far less.

Fiber is so important to health that the American Diabetes Association recently recommended that people who have diabetes or are at risk should strive for a whopping 50 grams a day. (Later in this chapter, we'll show you how to use a fiber supplement to help get there.) And the US Food and Nutrition Board recently set the first recommended daily intakes for healthy women and men. Consider these guidelines your minimum fiber requirement: Before age 50, men need 35 grams; women, 25 grams. After age 50, men need 30; women, 31.

- Eat foods rich in soluble fiber. Researchers suspect that it may play an important role in glucose control because it forms a thick gel that may interfere with carbohydrate and glucose absorption in the intestine. The result: lower blood sugar and insulin levels and more manageable diabetes. Gold-star soluble-fiber foods include orange and grapefruit segments, prunes, cantaloupe, papaya, raisins, lima beans, zucchini, oatmeal, oat bran, and granola. Other foods high in soluble fiber include barley, peas, strawberries, and apple pulp (the skin is insoluble fiber).

- To get the most nutrients, health benefits, and fiber, strive for five servings of veggies and four of fruit daily—and go for a rainbow of colors. It's not really difficult if you include a fresh fruit at breakfast, a generously sized salad (which counts as two servings) and fruit for lunch, and two veggies at dinner plus fruit for dessert. Visit the produce aisle for precut, quick-cooking fresh produce, and avoid frozen vegetables with breading or sauce, which tend to be high in carbohydrates, sodium, and trans fats.

GIVE PEAS A CHANCE

And other beans, too. They're the highest-fiber foods you can find, with the exception of breakfast cereals made with wheat bran. High-fiber diets are linked to less diabetes and heart disease, and one study showed that as little as 3.4 ounces of beans a day helped people with diabetes manage their blood sugar levels. Beans are especially high in soluble fiber, which lowers cholesterol levels, and folate, which lowers homocysteine, another risk factor for heart disease.

Ideally, eat beans five or more times a week. They add protein and fiber to any dish and can be used in salads, stuffed baked potatoes, and veggie chili. Or puree some to use as a sandwich spread. If you keep a variety of beans in your pantry, you'll always have the makings of a delicious, healthful dinner. If you use canned beans, remember to rinse them first—they're packed in a high-sodium liquid.

Here are a few ways to get your hill of beans.

- Keep instant bean soups on hand. In a national study of almost 10,000 people, eating beans, peas, or lentils four times a week cut heart disease by 22 percent. With instant bean soups, you have a heart-smart meal that's ready in about 6 minutes—and no dishes to wash. Good choices include Fantastic Foods Five Bean (240 calories, 1.5 grams fat, 12 grams fiber), Fantastic Foods Split Pea (220 calories, 1 gram fat, 9 grams fiber), and Knorr Hearty Lentil (220 calories, 2 grams fat, 8 grams fiber).
- Whip up a savory Southwestern omelet: Combine ¼ cup of canned or cooked black beans; 2 tablespoons each of corn kernels, minced red or green pepper, diced tomato, and minced scallions; 1 tablespoon of diced jalapeño pepper; 1 tablespoon of dried cilantro; and ¼ teaspoon of dried cumin. This is enough to stuff an omelet made with three eggs or 1½ cups of egg substitute.
- Top a homemade pizza with ½ cup of cooked kidney or black beans, 1 cup of shredded spinach, and sliced mushrooms. If you miss the meat, add a few slices of turkey pepperoni.

GO WITH THE (CEREAL) GRAIN

Sugar Solution

3

To your body, refined white flour is the same as sugar, making a diet high in white-flour foods the same as a high-sugar diet. Conversely, the evidence is accumulating that, besides cutting the risk of heart disease, stroke, and cancer, diets high in whole grains are linked to less diabetes.

In one of the most recent studies, Finnish researchers followed 2,286 men and 2,030 women ages 40 through 69 for 10 years. They found that those who ate the most fiber—not from fruits and vegetables but from cereal grains such as rolled oats, rye, barley, millet, and buckwheat—had a 61 percent lower risk of type 2 diabetes.

It's thought that cereal fiber may help fight type 2 in a couple of ways. Compared with simple carbohydrates like white bread, fiber-rich carbs are digested and absorbed slowly, leading to less insulin demand. Also, insoluble fiber speeds through the intestines, leaving less time for carbohydrates to be absorbed. However, it's possible that other components in whole grains, such as lignans, tocotrienols, and phytic acids, could be responsible for the reduction in risk.

Here are some speedy, tasty ways to prepare whole grains.

- If you already eat whole wheat bread and need a change, try whole grain rye bread, which is what most of the cereal grain eaters in the Finnish study ate.
- Select whole grain pastas—whole wheat, of course, but also those made with amaranth, quinoa, or buckwheat (including Japanese buckwheat noodles, known as soba noodles). You'll find them at upscale grocery stores or health food stores.
- Stuff peppers with a mix of cooked bulgur, beans, mushrooms, celery, and basil.
- Stir wheat germ into low-fat yogurt, or sprinkle it on salads.
- For a hearty, healthier meat loaf, mix 1 cup of cooked whole millet into each pound of ground meat.
- For a tasty cold salad, mix quinoa with chopped parsley, cucumbers, tomatoes, and minced garlic. Dress with olive oil and lemon juice.

KEEP TO YOUR FAT BUDGET

Despite the long-running low-fat food craze in the United States, the amount of fat in our diets has actually been increasing, with the average woman consuming about 65 grams a day. That's too much.

On an 1,800-calorie diet with no more than 25 to 30 percent of calories coming from fat, we should get 50 to 60 grams of fat. And that should be 50 grams of good fat, like the types in olive and canola oils (monounsaturated fat) and fatty fish (omega-3 fatty acids).

You've probably already switched to fat-free milk and low-fat dairy products. And you know you should trim visible fat from pork and beef and remove the skin from poultry. Here are some other fat-busting tactics.

- Spread your fat throughout the day. A little fat helps you absorb fat-soluble nutrients from vegetables and fruit.
- Use wine; lemon, orange, or tomato juice; herbs and spices; or broth instead of butter when cooking vegetables.
- Don't strip every gram of fat from your diet. Your body needs fat to function properly. Just focus on getting the right fats in the right amounts.
- Switch from high-fat meats such as ribs and sausage (with 8 grams of fat per small serving) and higher-fat beef, pork, and lamb (with 5 grams per serving) to leaner cuts like skinless chicken or turkey breast, fish, lean pork, or USDA Choice or Select cuts of beef—all of which have about 3 grams of fat per serving or even less.
- Flavor-test low-fat cheese. It doesn't taste like Styrofoam anymore, and ounce for ounce, the low-fat stuff could save you 5 grams of fat per slice.
- Use more egg whites, less yolks. Two scrambled whole eggs have a combined fat content of 5 grams; two scrambled egg whites, less than 1.
- Avoid the salad dressing ladle at the salad bar. One scoopful could contain 32 grams of fat! Instead, use a regular spoon—you'll save 24 fat grams.

GET THE SAFEST FATS FROM THE SEA

For years, we've heard that fat causes heart attacks, high cholesterol, and weight gain. But certain fats actually protect us
from high cholesterol, diabetes, and high blood pressure.

Omega-3 fatty acids help lower bad LDL cholesterol,
raise good HDL cholesterol, lower triglycerides (a type of blood fat), and
may reduce the risk of blood clots. That's good news for everyone, but
especially for folks with diabetes, who are more prone to heart disease.

Omega-3s aren't made by our bodies. We must get them from food,
specifically fish and plants. Fish provides important omega-3 fats called
eicosapentaenoic acid (EPA) and docosahexaenoic acid (DHA). Good
sources include salmon, mackerel, sardines, herring, anchovies, rainbow trout, and bluefish.

If you must have tuna, opt for cans labeled "chunk light tuna in
water." Although they have less healthy omega-3 fats than salmon and
mackerel, they averaged only 54 ppb of mercury. Besides its well-known
potential for damage to children's developing brains, accumulated mercury may impair adults' immune and reproductive systems and raise
heart attack risk. Try canned salmon or mackerel instead, say Purdue
University researchers who tested 272 cans of fish. They found that mercury levels averaged 45 ppb (parts per billion) in canned salmon and 55
ppb in mackerel, compared with as much as 340 ppb in tuna in oil.

According to the Environmental Working Group, which analyzed
the mercury content of popular fish for its recent report, "Brain Food,"
the following fish are low enough in the toxic metal for even pregnant
women to enjoy on a regular basis: croaker, farmed catfish, farmed
trout, fish sticks, haddock, mid-Atlantic blue crab, shrimp, summer
flounder, and wild Pacific salmon.

Ocean fish are less likely to contain high dioxin and PCB levels
than freshwater fish, since ocean waters tend to be cleaner. Before cooking fish, remove the skin, fat, internal organs, tomalley from lobster,
and mustard of crabs, all places where toxins are likely to accumulate.
Avoid frying fish; it seals in chemical pollutants. Grilling and broiling
allow toxins to drain away.

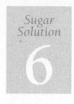

SAY NUTS TO BLOOD SUGAR PROBLEMS

Whether you like to crunch on walnuts, pistachios, or almonds or spread nut butters on whole grain bread, you're in luck. Nuts are packed with protein, fiber, and good fats that keep you feeling full and satisfied for a long, long time. Nut eaters can cut their risk for diabetes by 20 to 30 percent, Harvard Medical School researchers have found. And this may be why: An amazing group of studies has found that people who eat nuts tend to eat less the rest of the day, automatically.

Still, nuts are packed with calories—so go easy with these simple switches and strategies.

- Substitute 1 tablespoon of slivered almonds for ¼ to ⅓ cup of low-fiber cereal.
- Switch ¼ cup of cooked pasta for 1 tablespoon of pistachios.
- Use 1 tablespoon of chopped walnuts on your salad instead of ¼ cup of seasoned croutons.
- Avoid tagalong bad fats. Pass up snack bags of flavored nuts if the list of ingredients includes "partially hydrogenated oils"—shorthand for trans fats.
- Reuse that empty Altoids tin knocking around in a drawer. Put it to work helping you lose weight by filling it with almonds. Altoids boxes hold about 22 almonds—a 1-ounce serving (169 calories). That trick comes from Michelle Wien, DrPH, RD, who found in a recent study that almonds (in moderation) may help you stick to your diet.
- Cup a snack in your palm. A palmful of nuts is, in general, 1 ounce—the perfect snack size. Prefer to count 'em out? An ounce equals 14 walnut halves, 18 cashews, 20 pecan halves, 50 dry-roasted pistachios, 10 to 20 macadamia nuts (depending on size), or 24 filberts.

DISCOVER PLATE POWER

Unless you've been living underground the past few years, you know that protein has made a comeback and carbohydrates have lost favor. It's understandable that you might be tempted to jump on the pro-protein bandwagon—if you haven't already.

Don't do it. There's nothing wrong with carbohydrates like beans, whole grain cereal, or apples. It's highly processed carbs like cookies and cake that pack on the pounds.

To calculate your protein and carbohydrate needs, simply follow the "plate rule."

- Fill half your plate with vegetables and/or fruits.
- Fill the remainder with roughly equal amounts of starch and a high-protein food.

Eat this way, and you can watch the weight come off—along with lowering your risk of diabetes, cancer, and other diseases.

Here are a few examples of perfect plates.

Breakfast plates

- Whole grain cereal and milk topped with fruit
- Three-egg-white omelet with whole grain toast and fruit

Lunch plates

- Sandwich filled with two or three slices of lean meat, with a salad, fruit salad, or veggies
- Black bean, lentil, or other bean-based soup, with a salad or side dish of vegetables

Dinner plates

- Traditional meat and potatoes; salad or cooked veggies (half the plate); deck-of-cards-size piece of fish, poultry, or lean meat (one-third to one-quarter of the plate)
- Stir-fry: Three-quarters vegetables and one-quarter meat, poultry, or seafood. Fill three-quarters of your plate with stir-fry and one-quarter with rice.

GO ON PORTION PATROL

Most restaurants serve bowls of pasta as deep as mixing bowls or sandwiches almost as thick as a paperback. We pile our plates high at home, too. That's why many of us find it difficult to trim our waistlines. Mammoth portions aren't just adding extra calories to our diets. Chances are, they're also adding more fat, sugar, and salt.

One solution: Start reading the serving sizes on food labels. More often than not, the package of chips you have with lunch contains 2 or 2½ servings, not 1.

Also, learn what one serving of a particular food really looks like. For example, one serving of meat is 3½ ounces and fits in the palm of your hand; one serving of whole grain pasta is ½ cup and the size of a tennis ball. Here are some other ways to control portion sizes.

- Serve food from the stove rather than at the table. Having to get up for another plateful will remind you to pass up seconds.
- If you normally eat 2 or 3 cups of pasta at one sitting, stretch 1 cup with 1 cup of grilled or sautéed veggies.
- Instead of toting a whole bag of cookies or chips to the TV, measure out one serving and put the rest away.
- Keep portion control "tools" on hand. Put measuring spoons, a glass measuring cup for liquids, and smaller-cup measures for grains and such in a convenient spot in your kitchen. Use them for a day or so (or choose one meal a day for portion control checkups) to readjust your sense of proportion.
- Sip from a tall, slim glass. When researchers at the Marketing Science Institute in Cambridge, Massachusetts, asked grown-ups and kids to pour drinks and then estimate their contents, adults served themselves 19 percent more and kids poured a massive 74 percent more when using a short, wide glass than when the glass was tall and slim. Yet both assumed they were drinking less from a short glass and more from a tall one. Even experienced bartenders in the study overpoured by nearly 25 percent when the glassware was squat.

GIVE TRANS FATS THE BOOT

At last! Starting in 2006, food labels list levels of unhealthy trans fats, the "Frankenfat" that gunks up arteries and raises heart disease risk. But zero plus zero doesn't always equal zero. New US Food and Drug Administration labeling rules allow foods with less than 0.5 gram of trans fats per serving to claim "zero" grams of trans fats on their labels.

Under these guidelines, which went into effect on January 1, a food with 0.4 gram of trans fats can be listed as having zero trans fats. That means that Americans who consume three or four servings of these foods a day will have unwittingly eaten an extra gram or two of trans fats. And that's important because trans fats, like saturated fats, can raise the risk of heart disease as they increase levels of bad LDL cholesterol.

Currently, the FDA estimates that Americans consume an average 5.8 grams of trans fats per day. Barbara Schneeman, director of the Office of Nutritional Products, Labeling and Dietary Supplements for the FDA, says the reason the FDA is allowing foods under 0.5 gram of trans fats to be rounded down to zero is that current detection methods for trans fats aren't very reliable below 0.5 gram.

So, what's a concerned consumer to do? "If you see a food with zero trans fat, check the ingredient list for the words 'partially hydrogenated.' If you see 'partially hydrogenated,' that means the product contains some trans fats," advises nutritionist Samantha Heller from New York University Medical Center.

The FDA adds that products with shortening or hydrogenated oils in their ingredient lists also contain some trans fats, and the higher up the list you find those items, the greater the amount of trans fats the product contains.

Trans fats are created when liquid oils are transformed into solids, a process called hydrogenation. They're prevalent in many processed foods because they add to a product's shelf life and increase flavor stability. Heller said that most foods containing trans fats are foods you should eat in moderation, including deep-fried restaurant foods, doughnuts, cookies, cakes, and muffins.

GET THE SALT OUT

We believe in moderation when it comes to salt. So does Myron Weinberger, MD, director of the Hypertension Research Center at Indiana University School of Medicine in Indianapolis. "You don't need to drastically cut back on salt," he explains. "You'll benefit from a moderate sodium limit of 2,400 milligrams a day—1¼ teaspoons total from all sources." The average American gets about 3,400 milligrams of sodium a day, so that means cutting our usual intake by about one-third.

Cutting back can help lower high blood pressure and, if your blood pressure is normal now, cut your risk for developing it later in life. (High blood pressure often accompanies metabolic syndrome, prediabetes, and diabetes.) Easy ways to dial down the sodium:

- Omit salt from recipes. Or, reduce sodium 25 percent by using kosher or coarse salt instead—the coarse granules don't pack as tightly into a measuring spoon.
- Take the shaker off your kitchen table, or switch to a light salt (50 percent less sodium) or a salt substitute, which uses a stand-in such as potassium chloride.
- Use an alternative seasoning. Try a spice blend such as Mrs. Dash, or go with a squirt of lemon, crushed garlic (not garlic salt!), or thyme.
- Choose canned foods with low or no added sodium.
- Choose processed foods (such as frozen entrées) with less than 5 percent of the daily value for sodium in each serving.
- Give unsalted or reduced-salt pretzels, chips, and condiments a try.
- When buying low-fat cheese, go for a low-sodium variety.
- Check labels. Aim for foods with less than 200 milligrams per serving, and avoid those with more than 800. Convenience foods including frozen dinners, pizza, packaged soup mixes, canned soups, and salad dressings are often chock-full of sodium.
- Rinse canned foods, such as tuna and beans, to remove some of the excess sodium.
- Read over-the-counter drug labels. Some items, especially antacids, can be high in sodium. Ask the pharmacist about lower-sodium options.

THINK BEFORE YOU DRINK

If you have type 2 diabetes, it's okay to drink alcoholic beverages in moderation as long as your blood sugar is under control. The key is moderation: one drink a day for women, two for men. A drink is defined as one 4-ounce glass of wine, one 12-ounce bottle of beer, or a drink made with 1½ ounces of distilled liquor. Heavier drinking can worsen the complications of diabetes.

Also, if you've been diagnosed with diabetes, follow these guidelines for drinking alcohol, from the American Diabetes Association.

- Make an appointment with a registered dietitian or certified diabetes educator to create a meal plan. During this visit, ask how to best fit in a glass of wine now and then.
- If you drink alcohol at least several times a week, tell your doctor before he prescribes diabetes medication.
- Test your blood sugar to help you decide if you should drink and whether you need to eat something before or as you drink.
- If you take diabetes medications, drink alcohol with a snack or meal. You might nibble on popcorn, fat-free or baked chips, or raw vegetables with a low-fat yogurt dip.
- If you take insulin, drink alcohol with and in addition to your usual meal plan.
- If you've been told to calculate an alcoholic drink as part of your overall calories, fit it in by swapping out fat and carb servings. A 6-ounce glass of wine or a 1½-ounce shot of hard liquor equals two fat servings; a 12-ounce beer equals one starch and one fat.
- Opt for drinks that are lower in alcohol and sugar. Light beer and dry wines, which have less alcohol and carbohydrates and fewer calories, are good choices.
- Choose sugar-free mixers such as diet soft drinks, diet tonic, club soda, or water.
- If you have high triglycerides, as many people with diabetes do, you should not drink alcohol. Alcohol affects how the liver clears fat from the blood and encourages the production of more triglycerides.

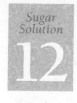

MAKE SMART SUBSTITUTIONS

To avoid insulin-spiking refined carbohydrates, try these substitutions in the kitchen and when you eat out. Dodge nearly 40 grams of carbohydrate by snacking on a cup of popcorn instead of a handful of pretzels.

INSTEAD OF	TRY	CARBS SAVED (G)
Bagel, plain (4")	Bread, whole wheat (1 slice)	25
Bread, white (1 slice)	Bread, light whole wheat (1 slice)	2
Cake, yellow, w/vanilla frosting (1 slice)	Cheesecake (1 slice)	18
Cola (12 oz)	Diet cola, seltzer, or club soda (12 oz)	38
Cranberry sauce, canned (¼ cup)	Cranberry sauce, made w/ Splenda (¼ cup)	22
Flour, all-purpose or whole wheat (¼ cup)	Flour, oat (¼ cup)	12
French toast (1 slice)	Omelet, ham and cheese (2 eggs)	12
Ice cream (½ cup)	Gelatin, diet (½ cup), w/ whipped cream (2 Tbsp)	14
Lasagna noodles (2 oz dry)	Eggplant or zucchini slices (1 cup)	35
Maple syrup, pure (2 Tbsp)	Maple syrup, low-calorie (2 Tbsp)	14
Milk, chocolate (1 cup)	Milkshake, chocolate, low-carb (1 cup)	26
Pancakes, from mix (two 6")	Eggs, large (2)	56
Potato, baked (1 med)	Corn on the cob (1 med)	34
Pretzels, hard twists (10)	Popcorn, air-popped (2 cups)	35
Spaghetti, cooked (1 cup)	Spaghetti squash, cooked (1 cup)	30
Sugar, granulated (½ cup)	Splenda (¼ cup) or stevia (⅛ tsp)	48
Tortilla, flour (6")	Tortilla, corn (6")	6
Yogurt, with fruit (1 cup)	Yogurt, plain, unsweetened (1 cup)	30

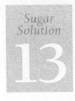

LEARN TO DECODE CARBS ON FOOD LABELS

While the Nutrition Facts label made great strides in clarifying nutrition information, the details of carbohydrate content can still be confusing. These tips will clear things up.

- Check the serving size first. This number is right at the top because all the figures below it are based on that serving size. If you're going to eat a larger serving, increase all of the nutritional figures, including the number of carbohydrates.
- Read the "As Prepared" figures. If a packaged food calls for the addition of eggs and milk, check to see whether the carbohydrates go up.
- Look at the total calories, grams, and milligrams that appear on the left side of the label. The "% Daily Value" on the right is based on 2,000 calories a day, which may not be the amount you're eating.
- Focus on the "Total Carbohydrate" figures. These are the most important figures to look at when you're watching carb intake. The total carbohydrate figure represents the sum of sugars plus starch plus soluble fiber plus insoluble fiber.

Specific figures for sugars and fiber may be listed underneath. If they are, you might notice that the numbers don't add up to the "Total Carbohydrate." This happens because sugars and fibers must be exactly measured in the laboratory and calculated separately from the total carbohydrate figure. Choose foods that will balance out your overall carbohydrate intake for the day or week.

- Strive for fiber. Fiber makes you feel full so that you don't overeat and helps to slow sugar absorption in carbohydrate-containing foods. Try to spread your daily fiber quotient across all three meals.
- Convert grams of sugar to teaspoons, which are easier to visualize. To convert grams to teaspoons, divide the number of grams by 4. For instance, if the label lists 8 grams of sugar, dividing by 4 tells you that the product contains 2 teaspoons of sugar per serving. Keep in mind that the total recommended amount of sugar you should eat each day is less than 10 teaspoons. Choose foods with the least sugar when you can.

BE PICKY ABOUT SUGAR-FREE FOODS

Some foods labeled "sugar-free" or "no sugar added" may actually raise your blood sugar nearly as much as the regular version. That's because some sugar-free cookies, cakes, or other sweet treats may contain nearly as many carbohydrates as the real, sugar-laden thing. Adding insult to injury, they may also pack nearly as many calories.

The fact is, not all sugar substitutes are the same—yet another reason to scrutinize a food's Nutrition Facts panel. Here's what you should know about them.

Sugar alcohols: Many sugar-free foods contain sugar alcohols like sorbitol or mannitol. These carbohydrate-based ingredients contain about half the calories of regular carbs, about 2 per gram. By law, they don't have to be counted as sugars on the Nutrition Facts panels, but they still add to the bottom-line carb count. Verdict: Many diabetes experts say these foods aren't of much benefit for diabetes control. You're better off with a small portion of the real thing.

Sugar substitutes: FDA-approved sugar substitutes such as acesulfame-K (Sweet One), aspartame (Nutrasweet), and sucralose (Splenda) contain no calories or carbohydrates. Foods sweetened with them may contain no calories (like diet soda), or they may contain some calories and carbohydrates from other ingredients (like hot cocoa mix).

Of all the artificial sweeteners, Splenda has drawn the least amount of controversy over its safety. It's one of the most-tested sugar substitutes, showing no harmful effects in more than 100 studies on humans and animals. And unlike some sugar substitutes, you can bake with Splenda, which is made from sugar but has no calories. For tips on how to bake with Splenda, as well as some delicious recipes, go to www.splenda.com.

Verdict: Check the carb content of any food sweetened with sugar substitutes. They may be a lower-carb way to enjoy a little treat.

CHOOSE CHOCOLATE THAT LOVES YOUR HEART

Adore chocolate? Fear heart disease? Start celebrating. Just 1 ounce of one brand of chocolate has more than twice the heart-healthy antioxidant punch of red wine or other dark chocolate.

Dove Dark, made by Mars, contains Cocoapro cocoa, a proprietary, specially processed cocoa that contains superhigh levels of antioxidant flavonoids called flavanols—so high that Dove Dark is used in medical research. Studies have shown that people with high blood levels of flavonoids have lower risk of type 2 diabetes and heart disease.

Researchers at the University of California in Davis compared the effects of 1⅓ ounces of high-flavanol Dove Dark chocolate with the same amount of low-flavanol dark chocolate on 10 healthy people. Only the Dove Dark reduced LDL oxidation and boosted antioxidant levels and HDL concentrations in the blood.

In the test tube, Cocoapro cocoa reduces blood clotting. It may also stabilize arterial plaque, making it less likely to travel and cause a stroke or heart attack. This effect is similar to that of aspirin. Some of the procyanidins in Cocoapro trigger the production of nitric oxide, which helps keep arteries flexible and increases bloodflow.

The chocolates with the highest cocoa content have the highest flavanol content. Two with superior levels of flavanol:

- El Rey Gran Saman Dark Chocolate, 1.4 ounces, 70 percent cocoa, 190 calories, 15 grams fat
- Scharffen Berger Bittersweet, 1-ounce bar, 70 percent cocoa, 170 calories, 11 grams fat

Several studies in animals and humans have shown the heart-healthy effects of chocolate's antioxidants—a boon for people with type 2, who are at higher risk for heart disease. One of these studies, led by Penny Kris-Etherton, RD, PhD, distinguished professor of nutrition at Pennsylvania State University in University Park, found that people who ate a diet rich in cocoa powder and dark chocolate had lower oxidation levels of bad LDL cholesterol, higher blood antioxidant levels, and 4 percent higher levels of good HDL cholesterol.

EAT EARLY AND OFTEN

If you commonly skip breakfast, skimp on lunch, gorge on a lumberjack-size dinner, and engage in lots of noshing in the hours before bed, it's likely that you're sending your blood sugar on a wild roller-coaster ride. Blood sugar plummets in response to the lack of food during the day and surges in response to that huge evening meal. Since the skip-and-gorge way of eating encourages overeating, it's not so good for your waistline, either.

There's a better way to control your blood sugar while you watch your calories and portion sizes: Consider having four to six minimeals of about 250 calories throughout your day rather than eating three big meals a day.

"By eating smaller, more frequent meals, with the correct proportions of proteins, fats, and carbohydrates, you may be manipulating your hormones in favor of reaching the weight you want," says Geoffrey Redmond, MD, director of the Hormone Center of New York in New York City and author of *The Good News about Women's Hormones*.

The minimeal strategy helps keep your blood sugar levels in check through what's known as the second-meal effect: The closer one small meal is to the next, the less your glucose levels will soar, which means lower insulin on a regular basis.

Minimeals might also help keep your weight in check, especially if you're a woman in midlife. In a study conducted at Tufts University in Boston, when healthy older women (average age 72) ate 500- and 1,000-calorie meals, their blood sugar and insulin levels remained high for up to 5 hours. (In young women, those levels quickly returned to normal.) But after 250-calorie meals, the older women's blood sugar and insulin did what they're supposed to do—rise, and then return rapidly to normal.

Just make sure your meals are truly "mini," however. Calories from small, frequent snacks and meals can add up fast, even if you're skipping fat- and sugar-laden snacks and opting for healthier fare.

BEEF UP YOUR DIET—SENSIBLY

Too much fat. Too many calories. A shortcut to heart disease. Many health-conscious people, especially women, have drastically curtailed their intake of red meat—but there's no reason to forgo meat if you go lean. In addition to being a very good source of protein, lean beef is an excellent source of vitamin B_{12} and a good source of vitamin B_6, which the body needs to convert the potentially heart-threatening chemical homocysteine into more benign molecules. Lean red meat is also packed with zinc, a mineral women often lack. One 3-ounce serving of beef has as much zinc as $5\frac{1}{2}$ chicken breasts. And one-third of the saturated fat in beef is stearic acid, a fatty acid that has a neutral effect on blood cholesterol levels.

The steaks, burgers, and roasts in today's supermarkets are leaner than ever. Here's how to get all the flavor without the extra calories and fat.

- To eat beef sensibly, look for the words "lean" or "extra lean" on the label; these cuts have 4.5 grams or less of saturated fat and 5 to 10 grams of total fat per serving. Or, look for these lean cuts: bottom, eye or top round, round tip, top sirloin, top loin, or tenderloin.
- Sauté thin slices of steak with onions, garlic, and fresh basil, then serve over whole wheat noodles or brown rice. You could also make beef kebabs (alternate meat with fresh veggies), brush with olive oil, and grill.
- In a rush? Try precooked and packaged lean beef. We like Louis Rich Seasoned Beef Steak Strips. They heat in just 3 minutes and work well in stir-fries or a salad of baby spinach leaves or wild greens with red peppers and thinly sliced purple onion.
- Add ground beef to tomato sauce and serve over pasta.
- Serve thinly sliced cooked tenderloin on toasted whole wheat French bread, and enjoy these open-faced sandwiches topped with roasted peppers and onions.
- Coat steaks with crushed peppercorns, then grill.

JUST SAY MOO

Extra body fat and too little exercise lull your body into resisting the efforts of insulin, the hormone that sends blood sugar into your cells.

Now researchers say that even if you're overweight, choosing more low-fat dairy products—such as a glass of 1 percent milk or a smoothie made with low-fat yogurt instead of a soda—could help preserve your cells' insulin sensitivity and cut short the first steps on the road to diabetes.

In a 10-year study of 3,000 people, those who were overweight but consumed lots of dairy were 70 percent less likely than dairy avoiders to develop insulin resistance. "The lactose, protein, and fat in milk all have the potential to improve blood sugar," says researcher Mark A. Pereira, PhD, of the University of Minnesota. "Milk sugar [lactose] is converted to blood sugar at a relatively slow rate, which is good for blood sugar control and reducing insulin levels. Protein helps fill you up. And fat may keep you feeling satisfied, too." Nutrients in dairy products, including calcium, magnesium, and potassium, also help.

Here's how to fight diabetes with dairy.

- Aim for at least two servings of low-fat dairy foods daily. Each serving cuts the odds of insulin resistance by 20 percent.
- Make smart switches. Have dairy products instead of high-carbohydrate, low-fiber snacks such as soda, sweets, or fast food.
- Team dairy with fruits, veggies, and whole grains. Add chopped fresh fruit to yogurt at breakfast. Snack on baby carrots with milk. Have a skinny grilled cheese sandwich—low-fat cheese melted on whole wheat bread.
- Add nonfat dry milk to casseroles, meat loaf, soups, and other dishes. Each teaspoon provides about 94 milligrams of calcium, and you can add up to 5 tablespoons to get 1,410 milligrams, an entire day's worth of calcium.
- Make supermilk. Add a couple of tablespoons of nonfat dry milk to your glass of milk to up the calcium and other nutrients.
- Make or buy fat-free pudding for dessert. Each ½-cup serving contains ½ cup of milk.

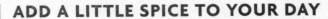

ADD A LITTLE SPICE TO YOUR DAY

Sugar Solution

19

Cinnamon does more than give a spicy lift to food: It also helps regulate blood sugar.

Cinnamon stimulates the production of glucose-burning enzymes and increases the effectiveness of insulin, says Richard A. Anderson, PhD, a chemist at the USDA Beltsville Human Nutrition Research Center in Maryland. Taking between ¼ and 1 teaspoon of cinnamon—the same kind you buy at the supermarket—every day helps control blood sugar levels.

Dr. Anderson's search for a natural way to keep blood sugar levels normal began more than a decade ago, when he and his co-workers tested plants and spices used in folk medicine. They found that a few spices, especially cinnamon, made fat cells much more responsive to insulin, the hormone that regulates sugar metabolism and thus controls the level of glucose in the blood.

Dr. Anderson and his colleagues found that the most active compound in cinnamon is methylhydroxy chalcone polymer (MHCP), which increased glucose metabolism by about 20 times in test-tube studies.

MHCP also prevented the formation of damaging free radicals. "That could be an important side benefit," notes Dr. Anderson. "Other studies have shown that antioxidant supplements can reduce or slow the progression of various complications of diabetes."

Experiment with adding cinnamon to foods such as meat loaf or oatmeal, suggests Dr. Anderson. His favorite way is to boil a cinnamon stick in water for tea. "Just one stick gives you the same benefit as 1 teaspoon of ground cinnamon," he says.

Here are a few other ways to enjoy this tasty spice.

- Stir it into low-fat yogurt, fruit smoothies, and low-fat cottage cheese.
- Slice up an apple, place it in a plastic bag with a teaspoon of cinnamon, shake, and enjoy.
- Add ¼ teaspoon of cinnamon to your morning oatmeal.

ENJOY A SPOT OF TEA

Love your cup of morning or afternoon Earl Grey or green tea? Now you can love it even more: Common teas boost insulin activity by more than fifteenfold, according to studies conducted by the USDA.

Researchers at the USDA Beltsville Human Nutrition Research Center in Maryland analyzed a variety of herbs, spices, and plants to see if they had any beneficial effect on insulin. They tested fat cells taken from rats—which they grew in test tubes—and "fed" the cells mildly radioactive sugar, insulin, and various tea extracts. (Radioactive sugar was easy to track.)

The result: Black, green, and oolong teas—both caffeinated and noncaffeinated—enhanced insulin activity the most. Herbal teas did not. Further, adding whole, fat-free, or soy milk or nondairy creamer seemed to dampen the tea's beneficial effect on insulin.

The chemical in tea that seems to most enhance insulin is called epigallocatechin gallate (EGCG). When green tea is oxidized into oolong and black tea, EGCG forms other compounds, called polyphenols, which are also strong antioxidants.

This insulin-boosting activity also might explain why tea seems to help prevent heart disease and high blood pressure. Medical investigators think high blood sugar damages blood vessels and increasing insulin activity lowers blood sugar levels.

You can drink from 1 to 5 cups of green, black, or oolong tea daily. If caffeine makes you jittery or you have a medical condition that prevents you from taking caffeine, feel free to drink the decaffeinated variety.

By the way, if you use tea bags and dunk the bag up and down while the tea brews, you get a huge bonus: The movement causes the tea to release vastly more of its polyphenols. In studies, tea bags dunked continuously for 3 minutes released five times more. If you use loose-leaf tea, you don't need to dunk; tea leaves release more of their polyphenols whether or not they get a workout.

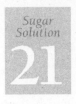

UNWRAP THE RIGHT BAR

What's not to love about snack bars? They're convenient. They travel well. They don't spoil or go stale. They taste great. And now, several companies are manufacturing bars formulated just for people with high blood sugar.

Among these specialty bars are ChoiceDM Nutrition Bar, Extend Bar, and Glucerna. In one study, people with diabetes ate a ChoiceDM Nutrition Bar with slow-digesting carbohydrates and an energy bar with standard carbs. One hour after they ate the ChoiceDM Bar, their insulin levels were 28 percent lower and their blood glucose was 16 percent lower than after the energy bar. (Elevated insulin and blood glucose levels are responsible for the damage diabetes can do.)

Many of these bars contain resistant starch, a type of carbohydrate that is digested and absorbed by the body at a slower rate. That means they don't raise blood glucose levels as quickly as other carbohydrate sources. The slow absorption also allows glucose to continue entering the bloodstream for a long time. This can help prevent hypoglycemia, especially in the middle of the night, when most of the carbohydrates consumed in a bedtime snack would normally be used up. As a bonus, these bars also contain vitamins, minerals, and fiber.

The bars are ideal almost anytime, including before, during, or after exercise; as an anytime snack; or as part of a quick meal when your schedule hits a snag and you can't eat a meal at the usual time.

If you want to try these bars, talk to your doctor first about fitting them into your meal plan. Once you have her okay, test your blood sugar levels frequently—before and after eating bars and in the morning—to see how you're responding to a particular bar.

One more thing: Don't use these bars to treat hypoglycemia. They may not raise blood glucose levels as quickly as the glucose in a glass of juice or piece of hard candy.

BRIGHTEN UP BREAKFAST

Researchers at the National Weight Loss Registry have been studying 3,000 people who've lost at least 30 pounds and kept it off for a year or more, looking for patterns to explain their success. One common trait is that 80 percent eat breakfast every day.

But there's even better news. You can eat virtually anything you want for your morning meal as long as it's healthy, from a bowl of soup to a healthy sandwich on whole grain bread. Here are a few ideas to get you started.

- Get creative with eggs. This excellent source of protein can be scrambled, hard-cooked, poached, fried, or even made into egg salad for breakfast. Add leftover vegetables, meats, and some reduced-fat cheese to eggs to make a quick omelet or frittata. Leftover quiche also makes an excellent breakfast dish in a pinch.
- Try whole wheat anything—crackers, a matzo, a tortilla, toast, half a medium bagel—spread with peanut, almond, or macadamia nut butter.
- Think outside the breakfast box. Who says you can't reheat leftovers from supper or have a bowl of soup? In Japan, it is customary to start the day with a bowl of warming soup. If you adore garden vegetable soup, indulge.
- In Mexico, Britain, and some parts of New England, beans are often served with breakfast. Beans are a terrific source of protein and make an excellent accompaniment to eggs. Try some seasoned lentils or kidney, pinto, navy, or northern beans.
- If you're a traditionalist and love your morning cereal, try a different (but still healthy) brand. There are dozens of varieties to choose from. Try a whole grain or high-fiber version such as All-Bran; oat bran or oatmeal; whole rolled wheat or rye; kasha (buckwheat); or unsweetened puffed grains such as brown rice, corn, or whole wheat. Top with fat-free milk and some blueberries or strawberries.

LOG ON, LOSE WEIGHT

The research is clear: People who track their daily intake of calories and nutrients find it easier to manage their weight and prevent weight gain. That's a good reason to take advantage of the many free diet analysis tools on the World Wide Web.

Below, you'll find some of the most reliable sites that can help you analyze and track your dietary intake and, in many cases, your physical activity. Most were cited in a report published in the *Journal of the American Dietetic Association.*

www.usda.gov/cnpp: Includes the popular Interactive Healthy Eating Index, developed by the USDA Center for Nutrition Policy and Promotion. Along with the ability to analyze food composition, this site will help you see how your daily diet stacks up against national standards.

www.fitday.com: One of the most popular sites, Fitday allows you to track your food intake as well as your physical activity. You can also monitor your personal diet and exercise goals. This site offers as many as or more features than some pay sites.

www.nutritiondata.com: This freebie site will give you a complete nutritional analysis of a single food or let you compare the attributes of several foods. In addition, it can help you track your calorie consumption and even analyze and suggest improvements for your favorite recipes.

http://www.ag.uiuc.edu/~food-lab/nat/: Developed and continually updated by faculty at the University of Illinois, Nutrition Analysis Tools and System (NATS) is recommended for consumers as well as professionals. In addition to nutrient analyses, this site offers an energy calculator that can determine daily calorie expenditures.

www.dietsite.com: This program includes a database of 5,600 foods to help in analyzing diets and recipes. Users can log on to track their food intake over several days and compare it to recommended daily intakes. This site also features nutrition news, message boards, and nutrition advice provided by a registered dietitian.

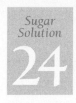

SNACK ON STOMACH-SATISFYING PROTEIN

Healthy, planned snacking can prevent you from loading up your plate for lunch and dinner. While many dieters turn to low-fat popcorn, pretzels, crackers, or sweets at snack time, research suggests that this carbohydrate load may be sabotaging weight loss. French researchers found that high-protein snacks keep you full longer and may reduce the amount you eat at your next meal.

"High-carbohydrate snackers got hungry as quickly as subjects who had no snack at all," says study author Jeanine Louis-Sylvestre, PhD. "But protein eaters, who snacked on chicken, stayed full nearly 40 minutes longer." Since it takes longer for protein to break down, you stay satisfied longer. (Note: Snackers ate 200-calorie snacks.)

Most of us don't think of chicken as a snack, but 2 ounces pack a powerful protein punch. Try prebaked chicken strips, such as 1 cup of Perdue's chicken strips (38 grams protein, 180 calories); a 3-ounce can of white chicken (14 grams protein, 70 calories); or a fast-food grilled chicken sandwich, minus the bun, mayo, and toppings (28 grams protein, 160 calories). Other options: 1 cup of low-fat cottage cheese (28 grams protein, 164 calories) or two string cheese sticks (14 grams protein, 160 calories). Other smart snacking strategies:

- Eat only when empty. "Your body is least likely to store fat if you eat only when you are physically hungry," says Dr. Louis-Sylvestre.
- Add carb snacks to your meals. If you absolutely have to have a cookie or chips, eat them with your lunch instead of between meals. Other food at the meal will blunt the carb's effect on blood sugar.
- Make your snacks an extension of all your meals. If you have a bowl of whole grain cereal and some fruit for breakfast but find you can't finish the fruit, save it for a midmorning snack. If you buy a sandwich, soup, and salad for lunch, eat your salad or half of the sandwich a few hours later.
- Prepack your snacks. Put 100 calories' worth of your favorite healthy snacks—low-fat cheese cubes, half of an apple smeared with 1 tablespoon of peanut butter—in small plastic bags. You'll know exactly how much you're eating.

EAT LIKE A WOMAN, NOT LIKE A MAN

25

When your partner helps himself to a third slice of pizza, it's tempting to do the same. But if you follow his lead, you may find that your pants grow tighter. Unfair as it may be, men can eat more than women without gaining weight. To keep his eating habits off your hips, try these tips.

- If he brings home junk food, ask him to keep it out of your sight. In fact, request that he hide it—you won't be able to succumb to temptation even if you want to.
- Take a trip together to the supermarket so when he goes solo next time, he can identify the healthy fare you'd choose. Go over takeout menus and circle healthy entrées; if he wants something else, get him to order a small portion of the marked item for you.
- It's sad, but true: You need only two-thirds of his helping, says Ellen Albertson, RD, cohost with her husband of *The Cooking Couple Show.* If you're currently matching his portions, start serving your meals on a salad plate and his on a dinner plate. To keep from finishing your scaled-down meal before he finishes his (and avoid going back for seconds), give him a head start while you sip half a glass of wine or ice water.
- Make it your job to prepare the salad. That way, you can have a tiny portion of his fat-laden entrée and fill up on a bowl of soup and some salad.
- Every few weeks, make it a point to suggest one change, such as leaving butter off the veggies or serving his rich favorites as side dishes. He may take the hint.
- Fire up the barbecue more. He can have his meat, and you can have your grilled fish or chicken—without a lot of extra dishes or fuss.
- Challenge him to a diet duel. Don't deal with pounds (men virtually always lose weight faster than women) but with food. For example, see which one of you is more likely to get in those 25 to 35 grams of fiber a day or nine servings of fruits and veggies. The loser has to do the other's chores for the next month.

DON'T BELIEVE YOUR EYES

In a surprising Swedish study, volunteers ate 22 percent less food when they were blindfolded yet reported that they felt just as full as usual. To harness this in-the-dark eating experience, you could travel to a trendy Parisian restaurant—Dans Le Noir (In The Dark), where patrons eat in total darkness—or to a spin-off planned for a 2006 opening in London. Or, simply pay more attention to your other senses when you sit down to a good bowl of homemade chicken noodle soup at your kitchen table.

Here are some practical ways to tune in to your body's hunger and satisfaction cues—and eat less.

- Clear the table. Place the mail and other clutter elsewhere. Set out just the dinnerware and a candle or simple flower centerpiece.
- Avoid distractions. Don't watch TV or read while you dine. When you do other things while you eat, you're less likely to notice when you're comfortably full.
- Go solo. Eating alone allows you to focus. If that's not practical, limit your number of dinner companions.
- Serve individual courses. Eat your salad first, then have your entrée. Leave the extras on the stove, and put only the food you're eating on the table. This will stretch out your meal so you'll recognize sooner when you've had enough.
- Close your eyes (for the first few bites). Taste what you're eating.
- Use the Five Ds. When you catch yourself eating more than you'd like, follow these steps.
  1. Determine what's going on.
  2. Delay your response by figuring out what's driving your urge to eat: Anger? Boredom? Loneliness?
  3. Distract yourself for at least 10 minutes.
  4. Distance yourself from temptation. Throw away the chips. Heck, bury them in the garbage if you have to.
  5. Decide how you'll handle the situation—will you stop eating or continue? It's okay to keep going, as long as you make a conscious choice to continue rather than being helplessly out of control.

DE-FANG YOUR DIET SABOTEURS

Want to really bring out the worst in people? Lose weight. The problem usually starts because you're in change mode (and darned happy to be there), but your friends and family aren't. In fact, in one survey, 24,000 overweight women reported that losing weight created problems in their relationships that regaining the weight would have resolved.

"Rarely would a real friend malevolently undermine your diet," says nutrition professor Audrey Cross, PhD, of Rutgers University in New Brunswick, New Jersey. "They just do unconscious things to keep the relationship the way it was."

There are lots of reasons why. Perhaps they feel guilty, or maybe they miss sharing food with you. Whatever the reason, you need to protect yourself from these often well-meaning saboteurs. Here are some healthier, lower-calorie options when friends or family are enticing you.

INSTEAD OF . . .	TRY . . .
Scarfing down wings and blue cheese with friends	Going to a restaurant where they can still get wings and you can get healthier food
Ordering dessert	Agreeing to share, then have only a forkful or two and spend lots of time marveling out loud about how wonderful it is
A 2-hour lunch	Eating a quick lunch, then go shopping or take a walk
Girls' night out at a restaurant or bar	Going to a spa for a manicure and pedicure; you can talk your heads off and have a great time
Guys' night out	Playing a pickup basketball game at the gym
Sharing a candy bar with your partner	Dipping strawberries in chocolate, giving his-and-her foot rubs, bringing home jewelry or play-off tickets

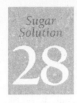

DON'T LET "FATITUDES" WEIGH YOU DOWN

It's true that diabetes and other conditions that affect your blood sugar, like polycystic ovary syndrome (PCOS), can make it more difficult to lose those stubborn pounds. But don't give up and let your good intentions be undermined by bad attitudes. To stay the course, adjust these common mental monkey wrenches.

The "fatitude": "I was born to be fat."

The reality: A USDA study found that women who think their gene pools preordain their jean sizes were more likely to be heavy. "Genes do have an impact on weight," says Thomas Wadden, PhD, director of the Weight and Eating Disorders Program at the University of Pennsylvania in Philadelphia. "But it's your environment that ultimately determines how fat you become."

The attitude adjustment: "The food and lifestyle choices I make shape my shape."

The "fatitude": "I won't be a happy or healthy person until I lose lots of weight."

The reality: "I see patients who set out wanting to lose 35 percent of their initial weight," says Dr. Wadden. "Then they're surprised at how good a 10 percent loss feels." They're probably basking in the glow of better health. The Diabetes Prevention Program proved that just a 7 percent weight loss and increased physical activity can delay or even prevent type 2 diabetes in high-risk people— and it did it so dramatically that the study ended a year early.

The attitude adjustment: "I'll be happier and healthier if I lose just 10 to 15 pounds."

The "fatitude": "I don't eat out much."

The reality: Maybe not in the special occasion sense, but every cafeteria lunch, take-out dinner, and vending machine snack still counts as food you don't cook at home. And that's dangerous because, for too many of us, dining out is tantamount to pigging out.

The attitude adjustment: "How many calories are hiding in this meal that I didn't make?"

USE YOUR COOKING STYLE TO EAT HEALTHIER

When 440 great home cooks took a personality test devised by food science researchers, most fell into one of five "kitchen types." Some dished out comfort food. Others were trendsetters. Still others followed recipes to the letter. Which of the gourmets listed below do you resemble?

Your kitchen type—innovative: You try new ingredients, new combinations, and new ways of cooking. Follow every step of a recipe? Never!

Cooking style: Like Jamie Oliver, the Naked Chef, you're a trendsetter who serves custard as part of the main meal and decorates the salad with edible flowers. You can cook healthy, but it's never a goal.

Healthy makeover: Add exotic, sophisticated ingredients packed with flavor and nutrition. Try farm-stand treasures such as heirloom veggies and those featured in ethnic cuisines (such as collard greens).

Your kitchen type—giving: Your meals are welcoming and nurturing. Think Betty Crocker or TV's *Two Fat Ladies*.

Cooking style: Cozy, creamy delights such as mac and cheese.

Healthy makeover: Go for small changes. Try roasted chicken instead of fried or baked potatoes with low-fat sour cream.

Your kitchen type—competitive: Ever flamboyant, you cook to impress.

Cooking style: Like Emeril Lagasse, you savor challenging recipes, leaping on trends and mastering them—whether the dishes are healthy or not.

Healthy makeover: Up your "oh, wow" factor by adding unique healthy ingredients such as gooseberries or Asian winter melon to perk up a boring meal.

Your kitchen type—methodical: You're a weekend Julia Child, following recipes to a T—with great results.

Cooking style: You use recipes from family and gourmet magazines.

Healthy makeover: Prowl the cookbook section of your local bookstore and select a healthy cookbook you'd normally never buy but that intrigues you. Then—let yourself go!

SUPPLEMENT YOUR FIBER INTAKE

If you just can't manage to eat the recommended nine servings of fruits and vegetables a day—or if you're trying to eat the American Diabetes Association's newly recommended 50 grams of fiber per day—consider taking a fiber supplement. In particular, people with diabetes or high cholesterol can benefit from extra fiber, says James W. Anderson, MD, professor of medicine and clinical nutrition at the University of Kentucky and chief of the endocrine-metabolic section at the VA Medical Center, both in Lexington.

Selecting a fiber supplement from the dozens on the shelves seems like a daunting task, but Dr. Anderson cuts down your choices. To improve cholesterol and blood sugar levels, reach for a soluble-fiber supplement like psyllium husk, such as that found in Metamucil products.

Another choice is to opt for guar gum, a natural fiber ingredient in Benefiber. It dissolves into drinks and soft foods with no gritty feel or strange flavor. Dr. Anderson, however, favors psyllium husk because it is the most extensively studied fiber on the market.

Many dietitians recommend powdered supplements, such as the types made from psyllium or beta-glucan, which you mix into a glass of water. That way, you're sure to have the water your body needs to feel comfortable with so much extra fiber on board.

When you first boost your intake, intestinal bacteria will interact with the fiber to cause excess gas and bloating. To minimize discomfort, start with a low dose and slowly work your way up. Or try Citrucel, which contains methylcellulose, a soluble fiber that doesn't interact with the bacteria. No interaction means no unwanted side effects.

When you take fiber supplements, it's crucial to drink plenty of water throughout the day. Take the majority of fiber products with an 8-ounce glass of water. Start with a single dose, and work up to twice daily if needed. Fiber supplements won't block absorption of most drugs, but to be safe, take them 2 hours before or after your medication, especially any for the heart or blood pressure, says Dr. Anderson.

CHAPTER 9

THE *SUGAR SOLUTION* KITCHEN

One of the best ways to start eating more healthfully is to reengineer your kitchen—the room that can make or break your best intentions for weight loss and healthy eating. If your refrigerator and pantry are bulging with store-bought cake, crackers, cookies, and other foods made with refined carbohydrates, now's the time to make room for the healthy building blocks of meals and snacks that will keep your blood sugar lower and steadier.

The strategy: Buy a rainbow's worth of in-season fruits and veggies, low-fat dairy and meats, and whole grain breads and cereals. Add a larder stocked with strategically chosen canned, dried, and frozen foods. Now your family is ready to eat well when most people have resigned themselves to take-out pizza, fast-food burgers, or cold cereal.

A key principle of *Sugar Solution* cooking: Accept help (in the form of healthy convenience foods, from sliced carrots to frozen broccoli to canned beans) when it's offered. That way, you can still have tasty, healthy, home-cooked meals even if your favorite fruits and veggies aren't in season yet or you simply ran out of time before you reached the bottom of your to-do list (and the final item was "get groceries").

You're ready if your fridge has a rainbow of color inside—prepared salad greens, those sliced carrots, roasted red peppers, spinach, broccoli, dandelion greens, asparagus, celery, carrots, squash, peas; your freezer's loaded with healthy protein (such as frozen shrimp and veggie burgers); and your pantry's full of canned goodies like vegetable-based soups, whole grains, and healthy oils. That's the *Sugar Solution* pantry. Here's how to bring it home—and cook it up.

IN YOUR CUPBOARDS

Start your kitchen makeover with your cupboards. Keep—and promise to buy more of—these easy-to-prepare *Sugar Solution* All-Stars.

Canned tomatoes and tomato sauces: They're the foundation for an endless variety of stews, soups, and pasta sauces. Look for varieties without high-fructose corn syrup or trans fats.

Dried fruit: Dried cranberries are among the best sources of proanthocyanidins, powerful antioxidants that also help prevent urinary tract infections. A ⅓-cup serving confers the same protection as roughly 8 ounces of cranberry juice cocktail. Dried plums (aka prunes) are among the fruits ranked highest in antioxidants, USDA research shows. And ¼ cup of apricots supplies three-quarters of the daily requirement for vitamin A. Just remember: A serving is usually ¼ cup, because dried fruits are calorically, as well as nutritionally, dense.

Whole grain cereals: Look for whole grain oats, wheat, amaranth, quinoa, or brown rice. The nutritional payoff: fiber, minerals, and beneficial plant compounds called phytochemicals. There might be a weight-loss payoff, too: One study found that people who ate oatmeal felt less hungry.

Beans: Staples in hearty soups and chilis, dried beans are superlative sources of iron, fiber, and heart disease–fighting folic acid. Some, such as white, great Northern, and navy, are also respectable sources of calcium. There's nothing wrong with using canned beans; just rinse to rid them of excess sodium, or try reduced-sodium brands. Keep dry beans in a cool, dry place in airtight glass or metal containers. If you have leftover cooked or canned beans, you can drain and freeze them for up to 6 months.

Soups and broths: They're not raw ingredients, but they're so versatile, you can use them as if they were. Try the creamy—but not fatty—vegetable-based butternut squash, portobello mushroom, broccoli, and tomato soups sold in resealable paper cartons by Pacific, Imagine, and Whole Foods. Add 2 tablespoons of whole wheat couscous, greens, and canned beans, and simmer for a few minutes. Serve with a little grated cheese.

Root vegetables: These include white or red onions, fresh garlic and ginger, and potatoes. Acquire a taste for sweet potatoes—they're more nutritious than white and lower on the glycemic index (GI), so they won't raise your blood sugar as high. Buy only as much garlic as you need for a week, thereby ensuring freshness. On the flip side, buy onions in bulk and use them often. Store fresh ginger and garlic in the fridge after they've been cut.

Whole wheat flour: It can be a satisfying supplement to your white flour. In baking, you'll get very satisfactory results by substituting up to half of the amount of white flour called for with whole wheat flour. As you grow accustomed to the taste and texture, swap out more white flour, or try recipes that call for only whole wheat flour.

Cooking oil: Truth is, all vegetable oils are a combination of good, bad, and in-between fats, but the balance varies greatly. The healthiest are highest in monounsaturated and omega-3 fats and lowest in saturated fats and contain moderate amounts of omega-6 polyunsaturated fats. The top two: olive oil for salad dressing and a quick sauté, canola for baking. Keep olive oil away from heat and light for the longest storage—up to 2 years. Store fine olive oils as well as nut oils that you use less often in the refrigerator. Don't worry if the oil becomes cloudy; its translucence will return when it reaches room temperature.

Throw out—or at least promise never to purchase again:

- High-sugar cereals. Consider tossing any cereal that contains 12 grams of sugar or more per serving.
- High-fat, high-salt processed foods. Canned pasta dishes, canned meat spreads, and even some tomato sauces are nutritional nightmares when it comes to fat and salt.
- Refined grain products. Are the only grains you have egg noodles and

white rice? It's time to expand into whole grains, such as semolina or whole wheat pasta.

- **Snack foods.** Check the labels and toss anything that has trans fats, is high in sugar, or has no fiber. And don't lead yourself into tempta-

LIVING THE SWEET LIFE

If you love to bake, try making healthier versions of your favorite recipes by using alternatives to white sugar. The sweeteners below either have fewer calories, a lower glycemic index, or additional nutrients. (Aspartame and saccharin cannot be used for baking and are not listed here.)

Brown sugar: A mixture of white sugar and molasses, it has a slightly lower carb content than white sugar. If you swap white for brown, you'll save 15 grams of carbs in every ¼ cup you use. Keep in mind that brown sugar is still a refined sugar and is not the lowest-carbohydrate sweetener.

Stevia: This herb has enormous sweetening power. The liquid form (it's also available in powder form) is the most convenient choice for cooking—it measures easily and stores in the fridge. But go easy. One-eighth of a teaspoon of liquid stevia is equivalent to ½ cup of sugar. Start out with less than you think you will need and gradually increase the amount. Unlike sugar, stevia doesn't aid in browning or provide textural lightening in baked goods, yet it works well in everything from pancakes to puddings. You'll find stevia in health food stores or large supermarkets.

Splenda: The primary ingredient in Splenda is sucralose, a sugar substitute processed from real sugar that has been modified so that it isn't absorbed by the body. Sucralose is calorie free, does not affect blood sugar levels, and maintains its sweetness across a broad range of temperatures. Splenda measures cup for cup like sugar and performs almost like sugar in recipes. When used in moderate amounts, it doesn't have the cloying aftertaste associated with artificial sweeteners.

Splenda is especially useful in baking, but it doesn't caramelize like sugar. One option is to use half sugar and half Splenda. You'll get the caramelizing and browning properties of sugar, but with fewer calories and carbs.

tion: Toss big bags of chips—the ones that are difficult to stop digging into.

- **White bread and rolls.** Give up the marshmallowy, low-fiber, low-nutrition types.

IN YOUR REFRIGERATOR

The top shelf of your fridge should be dominated by water, unsweetened iced tea, seltzer, and low-fat or fat-free milk. Also stock these.

Fruit and veggies: Keep enough fresh produce to last you at least a few days or the entire week (depending on how often you grocery shop).

Dairy: Go for reduced-fat, low-fat, or fat-free milk, cheese, and yogurt. Look for margarines with no trans fats, or, if your cholesterol is above normal, try a cholesterol-lowering margarine such as Benecol.

Eggs: Hard-cook extras to keep on hand for a day or two for a fast and nourishing snack or sandwich filling.

Peanut butter and other nut butters: All-natural peanut butter (stir it when the oil separates), as well as cashew, almond, and soy nut butters, should be kept in the fridge so they don't turn rancid. Packed with healthy monounsaturated fats, they're satisfying and healthy.

Healthy meats: Go for lean cuts of beef, skinless chicken and turkey, and lean pork. If it's not breakfast without bacon or sausage, try turkey bacon, all-natural chicken sausage, or soy hot dogs instead of pork varieties.

Condiments: Keep on hand low-fat canola mayonnaise (it has heart-healthy omega-3 fatty acids), low-sodium chutneys, mustards, ketchup, and relishes. Experiment with healthy, fiber-rich spreads from the supermarket deli section. One we love: hummus, a delicious, nutrient-rich chickpea and garlic spread that's great for sandwiches or as a dip for baby carrots.

Throw out—or at least promise never to purchase again:

- Sodas and sugary teas and fruit drinks. If you can't live without something bubbly or sweet in your cup, it's okay to have one diet soft drink per day.

(continued on page 110)

THE *SUGAR SOLUTION* SHOPPING LIST

Keep the items below on hand and you'll always be ready for quick, healthy meals.

In the Cupboard

Bananas

Garlic

Melons (cantaloupe, honeydew, watermelon)

Onions

Oranges

Plums

Sweet potatoes

Winter squash

In the Refrigerator

Apples

Bell peppers

Broccoli

Butter (preferably light)

Cabbage (green or red)

Carrots

Cauliflower

Celery

Cheese (Cheddar, mozzarella, Parmesan, Monterey Jack, cream cheese—preferably reduced-fat)

Cucumbers

Eggplant

Eggs

Fresh greens

Grapefruit

Grapes

Half-and-half

Lemons

Milk (1%)

Mushrooms

Nuts (almonds, macadamias, pecans, pine nuts, pistachios, walnuts)

Orange juice

Parsley

Raisins

Scallions

Seeds (sunflower, sesame)

Sour cream (reduced-fat)

Squash (yellow squash, zucchini)

Yogurt (low-fat, plain)

In the Freezer

Bacon (pork or turkey)

Beef (lean ground, tenderloin, various steaks)

Broccoli

Chicken (skinless, boneless breasts and bone-in parts)

Corn

Frozen fruit (no sugar added)

Green beans

Lamb (ground, chops)

Peas

Pork (chops, tenderloin)

Salmon

Sausage (pork or turkey)

Shrimp

Spinach

Tortillas (corn and whole wheat)

Turkey (cutlets, tenderloin, ground breast)

Unsweetened coconut

Veggie burgers

Whole wheat bread

In the Pantry

All-fruit spread (various flavors)

Apple juice (or cider in the fridge)

Brown rice

Brown sugar (or brown sugar substitute)

Canned broth (chicken, beef)

Canned chopped clams

Canned fish (anchovies, salmon, sardines, anchovies, trout fillets, tuna)

Canned fruit in fruit juice

Canned mild green chiles

Canned tomato products (whole, crushed, sauce, juice)

Canola oil

Cocoa powder (unsweetened)

Dried apricots

Dried mushrooms

Dry or canned beans (black, white, pinto, red kidney, chickpeas, brown lentils)

Hot-pepper sauce

Maple syrup (low-calorie)

Marinara sauce (low-sugar)

Mayonnaise (no added sugar)

Mustard

Oat flour

Oats

Olive oil

Olives

Peanut butter, natural (and other natural nut butters)

Peanuts, unsalted, dry-roasted (and other nuts)

Pearl barley

Pesto

Quinoa

Roasted peppers

Salt

Sesame oil

Soy flour

Soy sauce

Splenda

Stevia

Tea, herbal teas

Vinegar (cider, white wine, red wine, balsamic)

Whole grain crackers

Whole wheat couscous

Whole wheat flour

Whole wheat pasta

Whole wheat pastry flour

Worcestershire sauce

IN THE FREEZER

If you're lucky enough to be blessed with a large freezer, go crazy! The freezer is a marvelous tool for healthy eating. You can stock it with homemade meals that keep you on track and healthy convenience products for quick, satisfying meals. Frozen foods are designed for convenience and last up to a year. Have these on hand.

Frozen veggies: Flash-frozen at the peak of ripeness, they're often more nutritious than fresh stuff that's been languishing in the produce bins. Go for Asian stir-fry or other mixtures to capture the widest variety of healthful nutrients. Your pick should include one or more of the following: broccoli, carrots, cauliflower, and Brussels sprouts. For a fun change of pace, try edamame (young, green soybeans).

Frozen fruits: Like veggies, fruits are flash-frozen at their ripest. Your best-tasting and most nutritious bets: berries (loaded with antioxidants) and mangoes (with beta-carotene). Toss half a cup each of blueberries and raspberries into a smoothie or add to pancakes and breads.

Frozen soy foods: Veggie burgers and hot dogs cook in under 10 minutes—and some varieties of veggie burgers are even toaster-ready!

Frozen shrimp and scallops: They're as good as fresh; in fact, most "fresh" shrimp is actually defrosted before it's sold.

Nuts: Yes, we recommend storing nuts in your freezer. They'll last longer because the cold prevents the good-for-you oils from turning rancid.

Whole grain flours: Store tightly wrapped in the freezer. Bring to room temperature before using.

Throw out—or use up and don't buy again:

- High-fat, high-calorie, high-sugar frozen treats. (Keep one flavor of ice cream as a special treat, or make your own "sorbet" with frozen fruit and a splash of juice.)
- High-fat, high-sodium frozen foods.

COOKING TIPS

You've cleared your kitchen of unhealthy foods and replaced them with an array of nutritious, flavorful, blood sugar friendly alternatives. Now, just what should you do with them? Read on!

Beans: Magic Bullets for Blood Sugar Control

Beans come in a kaleidoscope of shapes, sizes, and colors, and each variety is stuffed with vitamins, minerals, and other nutrients. Beans are also rich in fiber, which gives them a low-GI rating. Here's how to use them.

- Add canned beans to salads and pasta dishes, or blend with herbs to make dips.
- Lots of time? Use dried beans for more flavor. Soups taste delicious when made with slow-cooked beans. Beans cook faster if you soak them overnight first, or try a slightly quicker soaking technique: Start the beans in a separate pot, cover with water, boil for 2 to 3 minutes, and then let sit for 1 to 4 hours. Add the beans to soup, and cook according to package directions.

Olive and Other Oils: From Everyday to Exotic

Most oils, like canola or vegetable, are healthier choices than saturated or solid fats like butter and bacon drippings. But while these oils have their place in healthy cooking, you should also make room for a fine olive oil—or something even more exotic. Fine oils cost more but yield wonderful flavor dividends. Here's how to showcase them.

- Extra-virgin olive oil is dark green and has a bold flavor that holds up best in uncooked dishes such as dressings, marinades, and sauces. You can also add it at the end of cooking to boost the flavor of pasta or vegetables, for example.
- Classic olive oil is more golden in color and mild in flavor. This is a good all-purpose choice for sautéing and cooking.
- Extra-light olive oil has a less noticeable olive flavor. Use it for sautéing, stir-frying, or baking. Among all the olive oil varieties, extra-light holds up best to high temperatures.
- Pure nut oils have a nutty flavor achieved by grinding whole or big pieces of nuts, roasting the ground nuts, and only lightly filtering the oil that's produced. Walnut oil, made from English walnuts, is topaz in color, with a delicate flavor. Cooking destroys its toasted-walnut

flavor, so use this oil for dressings and dips, or add it to hot dishes just before serving. Almond oil, which also has a mild flavor, holds up to heat better than walnut oil. It's a good choice for dressings, light sautéing, or baking. Try it in muffins or on green beans with almonds.

Nuts: The Healthy Indulgence

The ancient Romans often served nuts with or after dessert—hence the phrase "from soup to nuts." You can add nuts to almost any dish, savory or sweet, and they're loaded with healthy monounsaturated fats, protein, and other important vitamins and minerals. It's fine to snack on nuts right from the bag (stick with one palmful or less). Here are ways to take your nut presentation to the next level.

- Toast them to enhance flavor. Place nuts in a dry skillet over medium heat and stir frequently until lightly colored and fragrant. This should take only 2 to 3 minutes. If your oven is already on, place the nuts on a baking sheet and toast at 350°F for 3 to 5 minutes.
- Toss with pasta. Pasta dishes and casseroles are typically made with ingredients that have a high GI, like white pasta, potatoes, or bread crumbs. A tasty way to lower the GI is to add nuts. Pine nuts are terrific with pasta or couscous. Pecans, walnuts, and almonds work well with casseroles, vegetables, and rice dishes.
- Get beyond peanut butter. Cashew butter is exceptionally rich tasting and delicious on toast with fruit spread. Creamy macadamia nut butter makes a great sandwich spread. Almond butter is fantastic in sauces. You can use almost any nut butter to make a dip or sauce, including tahini (sesame seed butter), which is especially flavorful. You'll find these nut butters in most health food stores and some large supermarkets.

Whole Grains: Pasta and So Much More

It can be hard to give up white bread, white rice, or sugar-laden breakfast cereals. But as more Americans turn to whole grain products to cut their risk of diabetes and other diseases, a surprising thing happens:

They actually begin to prefer them. Here are some tips for using fiber- and vitamin-rich whole grains.

- Swap white pasta for whole wheat pasta and you'll get more fiber, a lower GI, and—believe it or not—more flavor. Whole wheat pasta has a more complex, nutty taste than your typical pasta made with white flour. Most supermarkets carry both strand and shaped whole wheat pastas, such as spaghetti, linguine, and rotelle. Look for them right next to the refined white pastas. Whole wheat couscous—a tiny, higher-fiber pasta—makes excellent grain salads and pilafs as well as a wonderful side dish on its own.
- Brown rice is higher in fiber and vitamins than white rice, and it has a chewier texture and nuttier flavor. Both short- and long-grain varieties work well in casseroles and as simple side dishes. Many grocery stores also carry whole grain rice mixes that include various types of wild and brown rice, with a taste that beats plain white rice hands down. If you must choose white rice, go for parboiled; it has a lower GI than regular white rice.
- Coat foods such as fish or chicken with whole grain bread crumbs. To make ½ cup of fresh whole wheat bread crumbs, place two slices of whole wheat bread in a food processor and process until fine crumbs form. Use immediately or freeze for another time.

Whole Grain Flours: Better than Bleached

Unless you've tried buckwheat pancakes or homemade whole wheat bread, you may shy away from giving up your all-purpose white flour. As a first step, mix whole grain flour with the all-purpose stuff, and use the combo to thicken sauces and dredge meats. Here's what you need to know about using the most popular whole grain flours.

- For delicate baked goods like cakes, use a combination of whole wheat pastry flour and oat flour to create a lighter texture. For instance, to replace 1 cup of all-purpose flour, use ½ cup of whole wheat pastry flour plus ½ cup of oat flour. You can also achieve a lighter texture with whole wheat pastry flour by sifting it a few times before using.

- Whole wheat pastry flour soaks up more liquid than all-purpose flour, so you might need to add a few extra tablespoons of milk, water, or juice to your recipe or use a few tablespoons less whole wheat flour than the recipe calls for.
- Try kamut flour. Pronounced ka-MOOT, this flour is an ancient relative of modern common wheat, with more minerals. The high gluten content makes kamut an easy substitute for white flour in your recipes. It tastes richer and nuttier and has more protein and fiber than all-purpose flour.
- Experiment with buckwheat and amaranth flours. Buckwheat flour is gluten free and works well in pancakes, breads, dumplings, and pastas such as soba noodles (buckwheat noodles). Amaranth flour tenderizes the final product somewhat and adds a pleasant nutty flavor. For recipes containing more than one type of flour, substitute 1 cup of amaranth flour for 1 cup of all-purpose flour.
- Lighten up baked goods. While most baked goods made with whole grain flours will be a little heavier than those made with white flour, you'll get a fairly light product if you sift the flour two or three times to incorporate some air.

Herbs, Spices, and Flavorings: Boost Flavor, Bust Fat and Calories

You can go way beyond squirting lemon juice on broccoli. Splurge on the most exotic flavorings you can find—saffron, real vanilla beans, fresh *herbes de Provence*. Here are a few ideas to get you started.

- The volatile oils in herbs are teeming with aroma. When using dried herbs, add them early in cooking so they have time to release flavor. Crush them before using for even more intense flavor. More delicate fresh herbs such as basil and parsley are best added toward the end of cooking.
- Citrus juices lend fresh flavor to everything from chicken and fish to pasta and vegetables. Or look to lemon, lime, or orange peel to bring out more flavor in baked goods like cookies and muffins. Vinegars brighten the taste of foods, too. Splash flavored vinegars

such as raspberry vinegar onto salads, vegetable side dishes, and beans.

- Dried foods are concentrated sources of wow-that-tastes-good flavor. A handful of chopped sun-dried tomatoes can really deepen the taste of pizza, pasta, and salads. Or add rehydrated dried mushrooms to rice dishes, soups, or casseroles. Dried porcini mushrooms are especially good. If you're making muffins, breads, or a dessert sauce, try dried fruit. When heated with almost any type of liquid, the rich, sweet flavor of dried apricots, dates, figs, and raisins blossoms beautifully.

- Kick it up! Nothing perks up a dish like hot sauce. Salsa, hot-pepper sauce, or even crushed red-pepper flakes may be just the thing to boost the flavor of a dish. There are dozens and dozens of hot sauces with amusingly quirky names, from Rigor Mortis Hot Sauce to something called Dave's Insanity Sauce.

CHAPTER 10

MAKING HEALTHY RESTAURANT CHOICES

At a popular pizza chain, the personal pan pizza with sausage packs 740 calories and 39 grams of fat. And at one major fast-food joint, a triple cheeseburger with everything has 810 calories and 47 grams of fat—two meals' worth of calories and more fat than most of us should scarf down in an entire day.

The bright spots in this grease-spattered scenario? First, you. Your power as a restaurant patron lies in your order. The waiter, cook, and manager want you to leave happy—just tell them what you want. Second, more and more fast-food spots, casual dining eateries, and even upscale restaurants offer healthier alternatives on their regular menus.

We believe that a meal away from home should be delicious and enjoyable—there's no need to order dry chicken breast, have only a glass of water . . . and sulk. The trick? A little preparation so that you can outwit the menu, sidestep temptation, withstand the siren song of enormous portions, and leave the table happy.

HAVE IT YOUR WAY

Eating out is, in a sense, eating blind. You don't usually have access to nutrition labels, so you don't realize how the cheese, butter, oil, sugar, and oversize portions are adding up. (That focaccia club sandwich? It packs 1,222 calories and 65 grams of fat!) The veggies may arrive dripping with butter and cream. The bread's heavenly, but it's white. That salad that seemed so healthy may have more calories and fat than a cheeseburger, thanks to fried chicken strips and an ocean of dressing.

And then there are the portions. When a pair of New York University nutrition experts weighed and measured the everyday foods served up in Manhattan's delis, bakeries, and sit-down restaurants, their

FAST FOOD OR FAT FOOD? IT'S UP TO YOU

An average fast-food meal can pack 1,000 calories or more and be full of refined carbs that will make blood sugar skyrocket. But if you keep the ground rules of good nutrition in mind, you can make healthy choices. A good rule of thumb: If you're having fast food for one meal, be sure your other meals that day contain healthier foods, like fruits and vegetables.

Breakfast. Choose a plain bagel, toast, or English muffin rather than a doughnut or muffin, which may be loaded with sugar and fat. Add fruit juice or low-fat or fat-free milk. Also good: cold cereal with fat-free milk, pancakes without butter, or plain scrambled eggs. Limit high-fat bacon, sausage, and cheese and the breakfast sandwiches made with them.

Lunch and dinner. Consider a grilled chicken sandwich or a plain hamburger—regular or junior-size rather than deluxe, and hold the mayo or the special sauce. Hold the fries. Most fast-food places now have soups and salads, too.

Salad bars. Go for the greens and veggies; limit your use of high-fat dressings, bacon bits, cheeses, and croutons, as well as offerings like potato or macaroni salad.

Mexican fast food. Stick with bean burritos, soft tacos, fajitas, and other nonfried items, and go easy on the cheese, sour cream, and guacamole. Choose chicken over beef, limit refried beans, and lay on the low-fat, spicy salsa. And don't eat anything in a taco shell—a taco salad can pack more than 1,000 calories.

Pizza. Order a thin crust with vegetable toppings, and have only one or two slices. Meat and extra cheese add calories, fat, and sodium.

results were amazing: Compared with government-recommended portion sizes, pasta servings were five times heftier, cookies were seven times larger, and muffins weighed three times more. Why you might not notice: Portions have slowly, slowly increased in size over the past 30 to 50 years. "What I found was appalling," says study author Lisa Young in her book *Portion Teller: Smartsize Your Way to Permanent Weight Loss*. "The foods we buy today are often two or three times, even five times, larger than when they were first introduced into the marketplace."

If you suspect that restaurant eating is a minefield, you're not alone. Even chefs have food issues when faced with a yummy menu— or the temptations cooking in their own kitchens. (If you were constantly surrounded by chocolate lava cake, fettuccine Alfredo, raisin nut bread, and bacon-wrapped filet mignon, what would you do?) "Having lunch at a restaurant is where I can get into trouble," confesses chef Sara Moulton, host of *Cooking Live with Sara Moulton* and *Sara's Secrets* on the Food Network, cookbook author, and executive chef at *Gourmet* magazine. Who wouldn't find it hard to resist the extras (like foie gras or a six-dessert sampler) that chefs often send to her table?

Yet Moulton stays slim—and even dropped a few pounds when she was about to start hosting a live television show several years ago. ("The camera really does add 10 pounds," she says.) Her strategy? Don't let yourself get too hungry, especially before a dinner out. "When you're hungry, your resistance to snack on tempting foods plummets," she says. She does splurge a little on weekly dinner dates with her husband. "Knowing I can have some cheese on Friday night helps keep me disciplined the rest of the week," she says. At lunch, Moulton sometimes can't resist eating an entire 714-calorie mozzarella, tomato, and basil sandwich. And yet, she believes in not letting a diet detour derail her successful efforts to maintain a svelte figure. She gets right back on the horse: "On those days, my dinner is a 300-calorie Lean Cuisine."

How can you achieve—and maintain—a lean silhouette while still enjoying a night out at a bistro? These strategies will help.

7 WAYS TO SURVIVE THE FOOD COURT

Endless food peddlers and long, frustrating lines can make the mall a disaster for healthy eaters who grow hungry and tired. Here's how to avoid stress and keep your waistline in check.

1. Start late. Avoid hectic weekend crowds. Take advantage of late shopping hours; head out after you've had dinner at home.

2. Dress casually. Wear comfortable walking shoes, and leave your coat in the car. You won't be as tired—or on the lookout for a snack to revive you.

3. Shop downtown or at an open-air plaza where you can stroll the streets and stop for a healthy bite at a local cafe.

4. Dine first. Instead of waiting until you're crazed with hunger, start your trip energized from a nice lunch at a sit-down restaurant.

5. Stop for a sample of soothing bath lotions, or try out a relaxing massage chair. You'll be less likely to eat from stress.

6. Hit the drugstore. Save calories and money by grabbing a bottled drink and a snack bag of pretzels that you can stow away for later.

7. Indulge—a little. At the candy store, a single, decadent truffle (0.4 oz) is just 60 calories—a perfect low-cal treat.

STEP 1: PREPARE YOUR PLAN OF ATTACK

It's amazing how much trouble you can get in even before your meal arrives. Take a proactive stance against the unhealthful food assault catapulting in from all sides.

Spoil your appetite. Before you leave for dinner, eat something substantial like a bowl of soup, a piece of leftover chicken, a piece of toast with low-fat cheese and leftover vegetables, yogurt with fruit and nuts, a hard-cooked egg, or apple slices sprinkled with cinnamon. Any healthy minimeal will be lower in calories and fat than an over-the-top restaurant appetizer.

Know where you're going. Become familiar with the dining guidelines for different kinds of restaurants (later in this chapter), and try to picture what you're going to eat before you even walk in the door. Don't let the menu sway you! If you've been to the restaurant before and can resist the temptation, keep the menu closed. Order what you'd like, and let the waiter sort it out. It's your meal—have it your way.

Avoid the bread basket. It's one of the leading causes of overeating at restaurants. Send the basket back—out of sight is out of mind. If that's unthinkable, take one slice of bread to enjoy with your meal. Bread can tack on an additional 500 calories to your meal's total—not even including the butter or olive oil that usually accompanies it.

Limit yourself to one alcoholic drink. Alcohol, whether in the form of a cocktail, wine, or beer, can weaken your resolve for exercising thoughtful moderation with your food. Plus, it dehydrates you and offers no nutritional benefit. When you go out, limit yourself to just one drink—or order a bottle of fancy water instead.

Because the body will use the alcohol for energy first (followed by carbohydrates, protein, and fat), when you drink and eat, the excess

---

FLYING? PACK—OR BUY—THESE TREATS

Don't put yourself at the mercy of airport and in-flight food: Even healthy choices can actually trip you up, thanks to extra sugar and fat and giant portions. Instead, pack some healthful snacks—almonds; dried fruit; a high-fiber, low-calorie energy bar such as a Luna bar—into your carry-on.

If you must buy food, be prepared to spend a little extra. Airport vendors often charge more for a bowl of fruit than for a cinnamon bun, but that extra $2 now is far less than the price you'll eventually pay if you routinely shortchange your health. At restaurants, stick to lean protein, and ask your waiter to double the vegetables and hold the rice or potatoes. With a little practice, your next trip won't be an excuse to take a vacation from a healthy lifestyle.

calories are often stored as fat. To keep the pounds from piling on, skip higher-fat entrées (such as duck and filet mignon) in favor of lower-fat fare (including white fish, pork, poultry, and venison) when having wine with dinner.

Drink water. You've heard this before, but we'll say it again: Drink water before, during, and after every meal, whether you're at a restaurant, at home, or anywhere else.

STEP 2: PLACE YOUR ORDER WITH CONFIDENCE

If you feel intimidated by servers, stop right now. Don't worry that you're holding them up with your questions and requests. Don't feel shy. Running interference between the kitchen and your table is a server's job, and he or she wants to please you. (There's a tip at stake here . . .)

Be constantly aware of portion sizes. Trust us: You likely won't need an appetizer *and* an entrée. Some restaurants have been known to serve up to seven times the normal portion for a meal.

Plan to leave food on your plate—or request that half of your meal be wrapped before it even comes to the table. Why you want to keep the extra food out of sight: In a Pennsylvania State University study, researchers found that all the volunteers who were given extra food on their plates ate it—without reporting feeling any fuller afterward.

Appetizers are generally more realistic portion sizes. Order your favorite as a meal with a side salad, or order two appetizers—one that is more vegetable-based.

Ask, ask, ask. Is it fried? What kind of sauce comes with it? What sides are served with each dish? Can I get brown rice instead of white?

Always request sauces and dressings on the side. You'll realize how little sauce and dressing you really need.

Don't order something new when you're very hungry. If you do, you'll likely order too much food, overeat, and regret it later. If you're starving, order a standby that you know is good for you (see the list below).

Order plenty of vegetables. Get a large mixed salad, or order vegetables sautéed in a bit of olive oil or steamed with sauce on the side (so you can lightly dip them in the sauce).

Sip some broth. Soup is a good high-volume food that will fill you up. Look for vegetable, broth-based, and bean soups. Avoid cream-based soups and chowders.

STEP 3: FINISH WITH A FLOURISH

Don't let down your guard after the server scurries off to the kitchen with your order. You'll still need to exercise some caution when your perfectly ordered meal arrives.

Stay alert. It's easy to get caught up in an engaging conversation and eat everything on your plate without even thinking about it. After you've finished your allotted amount, have the server wrap up your leftovers. The bonus is that you have tomorrow's lunch (or dinner) already prepared.

End your meal with refreshing green or herbal tea. Ginger tea can help with digestion, and green tea is good for your overall health. Many restaurants now offer a variety of exotic teas, so treat yourself to some! Some teas are so fruity that they're a perfect replacement for dessert.

Order a dessert for the table. Three bites of the chef's signature chocolate bread pudding with butterscotch sauce won't hurt—just make sure someone else will finish the rest.

HEALTHY EATING AROUND THE WORLD

Whether it's Italian, Chinese, Mexican, or any cuisine in between, our "best bets" will help you control your blood sugar—and waistline.

American

With all the ethnic food choices available to us today, plain old home-style American cuisine still ranks as our favorite. But this chow is loaded with fat and calories and focused on meat rather than healthier whole grains and vegetables. To cut through the fat trap, look for items that are grilled, marinated, or barbecued, says Joyce Vergili, RD, dietitian at the Northern Hudson Valley Dialysis Center in Catskill, New York.

Best bets

- Manhattan clam chowder
- Vegetable soup
- Shrimp cocktail
- Hamburger (4 to 6 ounces uncooked weight) with lettuce, tomato, onion, barbecue sauce, and mustard (hold the cheese and mayo)
- Blackened or Cajun chicken with steamed vegetables and baked potato (with less than 2 tablespoons sour cream)
- Charbroiled pork chops
- Shrimp scampi with rice pilaf

Chinese

Whether for takeout or dining out, Chinese menus are brimming with healthy choices if you know where to look. Steer clear of crunchy noodles and anything sweet and sour (just another phrase for"battered and fried"). Choose steamed rice or vegetable fried rice rather than pork fried rice. And before you pick up your chopsticks, check out the menu for lower-fat choices, says Vergili.

Best bets

- Egg drop, hot and sour, wonton, or Chinese vegetable soup
- Stir-fry chicken and broccoli
- Shrimp or vegetable lo mein (shrimp or vegetables over soft noodles)
- Chicken chow mein
- Vegetarian delight (steamed vegetables with tofu)
- Steamed vegetable dumplings
- One small egg roll with steamed white rice

French

French food fairly bursts with fat: cream sauces; duck legs roasted in their own drippings; pâté de foie gras. To get around all this fattening fare, look for entrées that are lightly sautéed, and avoid anything with aioli (a garlic mayonnaise made of eggs and oil), béarnaise sauce (cream sauce made with eggs and butter), or *beurre blanc* (white sauce that's heavy on the butter), says Vieira.

Best bets

- Bouillabaisse (seafood stew)
- Ratatouille (side dish of vegetables simmered in olive oil, garlic, and herbs)
- Crudités (marinated vegetables such as celery root, red cabbage, cucumbers, leeks, and tomatoes served raw or lightly cooked)
- Rouille (spicy sauce served with fish)
- En papillote (usually fish baked or steamed in parchment paper)
- Coulis (fruit or vegetable puree served over poultry or meat)

Indian

This cuisine is big on vegetables, basmati rice, and sauces based on legumes like chickpeas. Just stay away from korma (cream sauce) and dishes made with coconut. "Coconut oil is the most saturated oil known to man," Vergili says. Also pass on the *pappadam* (fried lentil chips) and go with chapati or naan breads instead of the fried *poori* or *paratha*.

Best bets

- Mulligatawny (lentil, vegetable, and spice soup)
- *Dahl rasam* (pepper soup with lentils)
- *Dahl* (spicy lentil sauce)
- *Raita* (side dish mixture of yogurt, cucumber, and onion)
- Vegetable *biryani* or *pullao* (similar to rice pilaf)
- Tandoori chicken or fish (marinated in spices and slow-roasted in a clay oven)
- Chicken or shrimp *saag* (spinach)
- *Saag panir* (spinach dish featuring cheese made with milk and lemon juice)
- Chicken or fish masala (red sauce, generally lower in fat)

Italian

Italian restaurants are known for their breads, salads, and pastas—all healthy foods in their original states. But smother the bread with butter or olive oil, drown the salad in creamy dressing, or drench a heaping 8-ounce portion of pasta in a creamy Alfredo sauce, and you can say ciao to healthy. "Pasta may be low in fat, but it still has calories," says Vergili. "A typical restaurant portion of pasta is 8 ounces, or about 4 cups cooked. Eat half and take half home, or ask for an appetizer [versus an entrée] portion, which is usually 3 or 4 ounces." Stick with angel hair, spaghetti, linguine, fettuccine, fusille, or ziti. Pass up Alfredo, carbonara, and cream sauces in favor of marinara, mushroom, wine, and clam sauces.

Best bets

- Minestrone
- Shrimp primavera (shrimp and vegetables in a flavored sauce)
- Mussels marinara
- Chicken cacciatore (make sure the chicken isn't breaded)

Mexican

The basic ingredients of Mexican food—corn, rice, chile peppers, and beans—are nourishing and low in fat and calories, as long as they're not turned into a deep-fried-loaded-with-cheese chimichanga or chili con queso, says Vergili. Skip the nacho chips, go for soft flour or corn tortillas over fried ones, and request black beans instead of lard-loaded refried beans. As for salsa—a tasty compilation of tomatoes, peppers, and onions—eat as much as you want. And don't worry; there are lots of great choices for an entrée.

Best bets

- Black bean or gazpacho soups
- Chicken, shrimp, or beef fajitas (grilled and sliced chicken, shrimp, or beef wrapped in tortillas and accompanied with veggie garnishes), but be moderate with the sour cream and Cheddar cheese
- Soft taco filled with beans, lettuce, tomatoes, and salsa, topped with a sprinkle of cheese
- Chicken enchilada (chicken in a softened—not fried—corn tortilla), hold the cheese
- Arroz con pollo (rice with chicken)
- Bean burrito with a sprinkling of cheese
- Seviche (fish marinated in lime juice)

CHAPTER 11

SWEETS, TREATS, AND CHEATS

Sweet, spicy cinnamon buns. Pizza dripping with cheese. Eat-'em-by-the-handful cheese twists. Our attraction to these foods is a hard-wired fact of life: Humans are born with a love of sweet and salty tastes.

Studies show that most babies prefer sweet tastes to those that are sour or bitter, and within 3 days of being born, some infants also develop a preference for salty flavors. And fat? Recent research suggests that humans can actually "taste" (and therefore savor) fat, much as we can distinguish among sweet, sour, bitter, and salty.

Sigh. We want them. We crave them. The world is packed with opportunities to grab 'em and eat 'em. Yet sugary, crispy, crunchy, salty treats aren't so great for your blood sugar or your waistline. The good news: If you make careful, smart choices, it is possible to fit these tempting treats into a healthy eating plan without jeopardizing your blood sugar.

SMART WAYS TO GIVE IN TO TEMPTATION

Allowing yourself an occasional sweet indulgence may make it more likely that you'll stick with a healthy eating plan. Here are four smart ways to indulge your sweet tooth.

- Pick your top five can't-live-without treats. Now, commit their carbohydrate count to memory. How many carbs in one serving of jelly beans? One serving of your favorite frozen yogurt? One slice of cheesecake? To find out, consult a book with carb counts, or check out the Nutrition Facts panel on a food's packaging.

- Half-size your servings. Often, just a bite or two of your favorite dessert will satisfy your sweet tooth. Some strategies to try: Split desserts with friends or your partner, or buy single-portion sizes. If your family loves sweets, ask your partner to stash them in an ingenious hiding place.
- Trade off. If you really want the brownie sundae, ignore the rolls and butter during dinner and eat high-calorie items sparingly (skip the sour cream and use just a sprinkle of cheese on your fajita, for example).
- Feel the burn. Take a 30-minute walk after your treat. Exercise can help regulate your blood sugar.

CHOCOLATE AND "THE CHANGE"

Before menopause, you could take chocolate or leave it. Now, you take . . . and take . . . and take some more. Why this late-blooming yen for sweets?

A recent Turkish study suggests that postmenopausal women's tastebuds undergo significant changes that make them crave sugar. Specifically, midlife women are less able to taste sweet foods and consequently are more likely to eat more or even sweeter foods in an effort to satisfy their tastebuds.

The researchers had 20 men and 20 postmenopausal women

(average age 60) taste a variety of solutions and identify them as salty, bitter, tasteless, or sweet. They found no gender differences when it came to identifying the first three, but for reasons they don't understand, the women were less likely to detect the sweet solutions.

The researchers also found that 35 percent of postmenopausal women had changes in their taste perception, and 45 percent reported that their diets had changed in middle age to incorporate more sweets.

HEALTHY CONVENIENCE-STORE PICKS

Convenience stores are filled with fatty, sugary, salty snacks that can spike your blood sugar and widen your waistline. Not so for the splurges below. All have less than 250 calories and contain nutrients your body needs.

Crunchy Peanut Butter Clif Bar	1 bar	240 calories	It's candy-bar delicious, but with 5 g of fiber plus vitamins and minerals.
Ultra Slim-Fast, Dark Chocolate Fudge	11-oz drink	220 calories	It tastes like a flavored shake but is fortified with 5 g of fiber plus vitamins and minerals.
Dannon Fruit on the Bottom Strawberry Low-Fat Yogurt	8 oz	210 calories	Sweet and creamy, it contains 300 mg of bone-preserving calcium.
Kraft Handi-Snacks Mozzarella String Cheese	1 oz	80 calories	As much calcium as half a glass of milk, it's great paired with V8 (see the next entry).
V8 Juice	10-oz bottle	70 calories	Richly satisfying, and you get a ton of cancer-fighting beta-carotene and lycopene.
Werther's Original	1 piece	20 calories	There are no vitamins, but this buttery morsel takes 10 minutes to melt in your mouth.
Planters Honey-Roasted Cashews	1.5-oz bag	230 calories	Treat your heart to mono-unsaturated fat and vitamin E.

WHEN YOU GET THE "CRUNCHIES"

The crunchies are a craving for fatty, salty snacks like potato chips or cheese curls. Like sweets, these treats tend to be high in refined carbohydrates and trans fats, so they're not for everyday consumption. Still, they're fine as an occasional treat. Here's how to satisfy those crunchies—in moderation.

- Indulge only in what you love. If kettle-cooked potato chips are what makes your heart beat faster, don't waste those calories on anything but.
- Time your treats. Give in to your cravings when you're least likely to overeat. Have a small bag of chips (not the "big grab" size) for lunch—but only if you had a healthy, satisfying breakfast that morning.
- Buy as you go. Purchase single-serving packages of salty treats. (That goes for sweet treats, too.) When we purchase jumbo packages, we end up eating jumbo-size portions. Researchers at the University of Illinois at Urbana-Champaign found that people ate 7 to 43 percent more food when serving themselves from larger containers.
- Consider substitutes. Save fat and calories by looking for lighter versions of salty snacks. The baked versions of potato chips and nacho chips are better than they used to be—some people can't even tell the difference! Just don't devour the entire package. "Fat free" doesn't mean "calorie free."
- Just go for the real thing. Substitutes don't always satisfy. If you hate the taste of low-fat cheese, for example, buy the real stuff, and eat it in small quantities that give you as much taste per calorie as possible.

CHAPTER 12

THE TRUTH ABOUT SUPPLEMENTS

Maybe you don't need supplements—if you are among the 7 percent of women who never, ever skip meals or eat popcorn for dinner once in a blue moon. For the other 93 percent of us, supplements are a great way to fill in nutritional missing pieces—including a few that can help you nurture your body's blood sugar control system.

Easier said than done. With all the pills and potions on the market—and the ever-changing headlines extolling the virtues of one supplement, the dangers of another—which ones do you really need? We've demystified the issue. The truth is, many supplements advertised as blood sugar busters don't work or haven't been tested carefully enough to earn our recommendation.

A better plan: Follow this guide for the latest news on daily supplements, based on the most recent safety and efficacy research. We've sorted through the evidence to find the basic supplements you need every day, and we offer a few add-ons that can help your body regulate blood sugar more efficiently—and safely.

START WITH THE PERFECT MULTIVITAMIN

All the nutrients on this list should be taken in a daily multivitamin with a meal. A multivitamin saves you money, compared with buying dozens of individual bottles, and the nutrients will work better as a team. These are recommended amounts for adults, not kids (we specify if doses are different for pregnant, breastfeeding, or menopausal women). Take this guide with you when discussing supplements with your doctor or when shopping for them. And remember, vitamins can't replace a healthy diet, but they can help compensate for what you're missing—and give you peace of mind as well.

Vitamin A/Beta-Carotene

Boosts immunity, maintains healthy tissue, aids in bone and tooth formation, and protects vision

How much: Up to 5,000 IU of vitamin A (higher amounts might cause birth defects); at least 20 percent as beta-carotene, which is nontoxic. The body converts beta-carotene to A but only processes as much as you need.

Look for: A mixture of vitamin A (such as retinyl palmitate or acetate) and beta-carotene

Food sources: Fortified milk, liver, egg yolks (vitamin A); dark green leafy vegetables, dark orange produce (beta-carotene)

Vitamin D

Strengthens bones and helps prevent osteoporosis; might lower risk of colon cancer, multiple sclerosis, and rheumatoid arthritis; may protect vision and curb PMS symptoms

How much: Ages 19 to 50 and pregnant or breastfeeding, 200 IU; 51 to 70, 400 IU; over 70, 600 to 800 IU

Look for: Vitamin D or cholecalciferol

Food sources: Milk, juice, soy milk, and cereals (fortified only); salmon; sardines; and egg yolks

Vitamin E

An antioxidant: counteracts DNA damage that ages cells and may help prevent heart disease, cancer, memory loss, and cataracts; boosts immunity

How much: 30 IU. Doses up to 400 IU are safe and possibly beneficial.

Look for: D-alpha tocopheryl ("natural" vitamin E), which is better utilized than synthetic dl-alpha tocopheryl

Food sources: Wheat germ, safflower oil, most nuts (almonds, hazelnuts, peanuts), and spinach

Vitamin K

Aids blood clotting, boosts bones, and may curb heart disease risk

How much: 90 to 120 mcg

Look for: Vitamin K, vitamin K_1, or phylloquinone

Food sources: Leafy greens

Folic Acid

Supports normal cell growth and prevents anemia and birth defects; may reduce risk of heart disease, high blood pressure, preterm delivery, memory loss, Alzheimer's disease, depression, and cancer

How much: 400 mcg. Pregnant women need 600 mcg; breastfeeding mothers, 500 mcg. Take no more than 1,000 mcg without physician approval.

Look for: Folic acid

Food sources: Leafy greens, orange juice, wheat germ, cooked dried beans, and fortified grains

Vitamin B$_6$

Helps produce hormones and brain chemicals; strengthens immunity; may lower risk of memory loss, heart disease, depression, and morning sickness during pregnancy

How much: 2 mg

Look for: Vitamin B$_6$ or pyridoxine hydrochloride

Food sources: Chicken, fish, extra-lean red meat, avocados, potatoes, bananas, whole grains, cooked dried beans, nuts, and seeds

Vitamin B$_{12}$

Helps prevent heart disease, memory loss, anemia, and depression; maintains nerve and brain function

How much: 2.4 mcg; pregnant, 2.6 mcg; breastfeeding, 2.8 mcg

Look for: Vitamin B$_{12}$, cyanocobalamin, or cobalamin

Food sources: Extra-lean red meat, poultry, shellfish, eggs, milk, and soy milk

Vitamin C

An antioxidant: maintains tissue, promotes healing, and boosts immunity; may reduce risk of cancer, sun damage, heart disease, cataracts, and tissue damage from secondhand smoke

How much: 75 mg; smokers, 110 mg; pregnant, 85 mg; breastfeeding, 120 mg

Look for: Vitamin C, ascorbic acid, ascorbyl palmitate, or calcium ascorbate

Food sources: Citrus fruit, Brussels sprouts, peppers, and leafy greens

Calcium

Reduces the risk of osteoporosis, high blood pressure, and possibly colon cancer; aids in blood clotting, muscle contraction, and nerve transmission; might reduce symptoms of PMS and help weight loss

How much: Ages 19 to 50 and pregnant or breastfeeding, 1,000 mg; over 50, 1,200 mg You will probably have to take calcium as a separate supplement to get enough—especially if you do not routinely consume three to four servings of low-fat dairy products daily.

Look for: Most forms of calcium are well absorbed. Avoid "natural" calcium from oyster shell, bonemeal, or dolomite, which may contain lead.

Food sources: Low-fat milk products, fortified juice and soy milk, sardines, tofu, leafy greens, and dried beans and peas

Chromium

Regulates blood sugar and may help lower blood sugar levels in those who are insulin resistant

How much: Ages 19 to 50, 25 mcg; pregnant, 30 mcg; breastfeeding, 45 mcg; over 50, 20 mcg

Look for: Chromium nicotinate, chromium-rich yeast, or chromium picolinate, which are better absorbed than chromium chloride

Food sources: Whole grains, wheat germ, orange juice, chicken, and oysters

Copper

Aids in nerve transmission, red blood cell formation, and bone maintenance, supports brain, heart, and immune function; regulates blood sugar and protects against birth defects

How much: 2 mg

Look for: Copper gluconate or copper sulfate

Food sources: Shellfish, organ meats, grains, nuts, seeds, soybeans, and leafy greens

Iron

Prevents fatigue, improves exercise performance, strengthens immunity, and maintains alertness and memory

How much: Women ages 19 to 50, 18 mg; pregnant, 27 mg. Men and menopausal women should look for a supplement with no iron.

Look for: Best absorbed as ferrous fumarate or ferrous sulfate

Food sources: Extra-lean red meat, fish, poultry, cooked dried beans and peas, dried apricots, leafy greens, raisins, whole grains, and fortified cereal

Magnesium

Aids in muscle contraction, nerve transmission, blood pressure regulation, immune function, and bone formation; might lower risk of heart disease and diabetes; helps control hypertension, headaches, and preeclampsia during pregnancy

How much: 400 mcg; may need to take separately. (See "Best Add-On Supplements for Your Blood Sugar" on page 136.)

Look for: Magnesium oxide, carbonate, or hydroxide

(continued on page 138)

BEST ADD-ON SUPPLEMENTS FOR YOUR BLOOD SUGAR

In addition to a good multivitamin, these supplements may help fill nutritional gaps that affect your body's regulation of blood sugar or cut the risk for complications tied to blood sugar problems, such as heart disease and memory problems.

Omega-3 fatty acids: Found in fish (especially cold-water varieties such as salmon), walnuts, and flaxseed, omega-3 fatty acids can lower risk of heart disease, memory loss, bone loss, and osteoporosis and may even ease mild depression and reduce symptoms of rheumatoid arthritis.

Best daily dose: 1 gram. People with high triglycerides should get 2 to 4 grams along with a physician's care. Look for a mixture of EPA and DHA (eicosapentaenoic acid and docosahexaenoic acid). Most potent source: fish-oil supplements.

Chromium: Found in beans, whole grains, and broccoli, chromium helps cells absorb blood sugar. While some studies suggest that supplementing with chromium helps keep blood sugar under control, the American Diabetes Association says only very low chromium levels cause problems and that for most people, supplements offer no known benefit.

Not everyone is so quick to dismiss chromium's potential for people with diabetes. "There are several lines of evidence suggesting that higher doses of chromium supplements may be beneficial," says William Cefalu, MD, associate professor of medicine and director of the clinical trials unit at the University of Vermont College of Medicine in Burlington. Diabetes experts say 600 micrograms a day have proven effective. Chromium nicotinate, chromium-rich yeast, or chromium picolinate are good sources.

Magnesium: This mineral is abundant in green leafy vegetables, legumes, nuts, wheat germ, and whole grains—but one in three people with diabetes is low on it. Research suggests that as magnesium intake goes up, the risk of developing type 2 diabetes goes down.

Experts say it's a good practice to make sure you're getting enough magnesium. (Most people, especially seniors, don't.) Supplements come in a variety of forms, including magnesium oxide, carbonate, and hydroxide. Look for one with 400 milligrams.

Alpha-lipoic acid (ALA): There are tiny amounts of this potent antioxidant in spinach and meat, but experts say you need more to help relieve a common diabetes complication known as diabetic neuropathy, which develops when high blood sugar levels damage delicate nerve endings. In Germany, ALA is a prescription drug used to treat diabetic neuropathy. It may also help control blood sugar in people with diabetes, possibly by lowering insulin levels and increasing the transport of sugar into cells.

"I recommend alpha-lipoic to my patients with diabetic neuropathy who haven't been helped by conventional treatments," says Aaron Vinik, MD, PhD, director of the Strelitz Diabetes Research Institute at the Eastern Virginia Medical School in Norfolk.

Look for a supplement with 600 to 1,200 milligrams. Talk with your doctor before taking ALA, as it may affect the dosage of your diabetes medications.

Food sources: Low-fat milk, peanuts, avocados, bananas, wheat germ, whole grains, cooked dried beans and peas, leafy greens, and oysters

Selenium

An antioxidant: may lower risk of heart disease, rheumatoid arthritis, and certain forms of cancer

How much: 55 mcg; pregnant, 60 mcg; breastfeeding, 70 mcg. Doses higher than 400 mcg can be toxic.

Look for: Selenomethionine and selenium-rich yeast

Food sources: Whole grains, nuts, seafood, and lean meat

Zinc

Speeds healing, boosts immunity, prevents pregnancy complications, and helps maintain strong bones and normal taste and smell

How much: 8 mg; pregnant, 11 mg; breastfeeding, 12 mg. Limit your intake to less than 40 mg per day.

Look for: Zinc gluconate, zinc picolinate, zinc oxide, or zinc sulfate

Food sources: Oysters, extra-lean red meat, turkey, nuts, cooked dried beans and peas, wheat germ, and whole grains

4

SLIM AND SLEEK: FITNESS FOR BETTER BLOOD SUGAR

CHAPTER 13

THE ACTIVE LIFE—
A PLAN FOR BUSY PEOPLE

What if you could dramatically improve the way cells throughout your body "grab" and process blood sugar—and, as a result, cut your odds for diabetes, heart disease, and even some forms of cancer? What if you could slim and tone your body's most troublesome spots at the same time, boost your energy, and raise your spirits—without using up more minutes than it takes to watch your favorite TV show?

You can—simply by lacing up your sneakers and heading out the door for a walk most days of the week; working your muscles just 10 minutes a day with a gentle strength-training routine; and taking advantage of opportunities to get more calorie-burning everyday activity such as washing the car, playing with the kids, or tending your rose garden.

Physical activity is a cornerstone of the *Sugar Solution* plan not only because it blasts calories and transforms puffy, jiggly fat into sleek, firm muscle—mountains of medical studies prove that exercise helps your body process blood sugar more efficiently. The exciting research:

Walking (or riding an exercise bike) reverses dangerous insulin resistance. In a University of Michigan, Ann Arbor, study, women who walked or biked every day for just 7 days improved their insulin sensitivity significantly—meaning their cells no longer ignored insulin's signals to absorb blood sugar. A University of California, Los Angeles, study of 31 men with metabolic syndrome or type 2 diabetes reported similar results: Daily treadmill walking, in 45- to 60-minute sessions, cut insulin resistance in half after 3 weeks. Why that's such good news: Insulin resistance raises levels of the hormone insulin in your body and, as a result, increases your risk for diabetes, heart disease, some cancers, and even memory problems and infertility.

Active fun offers serious protection against insulin resistance and prediabetes. A University of Buffalo study of 7,485 men and 5,856 women, ages 20 to 69, found that those who got the most activity during their leisure hours were half as likely to be insulin resistant—putting them at low risk for prediabetic conditions including high-normal blood sugar and metabolic syndrome (a combination of insulin resistance, slightly high blood pressure, slightly high levels of heart-threatening blood fats called triglycerides, and low levels of "good" HDL cholesterol). While some study volunteers engaged in intentional exercise, others simply played sports, gardened, and took walks for pleasure.

Strength training makes cells absorb and burn more blood sugar. In a small but well-designed study from Japan's Osaka City General Hospital, nine women and men with diabetes performed a short strength-training routine 5 days a week for 4 to 6 weeks. Their insulin sensitivity improved by 48 percent, while a control group that didn't pump iron saw no improvement.

Combining aerobic exercise and strength training is even better. A Greek study of nine women with type 2 diabetes found that after 4 months of regular strength-training and aerobic workouts (two sessions per week of each), study volunteers lowered their blood sugar by nearly 13 percent and insulin levels 38 percent—signs that muscle cells had become more insulin-sensitive.

THE EXERCISE RX

Physical activity works its metabolic magic in several ways. As your muscles contract and relax during exercise, they sip more and more glucose from your bloodstream and burn it for energy. But that's only the beginning.

Exercise also makes muscle cells more sensitive to signals from insulin, the hormone that tells cells to absorb blood sugar. In a University of Missouri–Columbia study, researchers found that sedentary lab rats had fewer insulin receptors on the surface of their muscle cells, giving insulin fewer opportunities to dock and relay its important message. Inside the muscle cells of couch potato rats, proteins that normally accept glucose and begin the process of converting it to energy were also less active. It's as if muscle cells fall asleep when they're not used—and it can happen fast. The researchers found that after just 2 days of inactivity, the animals decreased their insulin sensitivity by an amazing 33 percent. The same process occurs in human cells, too, the scientists note. Think about that the next time *American Idol* or the Home Shopping Network wins out over an evening walk or a trip to the gym.

Exercise also cuts intra-abdominal fat—the fat wrapped around internal organs deep within your belly. This nasty visceral blubber pumps out fatty acids and inflammatory compounds that raise your odds for insulin resistance and, ultimately, type 2 diabetes. You're at risk if your waistline tops 35 inches for women, 40 inches for men. But a brisk cardio workout, three to five times a week, can melt belly fat. "The length of time should be 40 to 60 minutes," says Syracuse University exercise physiologist Jill Kanaley, PhD, who found in a recent study that exercise trimmed abdominal fat better than a diet for women who already have diabetes.

THE *SUGAR SOLUTION* FITNESS PLAN

Our program combines an easy walking plan geared for your fitness level, a simple strength-training program even a beginner can master, and smart strategies for fitting more movement into your day even when you're not formally working out.

We believe this three-part plan gives you a distinct edge: You'll burn more calories; improve cardiovascular health; and build denser, stronger muscles that raise your metabolism so that you burn even more calories all day long. (Studies suggest that weight training can prompt your metabolism to burn 100 or more extra calories per day!) You've also got a built-in "fallback" for those busy days when time and your exercise schedule slip away from you. When you're in the habit of parking farther from the supermarket front door, taking the steps rather than the elevator at work, and playing tag with the kids instead of watching them from the kitchen window, exercise becomes a no-brainer—it's simply part of your day!

We'll also show you how to rediscover the pleasure of move-ment—and find ways to match your personality with fitness activities you'll truly enjoy. Take the quiz later in this chapter and find out whether you're a social butterfly or a thoughtful introvert, a competi-tor or an outdoorswoman—and which activities will best suit your fitness personality.

The details of the *Sugar Solution* fitness plan:

Walk! If you've never walked for fitness before, we'll show you how to start slowly for big results. By the end of the 28-day plan, walking rookies will be stepping out for 30 minutes of calorie burning every day. Walking veterans will learn how to gradually ramp up to 60 min-utes or more. (Of course, you can substitute or mix and match other aerobic activities such as jogging, biking, swimming, cross-country skiing, or an exercise class or video.) You'll find more information about our walking plan in Chapter 14.

Strength-train! Nine simple exercises—most of which use only your body weight to work your muscles—tone you from head to toe. You can choose to do your strength training in 10-minute segments 6 days a week, in 20-minute bouts 3 days a week, or in 30 minutes just twice a week. What could be more convenient—and you'll love the way this easy routine builds sleek muscle, whittles your waist, and slims your hips while boosting your metabolism so you burn more calories all day, every day. Read more about our strength-training program, designed by *Prevention* magazine Fitness Director Michele Stanten, in Chapter 15.

Everyday activity! Ever wonder why women, men, and even kids in 1950s-era snapshots and movies look so svelte? They weren't swimming laps or training for a 5-K charity run. They simply built

DON'T JUST SIT THERE . . . BURN MORE CALORIES!

Here's how various everyday activities stack up as calorie-blasters.

10 minutes of...	Burns this many calories...	
	If you weigh 175 pounds	If you weigh 250 pounds
Washing windows	48	69
Dusting	31	44
Washing floors	53	75
Gardening	42	59
Weeding	68	98
Pushing a mower	52	74
Preparing a meal	46	65
Washing or dressing	37	53
Shoveling snow	89	130
Painting your house	40	55
Chopping firewood	84	121
Working on your car	43	59
Caring for children (babies or toddlers)	41	63
Playing the piano	32	47
Dancing	60	80
Doing electrical work or plumbing	45	65

more activity into every moment of the day—by rolling up car windows by hand, "spin-drying" clothes through a hand-cranked wringer, washing dishes by hand, and walking to the bus stop and the grocery store. Thanks to modern technology, we've got automatic windows; a spin cycle on the washing machine; and a landscape of drive-thru doughnut shops, fast-food joints, banks, even (in some states) beer stores. The result: We've engineered about 700 calories' worth of activity out of every single day. Keep reading—we'll show you ways to put more calorie-burning movement back into your day wherever you can.

THE LIFESTYLE ADVANTAGE

Mayo Clinic endocrinologist James Levine, MD, burns a few extra calories every time he answers his ringing office telephone—because he keeps it stashed in a desk drawer, not out in the open. Dr. Levine, whose research has illuminated the dramatic calorie-burning potential of everyday movement, even hooked up his own computer workstation to a treadmill so that he can walk slowly while he works.

His strategy? Take full advantage of non-exercise-activity thermogenesis, or NEAT—physical activities that can burn hundreds of extra calories every day. In a recent study that monitored 10 overweight couch potatoes and 10 slim couch potatoes for 10 days, Dr. Levine discovered that while neither group bothered with formal exercise, the slim folks burned *350 more calories every day* simply because they moved around more. While slim folks walked around the house during commercials, twirled their hair, jiggled their knees, and fidgeted, the overweight folks sat very, very still for 150 minutes longer every single day.

"A person can expend calories either by going to the gym or through everyday activities," Dr. Levine notes. "Our study shows that the calories burned in everyday activities are far, far more important in obesity than we previously imagined." And while you don't have to hide your phone in the kitchen junk drawer, you can make plenty of small changes that get you up and moving. "Use your creativity when looking for ways to overhaul your daily NEAT expenditure," encourages Dr. Levine. "It's unlimited and will lead to success."

You might turn on the radio and dance while your morning coffee perks or vacuum one room of your house before breakfast. Plan a lunch-time excursion every day if you're home with the kids, or do some

(continued on page 151)

WHAT'S YOUR FITNESS PERSONALITY?

Whether you need a change from your current exercise routine or are ready to tackle exercise for the first time, the quiz below will help you identify activities you will enjoy and stick with, based on your personality, schedule, and workout goals. Take each section of the quiz and combine the results of the three parts to get a profile of your workout preferences—what we call your fitness personality.

Part 1: Personality and Hobbies

1. As a kid, the activities I liked best were:
   a. Gymnastics, cheerleading, jumping rope, or dance classes
   b. Playing outside—building forts, climbing trees, exploring the woods
   c. Competitive sports
   d. Playing with dolls, reading, coloring, or art projects
   e. Parties, playing with my friends

2. My favorite hobbies today are:
   a. Anything new and challenging
   b. Outside activities: gardening, walking the dog, watching the stars, etc.
   c. Tennis, card or board games, team and/or spectator sports
   d. Reading, movies, needlecraft, painting, or anything that provides an escape
   e. Group activities with friends— anything from a walking or book group to just talking

3. I get motivated to exercise if:
   a. I get a new exercise video or piece of equipment, or I try a totally new class
   b. I get a new piece of exercise equipment I can use outside, I discover a new walking or jogging path, or the weather is nice
   c. I'm challenged with some competition
   d. I find an exercise that I get really into to the point that I forget my surroundings
   e. I exercise in a group

4. I prefer to exercise:
   a. Indoors, in a gym or at home
   b. Outdoors
   c. Wherever there's a chance to win
   d. Wherever I'm not the center of attention
   e. In a gym or fitness center

continued

Interpreting Your Score for Part 1

Mostly a's or a mixture of letters: The Learner. "You're always trying something new—today you're painting; a few years ago you did photography," says Dr. Olson. You also welcome physical and mental challenges.

Choose activities that help you explore new moves, such as aerobics classes, African dance (or any form of dance), Pilates, Tae-Bo, tai chi, seated aerobics, in-line skating, skipping rope, fencing, or rebounding (aerobics on a mini trampoline).

Mostly b's: The Outdoorswoman. Fresh air is your energizer, so why not include nature in your exercise routine? Try hiking, biking, nature walking, gardening, or cross-country skiing. If you have a piece of home exercise equipment you love, drag it out to the patio on a nice day. Or sit and do yoga on your back porch.

Mostly c's: The Competitor. "You naturally like one-on-one, competitive types of activities," says Dr. Olson. Try fencing, cardio kickboxing, Tae-Bo, tai chi, or spinning classes.

If you excelled in or enjoyed a sport when you were younger, take it up again. "If you can't play anymore due to injuries, consider coaching—you'll stay active by demonstrating the drills and exercises, and you'll help others learn to play," says Dr. Olson.

Mostly d's: The Thoughtful Introvert. You're a "disassociative exerciser," meaning you fantasize or think of events in your life when you exercise, rather than the exercise itself. "Because you enjoy activities like reading, where you get lost in a story and forget your surroundings, you will like mind/body activities like yoga," says Dr. Olson.

Also try nature walking or hiking. "You'll probably prefer walking in a beautiful place out in the country or on a neat nature trail to treadmill walking," Dr. Olson says.

Mostly e's: The Social Butterfly. As a people person, you tend to prefer the gym to exercising in your living room. Try aerobics classes, kickboxing, seated aerobics, yoga, spinning classes, step classes, water aerobics, Tae-Bo, and tai chi classes. For weight lifting, find a buddy or two and do circuit training.

Part 2: Workout Style and Exercise Goals

5. My primary exercise goal is:
    a. To lose weight/tone up
    b. To relax and/or relieve stress
    c. To have fun
    d. It depends on how I feel

6. I prefer:
    a. A lot of structure in my workout
    b. Some structure, but not too much
    c. No structure
    d. It depends on my mood

7. I prefer to exercise:
    a. Alone
    b. With one other person
    c. In a group
    d. It depends on my mood

Interpreting Your Score for Part 2

Mostly a's: The Gung-Ho Exerciser. You don't mess around when you work out. "You'll benefit most from doing what I call volume-based exercise, where you spend an extended amount of time doing a specific activity, like cycling, aerobics, or using elliptical machines, treadmills, stairclimbers, etc., at a moderate intensity," says Dr. Olson. For optimal weight-loss benefits, you should burn 2,000 calories a week. One way to achieve this would be to perform 30 minutes of aerobic-based exercise daily and combine this with three sessions of weight training a week.

Mostly b's: The Leisurely Exerciser. Your main exercise objectives are to relax and de-stress. Studies have shown a direct relationship between physical activity and stress reduction. "If you're stressed and you have energy to burn, interval workouts work well," Dr. Olson says. Hop on the treadmill or head outside and walk for 5 minutes, then pick up the pace for a minute, and then return to your usual speed. Repeat this sequence several times.

Circuit strength training is another great option. Here, you do one set of an exercise for one muscle group and then follow up with one set of another exercise for a different muscle group. Continue until you've completed one set of each exercise, then go back through the series of exercises for a second set and perhaps even a third set. These types of workouts help reduce overall stress hormone levels, Dr. Olson says.

continued

Mostly c's: The Fun-Loving Exerciser. Fifty straight minutes on the treadmill is not your bag. You'll be most likely to stick to activities that are already an integral part of your schedule. "Instead of leaving your dog crying in the house while you head to the gym, run around with him in the backyard," says Dr. Olson. Grab your in-line skates and circle the neighborhood. Put on your favorite music CD and dance around the living room.

Mostly d's: The Flexible Exerciser. Exercise turns you on, but routine doesn't. You'd rather fly by the seat of your gym shorts—which is fine. "If you don't want to lift weights one day, go ahead and take a leisurely walk or yoga class instead," says Dr. Olson.

To add variety, use the elliptical machine one day, the treadmill the next, and the cross-country skiing machine the next.

Part 3: Your Lifestyle and Schedule

8. I have the most energy:
   a. In the morning
   b. In the middle of the day
   c. In the evening or at night
   d. My energy level fluctuates

9. I have the most time:
   a. In the morning
   b. In the middle of the day
   c. In the evening
   d. It depends on the day

10. I go to bed:
    a. Early and get up early
    b. And get up at the same time every day, but not particularly early or late
    c. Late and get up late
    d. Whenever I feel like it

Interpreting Your Score for Part 3

Mostly a's: The Morning Dove. You like to get chores out of the way as soon as you get up because that's when you have the most energy. "Exercising in the morning will fit better with your whole psyche," Dr. Olson says. Whether you go to the gym before you start your day or you head outside for a dawn walk, you'll have an edge over those who hit the snooze button a few more times.

Mostly b's: The Midday Duck. You'd rather plop down on an exercise bike than in front of a sandwich when noon rolls around. That's fine. Whether you're at home or work, exercise is a great way to break up your day.

Mostly c's: The Night Owl. You haven't seen a sunrise since that all-night party in 1974. If you have more energy at night, that's the time to exercise.

Mostly d's or an even mixture of letters: The Flexible Bird. The best time of day for you to exercise varies with your schedule. Just go with it. "In the summer, when I'm not teaching classes, I do all my exercise in the morning. But when my schedule changes in the fall, I do it in the afternoon—my body has to make a little transition, but it adjusts," says Dr. Olson.

---

stretches when you're stuck in a traffic jam. "Exercise doesn't have to be grueling to do you some good," says Michele Olson, PhD, professor of health and human performance at Auburn University in Montgomery, Alabama. "Research shows it's the accumulation of movement that counts—whether you walk the dog or do yoga, regular activity is more important than the specific activity."

One study conducted at the Cooper Institute for Aerobics Research in Dallas, for example, tested 235 formerly inactive men and women for 2 years; participants followed either a lifestyle activities program or a structured exercise program. Both programs produced the same improvements in fitness, heart health, and reduction of body fat percentage, indicating that an overall increase in lifestyle activity is just as effective as a structured exercise program.

How powerful is lifestyle activity? When researchers from the Medical College of Wisconsin crunched the numbers, what they found suggests that your house and garden deserve to be classed as "fitness equipment"—just like your sneakers, your bicycle, and your gym. To burn 100 calories without leaving home, they say, you could:

- Clean the house for 25 to 35 minutes
- Wash dishes or iron clothes for 45 to 50 minutes
- Mow the lawn for 15 to 25 minutes

- Dig your garden with a spade or tiller for 10 to 20 minutes
- Rake leaves for 20 to 25 minutes
- Wash and wax the car for 20 to 25 minutes
- Wash windows for 20 to 30 minutes
- Paint the walls or woodwork using a paintbrush for 35 to 40 minutes
- Shovel snow for 10 to 15 minutes
- Blow snow for 15 to 20 minutes
- Stack firewood for 15 to 20 minutes

More ways to keep your body moving (calorie burn is based on a 150-pound person; if you weigh more, you'll burn a bit more):

Chew sugarless gum. Moving your jaw muscles burns about 11 calories an hour.

Play tag with your dog. In just 5 or 6 minutes, you'll burn 40 calories.

Take the stairs, skip the escalator. Burn 16 calories on average per flight.

Window-shop while waiting for a bus or a friend. Burn 35 calories in 10 minutes.

Sing! Belting out "We Are the World" at a karaoke bar burns about 20 calories.

Play with kids. Impromptu games of basketball, touch football, or tag—or just jumping rope or throwing a ball—burn 80 to 137 calories every 10 minutes.

Dance, dance, dance! Turn on your favorite CD at home; hit the dance floor at a party. You'll burn about 50 calories in 15 minutes.

Join a kickball game. It's easier to kick a big ball with your foot than it is to whack a tiny, flying baseball with a stick anyway, so go for it—and burn 125 calories in a half hour.

Say yes to miniature golf. Getting your ball past the revolving windmill is as challenging as it was when you were 12 . . . and you'll burn 211 calories in an hour.

Move your own furniture. Time to rearrange the living room? Do it yourself and burn 100 calories in 15 minutes.

Dust off your musical skills. Play your piano; pick up your violin, clarinet, or flute. An hour of homemade music could burn 150 calories or more. (If you play drums, the burn's closer to 280 calories per hour.)

Be sporty at the next neighborhood picnic. Hit the lawn for a round of bocce, croquet, or horseshoes instead of hanging out on the chaise longue. You'll burn about 100 calories in a half hour.

Turn TV time into exercise time. Between the credits and commercials, at least 20 minutes of every television hour is stuff you don't really have to watch closely. Use this built-in downtime for a simple workout routine: Do warmups during the opening credits (try walking in place or jumping jacks). During the commercials, march or jog in place or do crunches, toe touches, and squats. You could even use TV time to do your strength-training routine (for details, see Chapter 15).

CHAPTER 14

THE NEW WALKING WORKOUT

Walking is about the most pleasant and nearly pain-free workout there is. It's also one of the most effective. It can not only help shave off pounds, which improves your health (and blood sugar levels), it can also relieve stress, brighten your mood, and rekindle energy. All this, and it's convenient, easy, and safe for just about anyone at any age.

While you could choose any aerobic activity as your basic form of exercise on the *Sugar Solution* plan—such as jogging, swimming, biking, hiking, aerobics classes, or videos—walking is our favorite. It's easy on joints; superconvenient (just head out the door!); requires little in the way of special gear beyond good shoes, a hat, and a bottle of sunscreen; and is beneficial whether you're a "beginner" fitness walker who does 15 minutes 5 days a week or a veteran putting in an hour a day.

The *Sugar Solution* walking workout is perfect for pound-the-pavement-every-day people and honorary members of Couch Potatoes Anonymous alike. Rookies start out walking 15 minutes a day and gradually increase to 30. Veterans start with 30 minutes a day in Week 1 and build to 60 minutes or more by Week 4.

Of course, even an exercise as simple as walking requires dedication and planning, and if you've been walking for a while, you may be looking for a new twist on this old favorite. Whether you're a beginner or have been at it for years, these six strategies will help you get the most out of your time on the trail, treadmill, road, or track.

STRATEGY #1: BEGINNERS—TAKE BABY STEPS

"It's all too easy to stress tissues by going a little too far, too fast," says Byron Russell, PT, PhD, chair of the department of physical therapy at

---

IF THE SHOE FITS . . .

When it comes to walking workouts, there's nothing more important than a good shoe. "Don't think that you can just go to the store and pick out cheap fitness shoes simply because you are a beginner or don't walk much," says Melinda Reiner, DPM, vice president of the American Association for Women Podiatrists. Different feet need different shoes. To find a perfect pair, keep these tips in mind.

Choose a walking shoe. Any old shoe may work, but a shoe designed for walking will decrease your risk of injury and boost performance. A good one will be flexible in the ball of the foot but not in the arch. (A shoe that bends in the arch will place increased stress on the plantar fascia.) The heel should be cushioned (you don't need a lot of padding in the forefoot) and also rounded to speed your foot through the heel-toe motion with ease.

Go offline for a fit. This is one purchase that must be made in person. Whether you have low arches or tend to overpronate, the salespeople in a good, technical running store will watch you walk barefoot and help you choose the features you need. Best to try: a store that's independently owned.

Buy big. People—women especially—tend to buy shoes that are too small. Ask the salesperson to help you check the fit, and don't get caught up in thinking that you have to buy a size 8 because that's what you've always worn. Athletic shoes can be sized quite differently from your dress shoes.

Toss 'em often. Don't skimp on your feet. Once the interior padding has lost its spring, it's time for a new pair. Generally, that means replacing your shoes every 500 miles—sooner if you have foot, ankle, knee, or back problems.

THE *SUGAR SOLUTION* WALKING PLAN

To start, simply choose the level that describes you best.

- You're a walking rookie if you do not walk regularly or rarely walk more than 15 minutes at a time.
- You're a veteran if you walk regularly for at least 25 minutes per session.

Turn to the *Sugar Solution* 28-day plan on page 215 for inspiring daily walking tips to help you burn more calories, tone muscles, and have more fun as you step toward fitness.

Week 1
Rookies: 15 minutes a day
Veterans: 30 minutes or more a day

Week 2
Rookies: 20 minutes a day
Veterans: 40 minutes or more a day

Week 3
Rookies: 25 minutes a day
Veterans: 50 minutes or more a day

Week 4
Rookies: 30 minutes a day
Veterans: 60 minutes or more a day

Eastern Washington University. "People think, `I'm just walking,' so they don't try to build up gradually. But if you're not yet in shape, your body can't tolerate longer distances or fast paces, especially if you have any existing health problems."

If you're getting started, walk just 10 to 20 minutes on mostly flat ground five times a week; then increase the time by 5 to 10 minutes each week. To get the best results, try to walk every day. If you skip a day, continue to increase gradually; don't walk twice as fast or twice as far during your next workout. Be sure to warm up your muscles by walking at a slower pace for 3 to 5 minutes at the beginning of your workout. Then stretch after your walk. (See our suggestions on page 158.)

To burn more calories, put your whole body into your stride. To make your stride shorter and quicker, roll from your heel through the center of your foot, then to the ball of your foot, and finally push off from your toes. And swing your arms as you walk. Keep them bent at about 90 degrees, and swing them forward and back—not out to the sides like chicken wings.

DON'T FORGET TO STRETCH

After you put foot to trail or road, do these simple stretches. Don't bounce when you stretch. Move slowly and stretch only as far as is comfortable.

Side reaches: Reach one arm over your head and to the side. Keep your hips steady and your shoulders straight to the side. Hold for 10 seconds, and repeat on the other side.

Knee pull: Stand against a wall. Keep your head, hips, and feet in a straight line. Pull one knee to your chest, hold for 10 seconds, and then repeat with the other leg.

Wall push: Lean your hands on a wall with your feet 3 to 4 feet away from the wall. Bend one knee and point it toward the wall. Keep your back leg straight with your foot flat and your toes pointed straight ahead. Hold for 10 seconds, and repeat with the other leg.

Leg curl: Pull your right foot to your buttocks with your right hand. Keep your knee pointing straight down. Hold for 10 seconds, and repeat with your left foot and hand.

Aim for invigoration, not exhaustion. Your walking pace should be neither so tough that you're gasping for air nor so easy that you don't break a sweat. On a scale of 1 to 10—10 being all-out exertion—aim for about a 7. At that level of exertion, you should be breathing harder than normal but still be able to carry on a simple conversation.

STRATEGY #2. STEP TOWARD FITNESS WITH A PEDOMETER

The secret to getting off the couch (once and for all)—or revving up your walking routine to a new calorie-burning level—is a beeper-size device that clips onto your waistband and may cost as little as $30. Studies show that sedentary people who wear a pedometer and have a daily step goal become more active throughout the day and see improvements in fitness and body fat comparable to those of people doing more structured workouts. And research into pedometer use proves that increasing your everyday activities—walking the dog and just getting up more often—can make a big difference.

The greatest power of the pedometer seems to be its ability to motivate. When you take a walk, it's satisfying to see your steps ticking away. It also cues you to be more active. When you see or feel the pedometer on your waistband, you're reminded to get moving.

Experts recommend at least 10,000 steps—or about 5 miles—a day for health. It may sound like a lot. But most people walk about 4,000 steps doing regular daily activities. (For example, if you are taking out the trash, picking up things around the house, or strolling at the shopping mall, you are probably taking around 85 steps per minute.)

The best way to get into pedometer walking: For the first 3 days, use it to see how many steps you walk naturally throughout the day. Then set small goals for added steps that will eventually move you to 10,000 steps per day. If you walk 4,500 steps during the normal course

THE GOLD STANDARD PEDOMETER

Whether you want to ramp up your regular walking routine or simply add more calorie-burning "lifestyle steps" into your day, a pedometer can help you get there faster. When *Prevention* magazine tested 38 different types of step-counters by asking 26 women to wear them, everyone moved more—whether they were veteran runners, committed walkers, or folks who exercise only by accident. One woman even jogged in place while brushing her teeth to build up her step count!

Choosing a pedometer can be a dizzying experience: You can spend $5 on a bare-bones model or $130 or more on a fancy version that also tracks calorie burn and heart rate—and lets you download your data into your computer. We suggest sticking with the very affordable, extremely accurate gold standard that researchers use when measuring the accuracy of other pedometers: the Yamax SW-200 Digi-Walker—a best buy at $22, from New-Lifestyles (www.new-lifestyles.com).

Accuracy matters: A 2004 University of Tennessee study found that some pedometers missed steps by as much as 25 percent, and others overestimated by 45 percent.

of your day, you might first increase your daily steps to 6,500. After a few weeks, move up to 8,500, and then to 10,000. Sounds huge? It's not. Every 2,000 steps is about 1 mile—a distance most people can cover in 15 to 20 minutes. You can bump up your daily steps by walking for a half hour at lunch and incorporating lots of step-filled activity into your day. At work or the grocery store, park in the spot farthest from the door. Do more errands on foot when possible. Walk around your house as you chat on the phone.

STRATEGY #3: VETERAN WALKERS—BURN MORE CALORIES AND FAT WITH INTERVALS

"Walking is great exercise," says exercise physiologist Len Kravitz, PhD, of the University of New Mexico. "But if you always do the same walking workout, it may not keep you as fit as you'd like. You burn more calories and improve fitness faster when you surprise your body with a variety of workouts that include some higher intensity."

A recent study of more than 15,000 men and women from the Fred Hutchinson Cancer Research Center in Seattle revealed that those who regularly walked fast or jogged were better able to keep off the pounds during middle age (when many of us gain) than those who stuck to the same slow pace.

If you're a longtime walker—particularly if your routine hasn't varied much for the past few months or even years—it's time to shake things up with interval training. Add several "sprints" of faster-than-average walking to your program, 2 or 3 days per week. The three interval routines below will all help burn more fat and calories and make you a faster walker; after about 4 weeks of regular interval workouts, all of your walks will go faster and seem easier. When that happens, you can boost your workout intensity by walking faster all the time and/or walking farther.

These intervals assume that you've been walking regularly for at least a few months. If you're a true beginner, your joints and ligaments need conditioning to handle the intensity, so do intervals only once a week for the first 6 to 8 weeks. Also, start with the easiest intervals and work up to the more challenging ones.

Steady intervals. Warm up for 5 to 10 minutes. Then increase your intensity for 1 minute so your work effort is a 7 or 8 on a 1-to-10 scale. After 1 minute, ease your intensity to a 5 for 2 minutes of active rest. Repeat throughout a 30- to 40-minute walk. Cool down for 5 to 10 minutes at the end of the workout.

This is a great interval for beginners; although you have less rest, you're not pushing the intensity as high. To make this more challenging, you can either increase your effort or extend the intense work portion to 90 seconds.

Brisk intervals. Warm up for 5 to 10 minutes. Then increase your speed for 1 minute so your work effort is an 8 or 9 on a 1-to-10 scale. After 1 minute, ease your intensity to a 5 or 6 for 3 minutes of active rest. Repeat throughout a 30- to 40-minute walk. Cool down for 5 to 10 minutes at the end of the workout. Note: You will have less "active recovery" during the "rest" sections of this workout, so each successive interval may feel harder. If need be, lower the intensity of your recovery so you feel completely ready for your next work effort.

High-intensity intervals. Warm up for 5 to 10 minutes. Then increase your effort (if you're outside, walk faster or jog; on a treadmill, walk faster or increase the incline) for 1 minute so your "work effort" is an 8 or 9+ on a scale of 1 to 10, with 10 being as hard as you can go. After 1 minute, ease your intensity to a 4 or 5 for 4 minutes of "active rest." Repeat throughout a 30- to 40-minute walk. Always end this workout with active rest or a 5- to 10-minute cooldown.

STRATEGY #4: FIT WALKING INTO THE BUSIEST DAY

"The number one reason people stop exercising is lack of time," says Harold Kohl, PhD, an epidemiologist with the Physical Activity and Health Branch of the Centers for Disease Control and Prevention (CDC). The answer for busy people? "Take a hard look at your day and figure out where you can substitute activity for inactivity," he says. "Think about exercise the way you think about substituting low-fat food for high-fat food." Any walking is better than none, he continues. "The key is to look for opportunities to be active in ways that aren't necessarily planned or structured. In other words, look beyond the stuff we typically think of as exercise."

Up your downtime. Once you adopt Dr. Kohl's thinking, opportunities for activity appear everywhere. Catching up on phone calls to friends or family? Walk in place or do some squats. For yard work, choose a push mower over a power one. If you're waiting at the school-bus stop, breeze up and down the block (keeping the stop in sight) until the bus pulls into view. Got mail? Scout out a drop box a 10-minute walk away. And when you get stuck at the airport, don't take the wait sitting down. Instead, hike through the terminal.

Leave the stands. Do you spend time schlepping your offspring to sports events? "Never just sit and watch," says Maggie Spilner, former walking editor of *Prevention* magazine and author of *Walk Your Way Through Menopause*. "Doing laps around the field gives you a workout as well as several vantage points to view the action."

Look for bite-size exercise. Instead of waiting until you have a free half hour—it might be next Christmas—dissect the goal into bite-size nuggets. Think of your daily exercise allotment as three 10-minute jaunts, six 5-minute spurts, or even fifteen 2-minute quickies (roughly equivalent to the number of commercial breaks in an evening spent watching television). "Studies show that you burn the same number of calories whether you exercise all at once or in short bursts," says personal trainer Liz Neporent, author of *Fitness Walking for Dummies* and *The Ultimate Body: 10 Perfect Workouts for Women*.

Use your indoor track. If all else fails, don't fight the four walls. Walking laps around the house may sound dizzying, but it works for women pressed for time or caring for young children, says Neporent. Best of all, you don't even have to make tracks. "You can walk in place while you're waiting for water to boil or watching television," she says. "The average person walks a mile in 15 to 20 minutes, and it doesn't matter if you're moving or standing in place." To make it more of a challenge, Neporent suggests adding some high knee lifts and big arm swings.

STRATEGY #5: TOO HOT? TOO COLD? OUTWIT HARSH WEATHER

Frigid winters or simmering summers needn't be a deterrent. Buy a treadmill or a gym membership; 25 percent of walkers use treadmills. Both

THE SUGAR SURVIVORS: Maggie Gallivan

Maggie Gallivan, 55, of Friday Harbor, Washington, struggled since she was 11 years old with an eating disorder that kept her ashamed and feeling like "an encapsulated weirdo" (as she wrote in her journal). "The possibility of ever experiencing exuberant physical activity or of connecting meaningfully with others seemed as remote as walking up on the moon," she says.

In March 2000, at 5-foot-4 ½, 227 pounds, she was prediabetic and taking antidepressants. "I couldn't look anyone in the eye," Gallivan recalls. "I didn't want to look at myself from the neck down. Most of all, I could no longer bear to think of never experiencing life as the happy, creative, and physically alive human being I longed to be. One month later, about to turn 50 and terrified of losing what life I had left, I became willing to accept daily help from members of an eating disorders support group, began working with an insightful therapist, and committed to walk at least 6 days a week."

Her first time out, on the YWCA track, Gallivan's knees and ankles screamed with every step. Stuffed into sweats two sizes too small, she fought back tears and stared at the floor the entire time. "I made it only once around the track, but I got myself to come back the next day and do it again. After 2 weeks, I was walking at a slow pace for 15 minutes—6 days a week. After a month, I was up to 30 minutes a day and started to swing my arms a little. I ventured outside the Y and began to walk around a nearby city lake in the May air, fragrant with crab apple blossoms." She treated herself to a new pair of sweats that fit.

Eighteen months later, Gallivan was walking an hour a day, 6 days a week, arms pumping, hair streaming back, cheeks rosy. She weighed 134 pounds and was eating three healthy meals a day. "I no longer needed antidepressants, and my blood sugar levels were normal," Gallivan says. "Today, my work involves singing and dancing with young children 5 days a week in my own playful music-and-movement classes. Walking is still the best medicine I know—and more delicious than dessert ever was."

can be expensive and, when it comes to the latter, childcare can be an obstacle. Beating the weather takes a little planning, however.

Weatherize your kid. As long as your child is dressed properly, there's no reason she can't be popped in a stroller and join you. The American Academy of Pediatrics says a good rule of thumb is to dress young children in one more layer of clothing than you would wear under the same conditions. For kids (and you), keep in mind that several thin layers (long johns, turtleneck, sweater, and coat) outperform a couple of hefty ones. For the heat, make sure she is well shaded, is wearing sunscreen, and has plenty of fluids handy.

Tune in. Spilner advises using walking videos. She likes Leslie Sansone, a walking guru with dozens of tapes to her credit. Or try *Prevention*'s *Walk Your Way Slim* video (available at CollageVideo.com). Pop in a video or DVD after you get home from work, during the kids' nap time, or while they're watching their favorite show in another room.

Be creative. No matter how you sidestep the weather, add variety to your routine. If you have children, play Twister, bounce on pogo sticks in the garage, or buy a few inexpensive jump ropes or a small indoor trampoline and institute daily recess for you and them. Each week, schedule weather-appropriate activities you can enjoy as a family, such as roller-skating, ice-skating, or a dunk in an indoor pool. Or you could combine culture with fitness by visiting your local museum or library and making the rounds through each floor of the building before you stop to peruse the collection.

Circuit-train. You don't need expensive equipment or a personal trainer to jazz up your workout. Create a minicircuit at home, says Spilner. Set aside 30 minutes or three 10-minute chunks and rotate through a few different activities, such as a walking video, moves with hand weights, a few yoga poses, and abdominal crunches.

STRATEGY #6: PAIN-PROOF YOUR ROUTINE

We all know that walking is the safest, easiest form of exercise there is, so why should you bother reading this section? Because left ignored, an innocent niggle can easily become a chronic problem. In fact, each year, nearly 250,000 hoofers are hobbled, thanks to a walking-induced pain or a nagging old injury that walking has aggravated. As bothersome as the initial problem can be, the real damage is what happens next: You stop exercising, misplace your motivation, and soon gain weight and lose muscle tone. Here's how to make sure you reach your fitness and weight-loss goals.

Tenderness on your heel or anywhere on the bottom of your foot
Possible diagnosis: plantar fasciitis

The plantar fascia is the band of tissue that runs from your heel bone to the ball of your foot. When this dual-purpose shock absorber and arch support is strained, small tears develop, and the tissue stiffens as a protective response. Walkers can overwork the area when pounding the pavement, especially when they wear hard shoes on concrete, because there's very little give as the foot lands. Inflammation can also result from any abrupt change or increase in your normal walking routine. People with high arches or who pronate excessively (walk on the inside of the foot) are particularly susceptible. You know you have plantar fasciitis if you feel pain in your heel or arch first thing in the morning (the fascia stiffens during the night). If left untreated, the problem can lead to a painful, bony growth known as a heel spur.

What you can do about it: At the first sign of stiffness in the bottom of your foot, loosen up the tissue by doing this stretch: Sit with ankle of injured foot across opposite thigh. Pull toes toward shin with hand until you feel a stretch in arch. Run opposite hand along sole of foot; you should feel a taut band of tissue. Do 10 stretches, holding each for 10 seconds. Then stand, and massage your foot by rolling it on a golf ball or full water bottle. To reduce pain, wear supportive shoes or sandals with a contoured foot bed at all times. Choose walking shoes that are not too flexible in the middle.

Soreness or swelling on the sides of your toes
Possible diagnosis: ingrown toenails

Tender tootsies can develop when the corners or sides of your toenails grow sideways rather than forward, putting pressure on surrounding soft tissues. You may be more likely to develop ingrown toenails if your shoes are too short or too tight. If the excess pressure goes on too long, such as on an extended hike or charity walk, bleeding could occur under the nail, and the toenail might eventually fall off.

What you can do about it: Leave wiggle room in your shoes; you may need to go up a half size when you buy sneakers because feet tend to swell during exercise. Use toenail clippers (not fingernail clippers or scissors) to cut straight across instead of rounding the corners.

Pain in the back of your heel and lower calf
Possible diagnosis: Achilles tendinitis

The Achilles tendon, which connects the calf muscle to the heel, can be irritated by walking too much, especially if you don't build up to it. Repeated flexing of the foot when walking up and down steep hills or on uneven terrain can also strain the tendon.

What you can do about it: For mild cases, avoid long uphill walks and reduce your mileage—or substitute non-weight-bearing activities such as swimming or upper-body training, as long as these don't aggravate the pain. In severe cases, limit or stop walking, and place cold packs on the injured area for 15 to 20 minutes, up to three or four times a day. When you return to walking, start with flat surfaces; increase your distance and intensity gradually.

Stiffness or soreness in your shins
Possible diagnosis: shin splints

Your shins have to bear as much as six times your weight while you exercise, so foot-pounding activities can cause problems for the muscles and surrounding tissues. The strain results from strong calves pulling repeatedly on weaker muscles near the shin.

What you can do about it: Cut back on your walking for 3 to 8 weeks to give the tissues time to heal. You might need a cold pack or anti-inflammatory, such as ibuprofen, to reduce swelling and relieve pain. In the meantime, keep in shape by cross-training with low-impact exercises such as swimming or cycling. You should also strengthen the muscles in the front of the lower leg (anterior tibialis) to help prevent a recurrence. Use this simple exercise: While standing, lift toes toward shins 20 times. Work up to three sets; as you get stronger, lay a 2- or 3-pound ankle weight across your toes to add more resistance.

CHAPTER 15

STRENGTH TRAINING IN 10 MINUTES A DAY

Looking for sleeker hips and thighs, a slimmer waist, a firmer "back view"—and lower blood sugar? Think strength training.

Working your muscles—using your own body weight, resistance bands, hand weights, or machines at the gym—won't turn you into Popeye or even a facsimile of Ms. Ironman 2006. This secret weapon in the war against flab boosts metabolism; turns on your muscle cells' fat-burning furnaces; and replaces soft, puffy fat with toned, shapely muscle.

The sugar advantage: In a 6-month study of 36 people ages 60 to 80, Australian researchers found that those who ate a healthy diet and followed a weight-lifting program saw blood sugar fall three times farther than those who simply dieted. (They also lost body fat!) Their 3-day-a-week program was quick and easy: nine exercises that targeted the major muscles in the upper and lower body, with 8 to 10 repetitions of each move. An American study confirmed the sugar advantage: When overweight people with above-normal blood sugar embarked upon a 16-week strength-training program, they ended up with better blood sugar control than nonexercisers.

Resistance training helps cells throughout your body become more sensitive to insulin, the vital hormone that sends blood sugar into cells. But that's not all. Strength training can increase your levels of glut-4, a compound that binds to the cell membrane and then helps move the glucose inside. People with high blood sugar often have suboptimal glut-4 levels (perhaps due to genetics and/or sedentary habits). Working your muscles boosts this important sugar-delivery service.

A bonus: Research also shows that strength training promotes heart health in people with high blood sugar. This is an important benefit because having high blood sugar doubles and can even quadruple your risk of heart disease. You get all this, plus a toned midsection, stronger bones, less cellulite, more energy, and a big confidence boost. (Researchers and personal trainers say that women who strength-train build greater self-esteem—probably the result of looking great and feeling wonderful.)

STRENGTH TRAINING THE *SUGAR SOLUTION* WAY

Our program, created by *Prevention* magazine Fitness Director Michele Stanten, author of *Prevention's Firm Up in 3 Weeks*, is designed to fit into the busiest schedules. This three-part plan includes a 10-minute lower-body workout, a 10-minute "core" workout to strengthen and tone your abdomen and back muscles, and a 10-minute upper-body routine. The goal? Do each segment two or three times a week for maximum results. How you get there is up to you: You can do one 10-minute segment each day, combine two for a 20-minute workout three times a week, or perform the entire 30-minute routine twice a week.

Most of the moves use your own body weight to work your muscles. You will, however, need light- to medium-weight dumbbells for the upper-body exercises. If you've never used dumbbells before, start with very light weights until you're accustomed to the exercises. To find a good starting weight, take this book with you to a fitness store, sporting goods shop, or a discount store with a sporting goods section. Starting with 1-pound dumbbells, "audition" weights by performing one of the upper-body moves described below. If you can easily lift the weight more than 12 times, it's too light. Go a little heavier. A weight is too heavy if you cannot lift it slowly and steadily 8 times—without jerking your body or arm. (If one weight is too light and the next is too heavy, choose the lighter weight for now. You can always get a heavier pair when your muscles are stronger.)

BUILD MUSCLE—AND SO MUCH MORE

The benefits of resistance training go way beyond reshaping your body.

Research conducted by Miriam E. Nelson, Ph.D., director of the Center for Physical Activity and Nutrition at Tufts University's Friedman School of Nutrition Science and Policy in Boston, and her colleagues found that 20 postmenopausal women who began a strength-training program *completely transformed their bodies*—inside and out. After a year of doing a five-exercise strength-training workout twice a week, the women were in the same physical condition as women 15 to 20 years younger. Among the benefits they gained:

Slimmer physiques. The women didn't diet but lost fat and gained muscle—so they looked leaner and dropped up to two dress sizes.

Higher metabolism. Metabolism tends to slow down as you age, making it more difficult to maintain your weight. There are ways to speed it up again like increasing the amount of muscle you have. Muscle tissue burns more calories than fat. One woman in the study gave her metabolism a major boost: She lost 29 pounds of fat and gained enough muscle to burn an extra 160 calories a day.

More energy. As the women became stronger, they felt more energized and began doing things they hadn't done in years—or had never done at all. They went canoeing, river rafting, dancing, biking, and skating. By the end of the study, the women in the strength-training group were 27 percent more active than a year before, while the non-strength training group became 25 percent less active in that year.

Improved mood. Lifting weights can lift your spirits. In another study, strength training was found to be comparable to antidepressant drugs at fighting depression, which affects far more women than men.

Added bone. After menopause, women typically lose 1 percent of their bone mass each year. The strength-training group in Dr. Nelson's study gained 1 percent of bone density, while those who didn't strength-train lost about 2 percent.

Better balance. Our ability to keep our balance deteriorates as we age, making us more likely to have a bad fall. The women in the study who didn't do strength training experienced an 8.5 percent decline in balance, but those who lifted weights improved their balance by 14 percent.

Follow these expert tips for successful strength training.

Work out between meals. Lifting right after a huge meal will make you feel uncomfortable; lifting on an empty stomach may make you light-headed. The optimal time to work out is midway between meals. Or have a light meal or snack an hour or so beforehand.

Warm up. Take 5 to 10 minutes to walk briskly, do jumping jacks, or march or jog in place. If you do an aerobic workout in addition to resistance training, you can do the aerobics first, in place of a warmup.

Tame the tension. When we contract one muscle, we have a tendency to tense the others as well. During strength training, though, only the muscles you're working should contract. Make sure that you're not clenching your teeth, furrowing your brow, or tensing your shoulders up around your ears.

Don't wait to exhale. Strange as it may sound, many weight lifters literally hold their breath, which can cause their blood pressure to spike. Exhale on the exertion—when you lift the weight or do the crunch—and inhale as you lower the weight or return to the starting position.

GEAR UP FOR SUCCESS

For hundreds of dollars less than a 1-year gym membership, you can buy everything you need to start our body-shaping program now. Here's what you'll need.

Dumbbells: Also called free weights, they are available in varying increments from 1 to 20 pounds.

Padding: A foam mat can turn any floor into a home gym. Mats are great for floor stretches, pushups, and crunches.

A good pair of athletic shoes: You need the stability when you're doing the exercises and some protection in case you drop a free weight.

Comfortable, functional clothing: You should wear comfortable clothes made of a breathable fabric like a cotton/synthetic blend. Avoid wearing anything that could impair your range of motion or is so baggy that a weight could become tangled in your clothing.

Take it slow. Fast, herky-jerky movements can cause injury. They can also cause you to use momentum, rather than muscle, to lift the weight. Slow, controlled movements are safer and take more effort, so you get more benefit. Each repetition should take about 6 seconds: 2 seconds to lift the weight, a 2-second pause, and then another 2 seconds to lower the weight.

Perfect your form. Good form—doing an exercise in exactly the right way—helps you get the most benefit from lifting and prevents injury. To watch your lifting form, stand in front of a full-length mirror. Make sure that your wrists are straight, not bent backward or forward, and that you are doing the exercise precisely as it is shown.

Pay attention to posture. Whether you're sitting or standing when you lift dumbbells, keep your back, neck, and head straight to prevent muscle strain and injury. Good posture doesn't mean standing stiffly, so stand tall but relaxed. If you're seated to do the exercise, sit up straight with your feet flat on the floor.

Be kind to your joints. Don't lock your elbows or knees when lifting weights. When you lock a joint, the joint bears the stress of the weight, not the muscle. To prevent joint pain, end the move just short of locking your knees or elbows.

Break between sets. Take a 1- to 2-minute break after you complete each set to give your muscles a chance to recuperate and prepare for the next set. To save time, you can do an exercise that works another muscle group. You might alternate between leg and arm exercises, for example.

Take a day off. Your muscles need at least a day to rest in between resistance-training sessions. It's actually during that time that your muscles get stronger. That's because lifting weights causes tiny tears in the muscle tissue. As your muscles repair that damage, they become stronger. If you choose to do 10 minutes a day, make sure you don't work the same group of muscles two days in a row—for example, if you do the upper body routine on Monday, be sure to do the core and lower-body routines next—on Tuesday and Wednesday—before performing the upper-body moves again. That gives each muscle group some crucial time off.

Finish with flexibility. Stretching after lifting muscles keeps them supple, which helps to prevent injury in the long run.

Work through soreness. You'll probably feel a little sore for the first few weeks of a resistance-training program. Don't increase the

---

SCHEDULE YOUR STRENGTH-TRAINING ROUTINE

Here's how to adapt the program to fit your schedule. (Note: On "off" days you won't strength-train, but you should continue with your walking program or another aerobic activity such as jogging, swimming, water walking, or biking.)

Option 1: 10 Minutes a Day, 6 Days a Week

You'll do each workout twice a week, with 1 day off for complete rest. Sample schedule:

Monday: Upper-body routine
Tuesday: Lower-body routine
Wednesday: Core routine
Thursday: Off
Friday: Upper-body routine
Saturday: Lower-body routine
Sunday: Core routine

Option 2: 20 Minutes a Day, 3 Days a Week

You'll do the entire workout twice a week, in longer sessions that give you 4 days off. Sample schedule:

Monday: Upper- and lower-body routines
Tuesday: Off
Wednesday: Lower-body and core routines
Thursday: Off
Friday: Upper-body and core routines
Saturday and Sunday: Off

Option 3: 30 Minutes a Day, 2 or 3 Days a Week

You'll do the whole workout at each exercise session, but you only have to work out twice a week. Add a third workout for faster results. Sample schedule:

Monday: Off
Tuesday: Upper-body, lower-body, and core routines
Wednesday: Off
Thursday: Upper-body, lower-body, and core routines
Friday: Off
Saturday: Upper-body, lower-body, and core routines
Sunday: Off

amount of weight you're lifting until the soreness subsides, and even then, add no more than a pound at a time. If the soreness is so bad that even everyday movement is painful, give yourself a few days of rest, then try again with less weight.

Pay attention to pain. Pain may be a sign that a muscle, tendon, or joint has been overworked or strained. If something doesn't feel right, stop. Rest a few days before trying your routine again. If pain persists, see your doctor.

THE MOVES

You'll repeat each exercise 8 to 12 times, rest for up to 1 minute, then repeat it another 8 to 12 times before moving on to the next. Or, you can do one set of 8 to 12 repetitions for each exercise, then repeat the entire sequence. Start with 8 repetitions in each set. When you can easily do 12, you can add a little more weight.

Lower Body
HALF SQUAT

1. Stand with your feet shoulder-width apart and your arms at your sides. Shift your weight onto your heels.

2. Keeping your abs tight and back straight, bend at your hips and knees and lower your buttocks about 6 inches, as if you're sitting into a chair. At the same time, raise your arms in front of you to help with balance. Hold for a second, then stand.

Where to feel it: Front and back of thighs; buttocks

Technique: When you look down, you should always be able to see your toes. If you can't, then stick your buttocks out and sit back more so your toes stay behind your knees. You can also turn your toes out slightly to improve your form.

Play it safe: If you feel any stress to the knees, make sure you're sitting back over your heels and not allowing your knees to go beyond your toes. If you have knee problems, check with your doctor before doing this exercise.

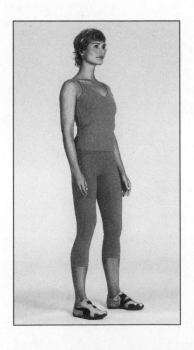 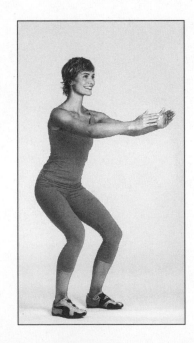

STATIONARY LUNGE

1. Stand with your right foot 2 to 3 feet in front of your left foot, arms at your sides. Shift most of your weight onto your right foot and lift your left heel off the floor.

2. Bend your knees and lower your body until your right thigh is parallel to the floor.

Where to feel it: Front and back of thighs; buttocks

Technique: When you look down, you should always be able to see your toes. If you can't, then you're leaning either forward or back as you lower. Make sure you keep your front knee directly over your ankle and lower straight down.

Play it safe: If you have knee problems, check with your doctor before doing this exercise.

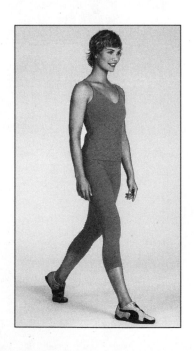 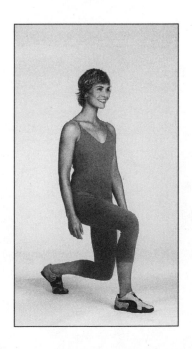

STEP UP

1. Stand in front of an exercise step or staircase, with your arms at your sides. Raise your left leg and place your foot on top of the step. (If you're using a staircase, place your foot on the first step.)

2. Shift your weight onto your left foot and press into the step, lifting yourself up onto the step. Tap your right foot on the step, then lower to the start position.

Where to feel it: Front and back of thighs; buttocks

Technique: Make sure your entire foot is on the step, and don't lean too far forward as you come up.

Play it safe: Keep your back straight as you step up and down, so that your legs do all the work.

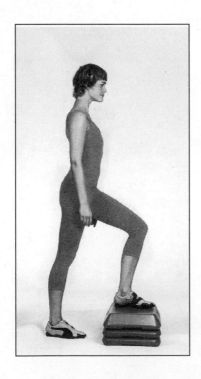 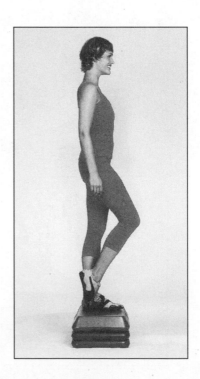

Upper Body
CHEST PRESS

1. Hold a dumbbell in each hand and lie faceup on the floor, with your legs bent and your feet flat on the floor. Position the dumbbells just above your chest, with your elbows pointing out.

2. Press the dumbbells straight up over your chest. Don't lock your elbows. Hold for a second, and then slowly lower

Where to feel it: Chest, back of upper arms, shoulders

Technique: If you feel any strain in your shoulders, rotate your arms so that your palms face in, the dumbbells are parallel to each other, and your elbows point toward your feet.

Mix it up: If you don't have a workout bench, try lying on a step bench designed for step aerobics.

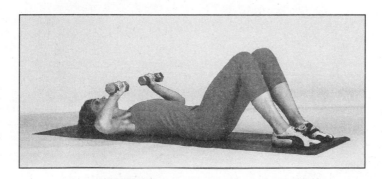

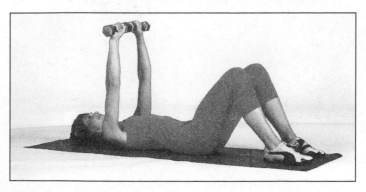

BENT-OVER ROW

1. Hold a dumbbell in your right hand and stand behind a chair, with your left foot about 12 inches in front of your right foot. Place your left hand on top of the chair and lean forward from your hips so that your right arm hangs directly beneath your right shoulder.

2. Keeping your abs tight, bend your right elbow and pull the dumbbell up toward your chest. Hold for a second, then lower.

Where to feel it: Midback, shoulder, upper arm

Technique: Keep the dumbbell close to your body and your elbow in, not pointed out to the side.

Play it safe: Practice this one first without weights to develop proper positioning.

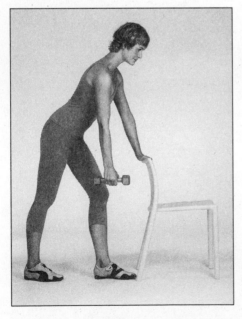
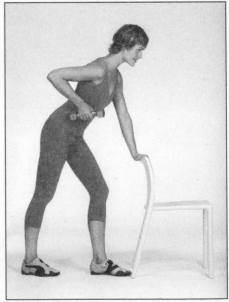

OVERHEAD PRESS

1. Hold a dumbbell in each hand and sit in a chair, with your feet about hip-width apart. Bend your arms out to the sides so that they form 90-degree angles.

2. Press the dumbbells straight up overhead. Don't lock your elbows. Hold for a second, then slowly lower.

Where to feel it: Shoulders, back of upper arms

Technique: If you feel any strain in your shoulders, rotate your arms so that your palms face in, the dumbbells are parallel to each other, and your elbows point forward.

Mix it up: Try changing the move slightly by starting with your palms and forearms facing in toward your chest rather than facing front. As you raise the dumbbells, rotate your forearms and palms so they face front when your arms are extended. Rotate and lower your arms back to the starting position.

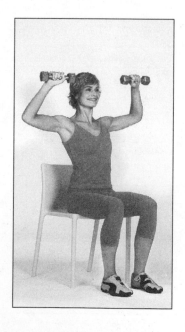 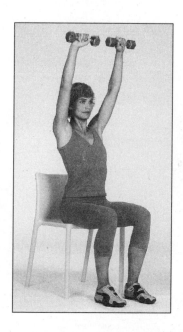

Core
CRUNCH

1. Lie faceup with your legs bent, your feet flat on the floor, and your hands behind your head.

2. Pull your abs in and slowly curl your head and shoulders off the floor. Hold for a second, then slowly lower.

Where to feel it: Front abdominals

Technique: Exhale as you lift, and imagine your rib cage sliding toward your pelvis. Inhale as you lower. Don't pull on your neck; you should always be able to put a fist between your chin and chest. Don't keep your eyes on the ceiling as you lift; as you curl up, your eyes should follow your head so at the top of the curl you're looking at your knees.

Mix it up: For a more advanced workout, try a reverse crunch. Lift your lower body toward your chest while keeping your head and shoulders on the floor. Your legs should be bent slightly at the knees, and your feet should be crossed at the ankles.

Play it safe: If you have lower-back pain, try the crunch with your feet and lower legs resting on a chair.

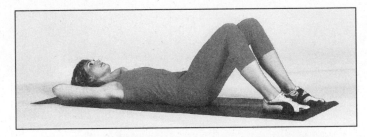

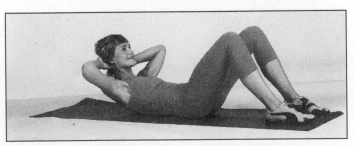

TWISTING CRUNCH

1. Lie faceup with your legs bent and your feet flat on the floor. Place your left hand behind your head and extend your right arm out to the side on the floor.

2. Pull your abs in and slowly curl your head and shoulders off the floor. As you come up, twist your torso to the right, aiming your left shoulder toward your right knee. Hold for a second, then slowly lower.

Where to feel it: Front and side abdominals

Technique: Don't pull your elbow across your body.

Play it safe: To avoid neck pain when performing crunches, place your hands on the sides of your head, or rest your fingers lightly at the back of your head and press your head lightly against them.

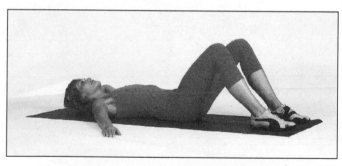

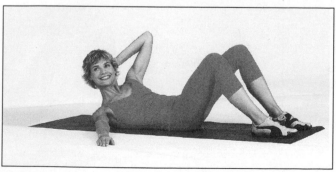

OPPOSITE ARM AND LEG LIFT

1. Kneel with your hands on the floor. Your knees should be directly beneath your hips, and your hands beneath your shoulders. Keep your abs tight and your back, head, and neck in line.

2. Simultaneously raise your left arm and right leg so that they are in line with your back. Hold for a second, then slowly lower.

Where to feel it: Back, buttocks, shoulders

Technique: Don't let your belly drop toward the floor and your back arch.

Play it safe: If you feel pain in your lower back while performing this exercise or after you've finished, talk with your doctor.

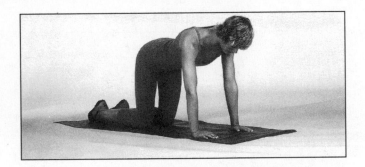

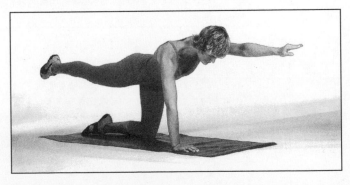

FINISH WITH A STRETCH

Follow your workout with these stretches to increase your flexibility.

LYING QUADRICEPS STRETCH ▥

Body zones stretched: Front of thighs, front of hips

Master the move: Lie on your side with your legs straight and together, one on top of the other. Support your head with the hand closest to the floor by resting your upper arm on the floor and bending it at the elbow. Bend your lower leg slightly if you need to for balance.

Bend the knee of the top leg so that your foot comes back toward your buttocks. Grasp your foot with your free hand and pull the heel in toward your buttocks until you feel a comfortable stretch in the front of your thigh. Hold it there for 20 to 30 seconds, then slowly release. Roll onto your other side and stretch the opposite leg.

STANDING HAMSTRING STRETCH▪

Body zones stretched: Back of thighs, inner thighs, buttocks

Master the move: Stand with your feet together and your arms at your sides. Take a very large step forward with your right leg. Keep your right foot pointing straight ahead and turn your back leg slightly so that your left foot points a bit to the left.

Bend the knee of your back leg, place your hands on the upper thigh of your front leg, and slowly lean forward with your torso as far as you comfortably can. Keep your back, neck, and head in a straight line. Bend your back leg farther while pushing your hips and buttocks down and back. Lift the front of your right foot off the floor while maintaining pressure on your front heel.

You should feel a comfortable stretch in your back and in the inner thigh of your outstretched leg. Hold for 20 to 30 seconds, then stretch the other thigh.

SHOULDER STRETCH

Body zones stretched: Chest, shoulders, arms

Master the move: Stand with your feet shoulder-width apart and your arms down at your sides. Extend your arms straight behind your body, stretching them back and upward as far as you comfortably can. If your hands reach far enough, clasp them together. Hold for 20 to 30 seconds.

SIDE BEND

Body zones stretched: Mid- and lower back, side abdominals

Master the move: Begin by standing with your feet shoulder-width apart and your hands on your hips. Without leaning forward, bend at the waist toward the hand on your left hip while slowly reaching over your head with your right hand as far as you comfortably can. Hold for 20 to 30 seconds, then stretch the other side.

BOWING SHOULDER STRETCH

Body zones stretched: Mid- and lower back, shoulders, arms

Master the move: Get down on all fours on an exercise mat, with your hands and knees about shoulder-width apart. Keep your back flat, your neck straight, and your eyes looking down at the floor. Sit back on your heels, extending your arms in front of you. Push down slightly with your palms and hold for 20 to 30 seconds.

5

SOOTHE STRESS, CONTROL BLOOD SUGAR

CHAPTER 16

THE HEALING POWER OF *AHHH*

Laugh. Love. Dance. Unwind with a long, slow yoga stretch. Calm your thoughts and come into the present moment with a mindfulness exercise. Or, simply lose yourself in the rhythmic clickety-click of your knitting needles as you create a sweater from silky, gorgeously colored yarn.

There are a thousand paths to relaxation and joy. And now, hundreds of medical studies prove that getting to *ahhh* isn't just an earthy-crunchy pastime. Cutting stress and boosting pleasure can reduce your blood sugar, make weight loss easier, and lower your risk for a long list of serious health concerns, including prediabetic blood sugar problems and diabetes itself. The mind-body link: Researchers know that when we *aren't* relaxed and happy—thanks to an overwhelming job, marital discord, financial worries, the demands of being a caregiver, or trepidation about the state of the world (or where your teenager is)—levels of the stress hormone cortisol rise. And so does your blood sugar.

Your body was designed for short bursts of stress—long enough to escape a marauding cougar, for example. Today, we've made tension and anxiety a 24-7 state of being—the new normal. We don't give our minds, bodies, or spirits space and time to recharge. "We need to step off the wheel," says Wayne Muller, an ordained minister and psychotherapist in Mill Valley, California, and author of *Sabbath: Restoring the*

Sacred Rhythm of Rest. "Life works in rhythm—the seas, the tides, the body, everything. If we're only on one track—producing and working, without time for reflection and regathering—we're doing harm."

It's time to step away from stress and move toward happiness. We're here to help.

THE *SUGAR SOLUTION* STRESS-BUSTING PROGRAM

We were so impressed by the growing body of research linking stress to weight gain, difficulty losing weight, and weight *regain*—as well as to high blood sugar and all of its related health problems—that we've made taming tension a key element of the *Sugar Solution* plan. De-stressing cannot take the place of a healthy diet or regular physical activity; it *can* help you stick with the other elements of your program, achieve better results more swiftly, feel great right away, and ensure that you've done all you can to sidestep blood sugar problems. Our smart, stress-stopping solutions:

- Develop resilience so that you can rise above daily stresses.
- Claim 15 minutes of "me time" a day for relaxation.
- Pursue and enjoy pleasure, in all its shapes and forms, every day.
- Get plenty of deep, refreshing sleep.

The Blood Sugar Benefit

Plenty of research shows that stress of all varieties can raise blood sugar by boosting levels of hormones that trigger the release of extra glucose from your liver. We looked harder, and found that the reverse is true, too: Cutting stress and building joy can lower blood sugar and shield you from the stress-disease-overweight cycle. Lower your stress, boost your happiness quotient, and your blood sugar will benefit.

In an encouraging study conducted at Duke University, 108 women and men with high blood sugar took five diabetes-education classes either with or without stress management training. After a year, more than half of the stress-relief group improved their blood sugar levels enough to lower their risk for the worst complications, such as heart disease, kidney failure, nerve damage, and vision problems. Study participants soothed their stress with a variety of techniques: progressive muscle relaxation, deep breathing, and positive mental imagery, as well as by stopping high-tension thoughts. (You can buy a compact disc and manual of the relaxation-training program used in the study at www. richardsurwit.com.)

Happiness counts, too, as researchers from England's University College London discovered when they tested the moods, saliva, and blood of 200 middle-aged Londoners. The result: Cortisol levels were 32 percent lower in the happiest people than in the most unhappy folks. "Cortisol is a key stress hormone related to a range of pathologies including abdominal obesity, type 2 diabetes, hypertension, and autoimmune conditions," says lead study author and psychologist Andrew Steptoe, MD. "The average difference in cortisol between the lowest and highest happiness quintiles is substantial and might contribute to health risk if it persists over months or years." Unhappy people also had levels of fibrinogen—a compound linked with clogged arteries and heart-threatening blood clots—12 times higher than the happiest people.

The Weight-Loss Bonus

Two-thirds of Americans are overweight, and chronic stress is part of the cause. Elevated levels of cortisol have been linked to increases in body fat and a decreased ability to sleep, so the body has less energy to exercise and craves more quick-fix snacks. Research has shown that big-league stressors—like a lousy marriage or messy divorce—compound weight issues, regardless of what you eat and how much you exercise.

Lowering stress can allow you to slip an ancient weight trap, say University of California, San Francisco, researchers who've found that tension compels mammals to eat sugary, fatty, high-calorie foods. In prehistoric times, anxious eating may have been a smart survival strategy. Your agitated ancestors grabbed berries after the tigers slunk away; you head for the candy machine after the boss roars. "You need to refuel for the next crisis," explains study coauthor Norman Pecoraro, PhD. Researchers found that stress prompts rats to release hormone signals for high-calorie eating. The eat-eat-eat signal stopped only when the rats had stored the extra calories as tummy fat. Pecoraro says it's a surprisingly similar scenario in humans.

Cutting stress can also help prevent dreaded weight regain. In a recent study, psychologists checked up on the moods, stress, and eating habits of 69 women who had just dropped pounds. Women who felt most stressed were most likely to have regained their weight within 18 months. "Incorporating stress- and mood-management techniques into weight-loss programs may help prevent or delay weight regain that occurs as a result of poor coping and/or increased high-risk or unhealthy behaviors," says researcher Paula Rhode, PhD, a psychologist in the University of Kansas School of Medicine's preventive medicine program.

LET GO, BE RESILIENT

Step 1 of our stress-busting plan: Cultivate the ability to bounce back—by calling on hope.

The key to practicing safe stress is to acknowledge that stress is part of daily living. Accept this, then develop healthy ways of coping. A stress-free existence is an unrealistic expectation fraught with frustration. Instead, aim for a stress-resilient lifestyle that allows you to bounce along with life's events, constantly adapting and adjusting.

Feel like your life is taking on a hectic pace? Think of stress as a flashlight. When you need your flashlight, you turn it on. When you're finished, you turn it off—or risk burning out the battery. The same is true for stress and your body. A little is good, but it's unhealthy, even lethal, to keep your stress levels elevated over time. When you feel helpless and defeated, your stress hormone levels skyrocket and stay there. As a result, you may neglect or even abuse your mind and body. That's unsafe stress.

Your weapon for controlling stress? Hope. The ultimate antidote to stress, it sends tension and anxiety plummeting. Where does hope come from? Most of the time, you must create it. If you're in the midst of a financial crisis, for example, it's easy to feel hopeless. But stress needn't overwhelm you. Instead, roll up your sleeves and dig in. Search for solutions to the problem. Devise a plan to save money, sell unwanted items, and create a schedule to pay off the debt. Your fear will begin to melt away. The end result: hope. Here's how to keep hope in your life.

Stay in the game. When a stressor hits, avoid the natural tendency to run away or feel defeated. See stresses as constant daily challenges in life. Embrace the challenges, and use whatever resources you have for support as you try to cope. Be patient with the process. Sometimes hope is hidden, waiting for you to discover it.

Open your mind, and know your options. You wanted to buy that house, but someone outbid you. Now you're disappointed and stressed. Try to remember that in the midst of difficulty lies opportunity. Take a moment to experience the more negative feelings. Then let them go, and move on. Another house may have just hit the market in a better location at the right price.

Explore ways to keep yourself excited and hopeful. How do you like to spend your time? What are your passions and dreams? If you are constantly stressed by a boring, dead-end job, create hope by taking classes in a field that excites and challenges you. If you're in a destructive relationship, you need to summon the courage to fight for yourself by calling it quits and moving on.

CLAIM 15 MINUTES A DAY FOR RELAXATION

There's stress we can control—and then there's everything else, from the weather to your morning commute, from your boss's mood to how your kid did in school today. Learning a proven stress-reduction technique—

GOT 5 MINUTES? YOU CAN RELAX

For a quick trip to calm, try this simple deep-breathing exercise.

1. Lie down, or sit in a chair.

2. Rest your hands on your stomach.

3. Slowly count to four and inhale through your nose. Feel your stomach rise. Hold it for a second.

4. Slowly count to four while you exhale through your mouth. To control how fast you exhale, purse your lips like you're going to whistle. Your stomach will slowly fall.

5. Repeat 5 to 10 times.

and practicing it for 15 minutes (or more) each day—means you're ready to cope with nearly anything life throws at you. We recommend these.

Mindfulness-Based Stress Reduction

Skip the mountaintop ashram, the guru with the scraggily facial hair, and the mystical mantras. Mounting evidence reveals that a thoroughly modern form of meditation called mindfulness-based stress reduction (MBSR) can make you happier *and* healthier.

Mindfulness—a buzzword among mind-body researchers—is all about simply paying attention to experience as it unfolds, without getting sidetracked by memories from the past, plans for dinner, or opinions about what's going on around you. The result: awareness, insight, and relaxation. Simple? Maybe. Profound? Without a doubt.

"As baseball's Yogi Berra once said, `You can see a lot just by lookin'.' If you pay close attention to your life as you live it, you notice all sorts of things. This leads to new insights and the ability to make changes," says Saki Santorelli, EdD, director of the Center for Mindfulness at the University of Massachusetts Medical School, in Worcester. "You may notice mental and physical habits that aren't really helping you anymore. You may also notice early signs of a migraine sooner or the conditions that set you up for a sleepless night or indigestion. And you can then do something about it."

But MBSR also does more, by putting the brakes on chronic stress and stopping the cascade of hormones that seem to make coping with—and treating—a wide range of medical conditions more difficult. At a National Institutes of Health conference on mindfulness and medicine in Bethesda, Marlyand, top researchers revealed the latest findings suggesting that adding MBSR to treatments can help people live better with everything from cancer to chronic pain to psoriasis.

"For a very long time in medicine, the mind was separated from the body by an artificial wall," says Dr. Santorelli, whose center has championed MBSR for more than 20 years. "Science is beginning to recognize that psychological and emotional well-being is linked with illness."

While MBSR is not a replacement for medical treatments, it's an effective add-on therapy. The procedure usually involves a series of exercises designed to help you focus on your experience in the present moment—breathing exercises, body scans to reduce physical stress, and a few yoga moves.

You don't have to travel to a special meditation center deep in the woods or to a faraway land to learn this simple, inexpensive technique. Hundreds of hospitals across the US offer classes to the public, as do psychologists and social workers trained in this easy technique. To find one nearby, type your zip code into the locater service at the University of Massachusetts Medical School's Center for Mindfulness Web site: http://www.umassmed.edu/cfm/mbsr/.

Or teach yourself with books developed by the center's directors. We recommend *Heal Thy Self: Lessons on Mindfulness in Medicine*, by Saki Santorelli, EdD, and *Full Catastrophe Living: Using the Wisdom of Your Body and Mind to Face Stress, Pain, and Illness*, by Jon Kabat-Zinn, PhD. Guided meditation tapes, including special tapes for people with psoriasis and with cancer, are available through the center's Web site at http://www.umassmed.edu/cfm/tapes/index.aspx.

"A class is great—you're in an environment with lots of energy and optimism and support," Santorelli says. "But if you can't do that, a book and tapes is a good way to begin. After all, there is an element to mindfulness that's solitary."

Yoga

Fast-paced, hot, and sweaty yoga can burn loads of calories, but gentler styles may do even more for your waistline (and won't hurt!). How? Yoga works on an emotional level to make losing weight easier. A survey that tracked weight gain in 15,500 adults from ages 45 to 55 revealed that the normal-weight people who practiced yoga at least 30 minutes a week for 4 of those years gained 3 fewer pounds (9.5 versus 12.6) than those who didn't. Even better, overweight yogis lost 5 pounds over the decade, while their non-yoga-practicing peers gained an additional 14.

"Yoga may not be a big calorie burner, but it helps you become more aware of your body, so you're more sensitive to feeling full from overeating," says lead researcher and yoga practitioner Alan R. Kristal, DrPH, of the Fred Hutchinson Cancer Research Center in Seattle. "Yoga also relieves stress, so you may be less likely to mindlessly stuff yourself." Taking a single yoga class can help you lower levels of cortisol.

Researchers at Jefferson Medical College took blood samples from 16 healthy yoga novices during a week when they took a daily 50-minute traditional class. The results: Cortisol levels dropped immediately—as soon as the first day. "This is very significant, because there's a vast amount of literature on how stress increases cortisol levels, but little is known about how to bring them down," says neuroscientist George Brainard, PhD, associate academic director of the school's Center for Integrative Medicine.

Yoga even rivals strength training. In one of the few studies that have compared these radically different exercise regimens, University of Pittsburgh researchers put 59 obese, inactive women, ages 25 to 55, on a low-fat diet. Everyone walked for 40 minutes 5 days a week, a third of the volunteers did additional strength-training exercises, and another third added a yoga routine 3 days a week. After 4 months, the yoga devotees dropped an average of 27 pounds, the strength trainers whittled away 23, and the walking-only group lost 20.

Another health benefit: lower blood sugar. When researchers at the Central Research Institute for Yoga, in Delhi, India, studied 149 people with diabetes, they found that practicing yoga every day for 40 days reduced blood sugar for 70 percent of the participants.

"Yoga is meant to be a nurturing form of exercise, not a rigid imitation of poses," says Richard Faulds, author of *Kripalu Yoga: A Guide to Practice On and Off the Mat*. "It's very possible to stretch and strengthen your body without having to touch your nose to your knees or your feet to your head." Here are some important issues for beginning yogis to consider.

Style guide: Look for gentle styles such as Kripalu, Viniyoga, or Integral Yoga. Bikram, Ashtanga, and Power Yoga are generally too vigorous for beginners and inflexible people.

Teacher training: Find an experienced, certified yoga instructor who asks about your physical limitations and will modify the pace or offer alternative poses to meet your needs. To find a certified instructor in your area, go to the Yoga Alliance Web site, or call them toll-free at (877) 964-2255 (from the US) or (610) 777-7793 (from Canada).

Sequence: Ten minutes of easy movements will increase circulation, lubricate joints, and ready your body to stretch. Poses should progress from simple to more difficult.

Postures: These poses can place tremendous strain on joints and disks: the plow, full shoulder stand, headstand, and full lotus. Beware!

Back protection: Keep knees slightly bent, and hinge from the hips when bending forward from standing positions. When arching backward in any pose, concentrate on opening the front of the body by lengthening from the navel to the sternum. Don't overarch the lower back, which compresses lumbar disks.

Knee savers: Don't lock your knees in standing postures, despite what a teacher may say. If you feel any strain during sitting or kneeling postures, place a cushion or folded blanket under your bottom.

Neck care: Always keep your neck in alignment with the rest of your spine when arching backward. Don't let it flop back or down.

Your limits: Get to know your body and its injury-prone zones. Back off from any movement that causes pain or cramping. Don't compare yourself with others.

Hands on—or off: Many teachers assist students during classes. In general, a light touch that brings your awareness to an area and allows you to make your own adjustments is safest. Teachers who adjust you by moving your body for you or forcing you into a posture may cause injuries. Just say no!

TAKE UP—OR REDISCOVER—A SOOTHING HOBBY

Creative, absorbing, meditative hobbies—anything that gets you into that timeless sense of "flow"—may banish stress as effectively as yoga, meditation, or staring at the kids' goldfish tank. That could be knitting, sewing, woodworking, gardening, perhaps even playing an instrument.

In a study that thrilled home stitchers coast-to-coast, a New York University psychiatrist measured signs of stress in 30 women before and after they sewed—and before and after they played cards, painted, read a newspaper, or played a handheld video game. Sewing lowered

(continued on page 198)

THE PLEASURE PRINCIPLE

Whatever it is that puts a curl in your toes or simply takes you outside the same old, same old for a few minutes, it's a good bet that you don't indulge in it often enough. If life is indeed a banquet, we have to start bellying up to the table, because pleasure keeps us healthy, both emotionally and physically.

The more we seek pleasure, the less irritable and uptight we are, says Stella Resnick, PhD, a psychologist in Los Angeles and author of *The Pleasure Zone: Why We Resist Good Feelings and How to Let Go and Be Happy*. "Our bodies become more relaxed. We breathe easier. Our blood flows freely. And we're less susceptible to illness," she says.

The good news is, with a little creativity, we can return to that guilt-free, cartwheeling sense of fun, play, and enjoyment we had as children—while still accomplishing all that our frantic work and home obligations demand. The tips below can help you reconnect with your inner kindergartener—and grant yourself permission to enjoy your own life.

Laugh long and loud. Japanese researchers have found that people with diabetes who watched a comedy show had a smaller rise in postmeal blood sugar than when they listened to a nonhumorous lecture. The effect occurred in people without diabetes as well.

Date your spouse. Forget the bills, the chores, the home renovation plans, and the kids' orthodontia. Rediscover the passion and thrills that brought you together in the first place. Shared pleasure enhances the sense of being a happy couple. Time spent with your partner that doesn't involve the kids, errands, bills, or dishes fosters a closer bond. The added bonus of intimacy: "With more relaxed enjoyment in your life, there will be more hugging, kissing, smiles of appreciation, and better sex, all of which help us chill out and de-stress," says Susan Heitler, PhD, a clinical psychologist in Denver and author of *The Power of Two: Secrets to a Strong and Loving Marriage*.

Take a mental health break—at a spa. One of the fastest-growing segments of the beauty industry is the day spa, with facials, massages, and other forms of pampering becoming a regular part of the routines at many beauty salons.

Get a long massage. Yield to your

need to be kneaded. It feels amazing. And although you may not care while in the midst of having your feet rubbed, research suggests that massage strengthens immunity by helping your body produce more disease-fighting white blood cells, lower blood pressure, reduce stress hormone levels, and improve your mood.

Try aromatherapy. Sweeten the atmosphere in your home and office with fresh flowers; gorgeous green plants; potpourri; and aromatherapy sprays, candles, or oils. There's some science behind the scents: In a study published in the *International Journal of Cosmetic Science*, researchers at the industry trade group International Flavors and Fragrances reported that the majority of the 100 women who took scented baths felt more relaxed than those who took unscented ones. Scientists looked at electronic images of the trapezius muscles (the ones in your upper back that turn to stone when you're stuck in traffic) to measure tension levels. Another recent study found that the citrus smell of clementines made people feel happiest; vanilla made them feel most relaxed.

"Collect" positive emotional moments. Make it a point to recall times when you experienced pleasure, comfort, tenderness, confidence, or other positive emotions.

Get a puppy. Research points to happiness as one of the top three benefits of owning a dog. (Companionship and protection are the other two.) One reason for this could be the play factor: Adult dog owners spend 44 percent of their time playing with their pooches. Those who are age 65 and older take twice as many walks as people in the same age group who don't have dogs. They're also significantly more satisfied with their social lives and physical and emotional health than their dogless peers. "Pet people describe themselves with more positive adjectives than nonpet owners," says Lynette Hart, director of the Center for Animal Alternatives at the University of California in Davis.

But then, it's easy to feel good about yourself when you're around someone who shows love so easily and doesn't care about your social status, dress size, or bank account.

heart rates by 7 to 11 beats per minute, while the other pastimes raised heartbeats by about 4 to 8 beats per minute, reports study author Robert H. Reiner, PhD. "The importance of a hobby or creative pursuit cannot be overemphasized," he says. "If we don't allow our bodies to rest from the pressures of everyday life, we are placing ourselves at risk for heart disease or other illnesses. Creative activities and hobbies—like sewing—can help a person focus on something productive and get away from worries for a while."

Women seem to be getting the message. According to the Craft Yarn Council of America, 36 percent of American women—53 million—know how to knit or crochet, a 51 percent increase over the past 10 years. The most-cited motivation? Relaxation and stress relief.

Why meditative, repetitive hobbies seem to bust stress best: "The body has an inbuilt relaxation response. When you bring about this response, you are essentially blocking the stress hormones adrenalin and noradrenalin. Slower brain waves also occur. It's fairly straightforward. When you do something meditative like knitting, you decrease metabolism, heart rate, blood pressure, and the rate of breath," notes Herbert Benson, MD, a professor at Harvard Medical School and the author of *The Relaxation Response*. "The repetitive practice breaks the train of everyday thought and allows the body to remember a quiet state. And this has been proven over and over."

Handwork isn't just a solitary meditative experience. Many knitters have discovered the joy and stress-busting benefits of informal knitting circles—and hip new knit cafés where you can knit, purl, sip cappuccino, and chat. "You let your hair down, and people start to open up," one knitter at a Manhattan knit café called Knit New York told *US News and World Report*. "And let's face it, we all need a little group therapy."

CHAPTER 17

BEYOND BUBBLE BATHS: TENSION TAMERS THAT WORK

Got stress? Of course you do. And even if you were one of the few American women who don't occasionally feel like ripping their hair out, you'd probably be ashamed to admit it. Like it or not, stress has become a status symbol, the badge a woman wears to prove she has a full, active life. But too easily, stress can overwhelm. In a recent survey of 1,000 harried Americans by the National Consumers League, over half said their stress was higher than they'd like it to be. Top causes:

1. Work: Forty-one percent said they're really burned out on the job.
2. Not enough time: Twenty-five percent said they can barely juggle their commitments at home, at the office, and in their communities.

Meanwhile, other studies shed light on more of the big stresses facing Americans.

We're rushing 24-7. A poll of 1,000 Americans by Princeton's Opinion Research Corporation International found that 56 percent had trouble managing the time demands involved in balancing work and private life.

We're taking care of ill partners, spouses, and other relatives. A survey of 1,247 women and men by the National Alliance for Caregiving and the American Association for Retired Persons estimated that 44.4 million of us are unpaid caregivers—and more than half hold down jobs while taking care of a sick relative.

Our marriages could be better . . . if we just had the time. A series of landmark University of Minnesota studies of more than 15,000 couples finds that 65 percent are unhappy—wrung out by conflict and disappointment. (And even among the contented 35 percent, one in four wives said she contemplated divorce at one point or another.) We're caught in a bind: We want better marriages, yet most American couples spend barely 4 minutes a day really talking together about things other

UNDER STRESS, DO YOU STARVE OR STUFF?

Why do some women lose their appetites when they're upset, while others turn to food?

Most people initially stop eating during severe stress, due to an appetite-suppressing action upon the release of the first stress hormone, corticoid-releasing factor (CRF), says Elissa Epel, PhD, assistant professor of psychiatry at the University of California, San Francisco. If the story ended there, we would all just avoid food during times of stress, yet stress eating is a tremendous problem for many people. Stress eating as a coping method to reduce negative emotions is a strong conditioned behavior and may override any

hormonal effects, leading to excess calorie intake and weight gain.

What's more, stress hormones may vary among individuals, which explains why some are stress undereaters and others are stress overeaters, says Pamela M. Peeke, MD, assistant clinical professor of medicine at the University of Maryland School of Medicine, Baltimore. And according to one theory, women who produce more of the appetite-boosting stress hormone cortisol may tend to eat more under stress, possibly because they are producing more appetite-stimulating cortisol relative to appetite-suppressing CRF.

than the kids, the chores, the mortgage, and who's taking out the trash.

In this chapter, we've got the nitty-gritty, practical advice that can help you cut the stress and find solutions for some of life's most common stresses.

MAKE HOME AN OASIS OF CALM

Forgotten lunch bags, burned breakfasts, errant keys—weekday mornings can make you feel like Lucy Ricardo in the candy factory. Preparing your family and yourself to meet the day will never be effortless, but keeping your own needs in mind will make it less stressful. These strategies can help.

Greet the day with exercise. It burns up the toxins of the stress response, boosts feel-good endorphins, and lowers cortisol, which makes it an excellent stress reliever. Morning exercisers are more likely to stick to a regular routine; the stress of the coming day can't interfere, and accomplishing a major goal before hitting the shower helps you feel in control all day. Get up 20 minutes earlier to walk the dog at sunrise, or do some yoga in the backyard. (Go on, let the neighbors gawk.)

WRITE OFF YOUR STRESS

Keeping a journal, even sporadically, is an effective way to cope with the storm of stress in our lives. In one study conducted on college students, journaling just 20 minutes once a week improved their moods and overall health—in just 3 weeks. Try to set aside 3 or 4 days and write for about 20 minutes. You don't need to write regularly. Just do it as you need it.

While your first entry may leave your emotions topsy-turvy, those feelings will pass, says James W. Pennebaker, PhD, professor in the department of psychology at the University of Texas at Austin and author of *Opening Up: The Healing Power of Expressing Emotions*. "The more you write, the less impact an event has," he says.

Working up a sweat can be particularly helpful if you're a chronic worrier who frets about everything. In a study of 118 college students, researchers from California State University, in Chico, found that chronic worriers who exercised long enough to get their heart rates pumping and break a sweat during stressful final exam weeks felt better and had fewer depressive symptoms than those who didn't exercise.

This research suggests that exercise can provide special benefits to people prone to chronic worrying, especially when they're under stress, says lead researcher Warren R. Coleman, PhD: "We're not sure why it works, but it's definitely worth trying."

Make breakfast a breeze. For breakfasts on the run, buy a week's worth of single-serving yogurt, cottage cheese, applesauce, baby carrots, raisins, and nuts. Prebag portions of high-fiber cereal. Hard-cook a dozen eggs on Sunday and store them in the fridge, then dump a peeled egg and a pinch of salt in a resealable bag.

CALM YOUR DAILY COMMUTE

Daily traffic jams—second only to teenagers in the category of "things I'll never be able to control"—can frustrate even the most intrepid driver. When your commute starts to take its toll, try these mobile attitude adjusters.

Prepare for your entrance. Time your average trip, then allow 5 minutes extra. When you get to work, park in a low-profile spot and spend 5 minutes meditating before you charge inside to your office. Meditating every day may even contribute directly to weight loss. In a preliminary pilot study, Elissa Epel, PhD, assistant professor of psychiatry at the University of California, San Francisco, found that after 3 months, men who had meditated lost more belly fat than those who hadn't. Most likely, women benefit in the same way.

Reclaim your time. Make a long commute more enjoyable by filling your car with birdsongs, classical music, or mariachi. Listen to books on tape from your local library, or start a lending pool with your fellow commuters. Don't subject yourself to the morning shock jock unless you're absolutely addicted.

Listen to yourself. Stress often begins with unconscious beliefs such as "I'm letting everyone down." Start changing that inner nag by making a cassette of five positive affirmations in your own voice. Ann R. Peden, DSc, a psychiatric nurse, professor at the College of Nursing at the University of Kentucky in Lexington, and lead researcher for a study of affirmations for the National Institute of Nursing Research at the National Institutes of Health, suggests starting with your negative message and reversing it. For example, "I can't keep up" becomes "I am calm and in control." Say each affirmation three times, and listen to your tape twice a day. Dr. Peden's research shows that practiced regularly, affirmations strike a major blow at negative thinking.

HOUSE AND HOME: DON'T SUCCUMB TO "MARTHA-ISM"

The fantasy: This year, for sure, you'll do that cute Christmas wreath you saw in that fancy home magazine—the one where you hand-gild each tiny, perfect holly leaf. The reality: Your laundry hamper is overflowing. Just accept that your home probably won't ever look Martha Stewart perfect—and try these tips to keep on top of the chaos.

Delegate, delegate, delegate. Before dinner, have everyone sweep through the house—one room at a time—to claim all their stuff and take it back to their rooms. Train your kids early on to help set the table and clear and clean the dinner plates. Praise them for pitching in.

Use chores as mini meditations. Instead of rushing through the dishes to watch another hour of mind-numbing TV, concentrate on the feeling of your hands in the warm water and appreciate the sparkle of clean glasses in the drying rack.

Designate a master control center. Instead of mentally scrolling through your to-do list, hang a huge wipe-off board in the kitchen. Write each family member's name across the top and the days of the week down the side. Fill in soccer games, drama practices, parent-teacher conferences, and dentist appointments, noting chaperoning or shuttling duties. By managing your own time publicly, you also teach that skill to your kids (and spot where you need help).

Do "homework" on Saturday. Don't fritter away your precious weekends on chores that you "should" do but aren't really necessary. To combat time-wasting perfectionism, set an alarm clock for 3 hours, make a list of priorities, and attack it with gusto. Once the bell rings, walk away and let it go. By giving yourself a deadline, you can focus all your energies without getting distracted by perfectionism.

Drop whatever chore you're doing for a nonnegotiable stress break. A daily half hour spent alone can make the difference between burnout and relative bliss. Deputize your eldest to shield you from incoming calls and sibling spats, then lock the door and focus on letting the bathwater absorb your troubles.

Commit to a bedtime. No basket of laundry or dirty dish is more important than 8 hours of sleep. Sleep banishes the fatigue that hamstrings your willpower. Face it: The laundry will never be 100 percent done. Admitting this can be very freeing. Make peace with lower expectations, and get to bed.

MAKE WORK MORE MANAGEABLE

Is "mind reader" listed on your business card? Not likely. When massive deadlines loom, the biggest stress is trying to divine what your boss expects from you. The following tricks reduce your reliance on guesswork.

Ask questions. Begin each project with a set of standard questions: When is this due? How long should it be? What information do you want included? Anything you don't want to see? Try to get a good mental picture of the finished product before you put your fingers on the keyboard.

Break it down. Working back from the deadline, break down the entire process into minigoals, each with its own target completion date. If you miss any of the goals, reevaluate the entire project and shift the deadlines appropriately so you don't find yourself caught short at the end. Achieving one goal every day will give you a sense of control.

Own your breaks. Lewis Richmond, a former Buddhist monk and author of *Work as a Spiritual Practice*, recommends using your bathroom breaks as opportunities to regroup and center yourself. Breathe in for four steps, out for four steps. Try a workplace mantra like "Plenty of time, plenty of energy" or "Plenty of time, plenty of care."

EASE CAREGIVER OVERLOAD

When you open your home to an aging parent, emotional baggage can take up more space than her ailing body. One national survey found that 25 percent of female caregivers endure emotional stress from their caregiving roles. Try the following tips for relief.

Establish realistic expectations. When a loved one needs you, you may have a hard time saying no, but if you're not careful, your big heart will overcommit your limited hours. Sit down together and talk about what each of you wants. Focus on the overlaps ("We eat meals together") and negotiate the disparities ("I keep you company all weekend"). After you've fulfilled your agreed-upon expectations, you can always commit more time—but on your own terms.

Look for social proxies. You don't have to shoulder the burden alone. Thousands of services have popped up to help with the growing numbers of elderly who need social outlets, not nursing care. Look into senior day care, community programs, bus tours, library book groups, and Web TV. Ask helpful neighbors to check in on your parent, or swap "sitting time" with a fellow caregiver.

Hire some help. If your parent has moved into your home, you not only have another mouth to feed, you also have more laundry, dishes, and so on. That extra work translates into time: Two-thirds of caregivers actually lose money from their paid jobs while scrambling to meet everyone's needs. Rather than being resentful, tell your mom you could spend more time with her if you had less to do, then ask her to pay for cleaning help. She'll probably welcome the chance to make a contribution, and she'll definitely be grateful for a less stressed, more present you.

TAKE THE STRESS OUT OF SPOUSAL SPATS

Living with someone for several decades is bound to involve a few tense moments. The key is to remember how much you love each other, despite each other's faults.

Chart your course. Once a year, around the holidays, talk about what you'd like to accomplish together the following year. Being very specific, write down your goals as a couple, as a family, and as individuals. Keep the document in a special place, and celebrate each goal reached with a dinner for two or a family picnic. Your shared mission statement will give you a chance to literally work off the same page and buffer you from periodic conflicts over money and plans, says Ronald Potter-Efron, PhD, a psychologist and author of *Being, Belonging, Doing: Balancing Your Three Greatest Needs*.

Divide the labor. Once you know your goals, you can split up the work. Is "keep a clean home" among your goals? If so, what does that mean? How often will you clean, and who will do what? Write down every chore in the house and give each to a specific family member. Knowing who's responsible for what will remove a tremendous amount of stress and resentment.

Show appreciation. Thank him, even if the chore he's done is on his list of things to do. If he washed the car, tell him it looks great. When he does his share of the laundry, thank him—not because he's "helping you," but to say, "I appreciate you." Chances are, he'll reciprocate; appreciation is a gift that keeps on giving.

CHAPTER 18

A GOOD NIGHT'S SLEEP, AT LAST

Sleep deprivation steals your energy, sours your mood, and turns your brain to mush. And then there's the toll it takes on your appearance. There's virtually nothing more irritating than having your colleagues inform you of what you already know—that you look exhausted.

Lack of sleep—whether from insomnia or just staying up way too late—also makes it more difficult for every cell in your body to properly absorb blood sugar. Getting insufficient shuteye blunts your body's sensitivity to insulin. In one study, people who got 5½ hours or less of sleep were 40 percent less sensitive to insulin than those who got nearly 8 hours a night. In another, researchers found that people who averaged only 4 hours of sleep demonstrated the kind of insulin resistance usually found in old age. Over time, insulin resistance leads to metabolic syndrome—the prediabetic condition that hurts your cardiovascular system, your memory, and even your fertility—and to diabetes itself.

Another reason we continue to toss and turn: There's plenty of false information out there about how to pursue a good night's sleep. Read on as we bust some of the biggest sleep myths and give smart solutions to common sleep problems.

MYTH #1: EVERYONE NEEDS AT LEAST 8 HOURS OF SLEEP

Think most experts agree on this one? Wrong! "Asking how much sleep a healthy adult needs is like asking how many calories a healthy adult needs," says Michael Perlis, MD, director of the University of Rochester's Sleep and Neurophysiology Research Lab. "It depends." Since our sleep requirements are partly inherited, some of us need more—or less—than others.

It's one of the most contentious issues in sleep research today. When sleep researcher Daniel Kripke, MD, from the University of California, San Diego, argued at a recent conference that getting less than 8 hours a night might be beneficial, "it practically started a food fight," recalls Phil Eichling, MD, an eyewitness at that conference and a sleep researcher at the University of Arizona College of Medicine.

Dr. Kripke has good reasons for giving the thumbs-down to the 8-hour rule. He conducted one of three studies that found that people who slept either 8 hours or more—or 6 hours or less—ran significant risks of dying of heart disease, stroke, or cancer. The highest risk was found among those who slept the longest. (Critics say long sleepers probably have underlying health problems that are the real problem, such as diabetes, depression, heart disease, or even cancer.)

Your best bet is to figure out what *your* body needs. Keep a diary for the next week or two, logging how much snooze time you get at night and how alert you feel the next day—without the use of stimulants such as a caffe latte or a splash of cold water on the face in the afternoon. If you need stimulants to keep you awake, you're not getting enough sleep.

MYTH #2: NODDING OFF—ESPECIALLY IN THE MIDAFTERNOON—IS PERFECTLY NORMAL

It's normal to feel slightly less energetic in the afternoon, due to your circadian rhythms of sleepiness and wakefulness. But if your head starts drooping while your boss is going over last month's figures or your adorably earnest preschooler is explaining why Superman bests Batman, you need more sleep. The difference between less energetic and downright drowsy? If your eyelids feel heavy, you're tired, says William C. Dement, PhD, the Stanford University scientist known as the father of sleep research.

You may even be running a significant "sleep debt." That's sleep research lingo for the total hours of sleep you've lost, one sleep-deprived night after another. Here's how it happens: If you need 8 hours of sleep and get only 7 each night, after a week you've lost the equivalent of almost a full night's sleep. That's your sleep debt. And it's cumulative. One expert estimates that the average sleep debt among Americans is 500 hours a year!

After losing the equivalent of 1 night's sleep over the course of a week, however, your body will respond as if you'd pulled an all-nighter: You may experience waves of extreme fatigue; itchy, burning eyes; emotional fragility; loss of focus; even hunger as your body tries to find a way to become energized and stay upright. Sleep debt can also cause serious health problems down the line. Some recent studies suggest that decades of chronic sleep deprivation may increase your risk of high blood pressure, heart disease, and diabetes—by speeding age-related changes in the way your body uses glucose.

If you're like millions of time-starved Americans, you're stealing sleep time to finish work from the office, answer e-mails, pay bills, do laundry, or just have some quiet time. This bad habit is the number one cause of daytime sleepiness in the United States, says Carl E. Hunt,

SNORING'S HIDDEN DANGERS

If you snore every night and you're overweight, see your doctor. A study of almost 70,000 nurses found that those who sawed wood regularly had more than twice the normal risk of developing type 2 diabetes, regardless of their weight. Regular deep snoring triggers the release of catecholamines, hormones that can promote insulin resistance, notes researcher Wael K. al-Delaimy, MD, PhD, of the Harvard School of Public Health. Sleep apnea, a condition in which you actually stop breathing numerous times a night, may have the same effect, he says.

MD, director of the National Institutes of Health National Center on Sleep Disorders Research in Bethesda, Maryland.

To repay your sleep debt—and avoid future problems—your first step is to determine what's behind it. The remedy will depend on the right diagnosis. Consider these questions.

- Do you take more than 30 minutes to fall asleep at night?
- Do you awaken in the middle of the night and have trouble getting back to sleep?

If the answer to either or both is yes, and it's happening 3 or more nights a week, insomnia is piling up your sleep debt. Skip the rest of this section and go straight to myth #3 for advice, because the Rx for insomnia is very different from remedies for other sleep problems.

Not an insomniac? Lots of things could be keeping you up or interrupting your sleep occasionally: worry, a child with nightmares, a pet hogging the pillow, a snoring spouse, even tree branches brushing against your house. One good night's slumber will correct that. But if you're cheating yourself of sleep time "to get things done," it's time to pay up . . . and stay out of debt.

Take a week or so to experiment. Keep your rising time the same, but move your bedtime ahead an hour for 3 or 4 days—say, from midnight to 11 o'clock. If you're still waking up tired and lurching to Starbucks in midafternoon, move your bedtime another 45 minutes to an hour earlier. Staring at the ceiling for 30 minutes before you drift off? Shift your new bedtime later in 15-minute increments until you hit your magic hour. How will you know? You'll wake up refreshed, you'll feel in top form at work, and decaf will do.

MYTH #3: IF YOU HAVE INSOMNIA, YOU NEED TO GO TO BED EARLIER, SLEEP LATER, OR NAP

Step away from the bed! If you suffer from insomnia, all three of those "remedies" could make your tossing and turning much worse, says Kimberly Cote, PhD, a sleep researcher at Brock University in Ontario.

Blame it on something called the sleep homeostat. A hardwired system controlled by brain chemicals, it's not unlike your appetite. Your

WHEN THE PROBLEM IS YOUR PET

Fluffy curls around your head all night. Fido's bladder demands outdoor bathroom trips at 3:00 and 5:00 a.m. Up to 25 percent of insomniacs may be able to blame their pets for their sleep problems, conclude researchers at the Mayo Clinic Sleep Disorders Center in Rochester, Minnesota, who surveyed 300 patients. How to stop pet-induced insomnia:

- Invest in a white-noise device or turn on a fan or air conditioner to help disguise your pet's night noises.
- Provided your pet is healthy and has no bladder or urinary tract conditions, she should be able to wait until sunup. Take away her water bowl a few hours before bedtime, and make sure she "goes" before bed. Then, when she asks to go out, delay taking her for 10 to 15 minutes. Every 3 or 4 nights, delay an extra few minutes.
- Invest in an animal crate—talk with your veterinarian about the best size for your pet and how to introduce Fido to his new night spot.

homeostat builds up a hunger for sleep based on how long you've been awake and how active you've been. The more sleep hungry you are, the faster you nod off and the more soundly you doze. But just as you're not eager for a big meal at night if you pig out all day, you're not going to feel tired if you go to bed earlier or nap.

Instead, try going to bed an hour *later* than usual to make yourself more tired. If you absolutely must nap—perhaps because you're exhausted and have a long drive ahead of you—make up for it by postponing bedtime for the amount of time you napped. Feeling anxious about sleep—or other worries? Try counting long, slow breaths while you lie in bed. Or visualize a pleasant and relaxing experience, such as lying on a deck chair on a cruise ship in the Caribbean. Still can't settle down? Leave the bedroom. The idea here is to break the association between bed and anxiety. Try reading or doing some other enjoyable but low-key activity. Other sleep tricks that work:

Take a warm bath just before you go to bed. Bathing will elevate

TAKE A POWER NAP

A 10-minute nap is your best midday recharger. In an Australian study, 12 university students had either no nap, a 5-minute nap, a 10-minute nap, or a 30-minute nap following a short night's sleep. Ten minutes is perfect because you recharge without falling into a deep, tough-to-wake-up slumber.

your body temperature, but lying down will make it drop because your muscles relax and produce less heat. Sleep tends to follow a steep decline in body temperature.

Exercise. In a number of studies, exercising 30 to 45 minutes during the day or evening helped insomniacs enjoy better and somewhat longer sleep. Why exercise seems to help is still unclear, though one possibility is that it has effects similar to sleeping pills. If exercising in the evening seems to get you keyed up, move your workout to earlier in the day.

See your doctor. If your insomnia is chronic, make an appointment with your family doc. He can diagnose and treat any contributing health problems or refer you to a sleep center.

6

PUTTING IT ALL TOGETHER: THE *SUGAR SOLUTION* LIFESTYLE MAKEOVER

CHAPTER 19

28 DAYS TO BETTER HEALTH AND A SLIMMER YOU

I f you're ready to tame high blood sugar and smooth out sugar "spikes"—and lose weight, get active, and send your stress levels south at the same time—here's the perfect plan. It's simple, effective, and delicious.

For the next 4 weeks, you're in the care of Ann Fittante, MS, RD, certified diabetes educator, nutrition educator, and exercise physiologist at the renowned Joslin Diabetes Center at Swedish Medical Center in Seattle. She's created this exclusive plan just for us—and for you. It's based on three core health principles—good nutrition, regular physical activity, and stress management.

Each day of the plan contains three components.

- **The menu plan.** While you lose weight, you'll eat more than you ever thought possible, including lots of your favorites—pasta, chocolate chip cookies, ice cream. (Yes—even on a low-glycemic-index diet, you don't have to forgo these treats!) In the recipe section, which starts on page 226, you'll learn how to create dishes featured in the plan. (Note: This meal plan is not adequate for meeting nutritional needs during pregnancy or for those who have been diagnosed with gestational diabetes.)

- **A motivational tip to make your walking program more inspired, exciting, comfortable, or effective.** You'll also follow weekly walking goals for rookies and veteran walkers ("Walk This Way").
- **A tip on how to de-stress and take some "me time" each day ("Take a Tranquility Break").** We know your time is tight, but we're talking 5 minutes a day. (Of course, take more time if you have it.) It may be hard to believe now, but those 300 seconds can add up to a calmer, less stressed you. Feel free to use our tips or make up your own.

If you're dreading yet another diet, be prepared to be pleasantly surprised.

YOU WON'T GO HUNGRY ON SIX MEALS A DAY

Like pasta? Burgers? Peanut butter? Baked potatoes? A glass of wine or beer with dinner? On this plan, it's all allowed. Here's a snapshot.

MUST-HAVE CONDIMENTS AND SEASONINGS

You probably have some of these in your spice rack right now, but if you don't, invest in them. You're sure to love the sweet, spicy, or piquant flavors they add to healthy cooking.

- Asian plum sauce
- Basic seasonings: bay leaves, cinnamon, cumin (whole seeds), Italian seasoning, nutmeg, oregano, paprika, parsley (dried and fresh), rosemary, thyme
- Capers
- Chili sauce
- Cooking wine
- Dijon mustard
- Flax oil (store in refrigerator)
- Horseradish
- Hot-pepper sauce
- Low-sodium soy sauce
- Natural sweeteners: honey, apple butter
- Olive and canola oils
- Salsa
- Sun-dried tomatoes
- Tahini
- Vinegars: balsamic, red wine, rice wine
- Worcestershire sauce

MAKE-AHEADS FOR EACH WEEK

Sunday afternoons are the perfect time to prepare one or more of the menus for the coming week. Below, you'll find a schedule of the tasty offerings for the following week. If you'd like to prepare one recipe scheduled for that week—such as the Mexican Lasagna—and eat that as a substitute for other dinner meals, go ahead. Simply stick to one serving.

- Each week: Mix up a week's worth of salad dressing. (For one to try, see "Dress for Success" on page 221.) Wash, dry, and mix a week's worth of salad greens in an airtight container and refrigerate them.
- The week before you begin the plan, for Week 1: Greek-Style Lentil Soup (page 335), Multigrain Cereal (page 319), Not Your Mother's Meat Loaf (page 372).
- Week 1 Make-Ahead, for Week 2: Chocolate Chippers (page 405), Quinoa with Peppers and Beans (page 354), Barley with Spring Greens (page 351), Garlicky Spinach Dip (page 327).
- Week 2 Make-Ahead, for Week 3: Tuscan Bean Stew (page 334), Blueberry-Yogurt Muffins (page 320), Chicken and Mushroom Pasta Casserole (page 397), Country-Style Potato and Green Bean Soup with Ham (page 340).
- Week 3 Make-Ahead, for Week 4: Spicy Meatballs with Coconut Milk (page 371), Shrimp and Crab Cakes (page 387), Mexican Lasagna (page 396).

- You eat 1,500 to 1,600 calories a day (50 to 60 percent carbohydrate, 15 to 25 percent protein, 25 to 30 percent fat). Meals and snacks are low fat and do not contain trans fats.
- Meals are divided between three meals and three snacks (two 80-calorie snacks and one 150-calorie snack). To decrease calories to 1,300 to 1,400, choose the meals plus two "free" snacks and one 80-calorie snack.
- To increase calories to 1,700 to 1,800 calories, choose the meals plus three 150-calorie snacks.
- On days that feature higher-calorie breakfasts (for example, Puffy Frittata with Ham and Green Pepper, Asparagus and Goat Cheese

(continued on page 220)

HELPFUL HINTS AND YUMMY SUGGESTIONS

Lowering your blood sugar doesn't have to be hard on your tastebuds or your pocketbook. Read on for ways to save time and money while you're on the plan, as well as for tips on choosing and using some of the featured foods.

The Helpful Hints

- Whole foods are those that are minimally processed and/or have one ingredient, like apples, barley, rolled oats, beans, carrots, and nuts. Choose them whenever you can.
- Choose organic foods to limit pesticides.
- Buy foods in bulk to save money.
- On labels and in recipes, subtract grams of fiber from the total amount of carbohydrate.
- Flax oil is a rich source of heart-healthy omega-3 fatty acids. It's also highly vulnerable to heat and light, so store it in the refrigerator and use it in salad dressings or drizzle on cooked food. Don't use flax oil to cook; use canola or olive oil instead.
- Some of the recipes call for flaxseed. You can buy it already ground in health food stores, or grind it yourself in a food processor or coffee grinder.
- Unlike flax oil, flaxseed is more stable when heated, so you can stir it into oatmeal or other cooked foods. You can bake with it as well.
- When you buy peanut, cashew, or almond butters, buy all-natural brands that do not contain hydrogenated oil. With natural nut butters, oil separation is normal; just stir before use. Keep the opened jar in the refrigerator.
- Rinse canned beans in cool water to wash off excess sodium.
- If you have a pressure cooker, consider cooking dried beans yourself. Most varieties take only 10 to 15 minutes, and beans prepared this way contain significantly less sodium than canned beans.
- When you choose whole grain breads, look for "100 percent whole wheat or stoneground wheat" as the first ingredient. Most will have at least 2 grams of fiber.

The Yummy Suggestions

- Homemade low-fat muffins can be a healthy choice for breakfast or snacks. In recipes, you can replace half the flour with whole wheat flour, use safflower or canola oil, use ¾ cup of sugar or less, and add nuts. A 1-ounce muffin is roughly 130 calories. Most commercial muffins are 4 to 6 ounces and pack 500 to 800 calories.

- If you enjoy breakfast cereal, have it. But opt for high-fiber brands, and limit the total amount of carbohydrate—including milk—to 60 grams. Avoid fruit with dry cereals unless the carbohydrate content of the cereal is around 25 grams per serving.
- Use a variety of greens in salads. Darker leaf lettuce is higher in nutrients than iceberg, and it's a delicious change. Try a combination of spinach, kale, Swiss chard, collards, mustard greens, and/or arugula for added flavor and more beta-carotene, folate, and magnesium.
- Whole wheat pastas have been used in the meal plans. You can substitute other whole grain pastas like corn, buckwheat, soba, quinoa, spelt, lentil, and brown rice pastas. Check your local health food store for different varieties.

- Edamame (ed-ah-mah-may) are green soybeans. Cooked, they have a sweet, nutty flavor. In China and Korea, they're traditionally eaten as a vegetable in stir-fries; in Japan, edamame are eaten as a snack, much as we eat peanuts. To make Edamame Salad, combine ⅔ cup cooked edamame and chopped onions, garlic, peppers, and carrots. Dress with 2 tablespoons of any low-fat dressing or Flaxseed Vinaigrette on page 221.
- Quinoa is a grain that comes from the Andes Mountains in South America and has the highest protein content of the grains. It takes 15 to 20 minutes to prepare and forms tiny spirals when fully cooked. Rinse quinoa before cooking to remove the saponin, a naturally occurring coating that has a bitter taste. You'll find quinoa at your local health food store.
- Steel-cut oats (also called Irish oatmeal) have a nuttier taste and chewier texture and are a tasty alternative to old-fashioned rolled oats. Avoid instant oatmeal, which is highly processed and contains a fair amount of sodium and sugar.

BUY NOW FOR LATER

While you'll want to shop weekly for fresh fruits and vegetables, breads, meat, and dairy, you can buy the following items now for the entire month.

- 1 pound raisins
- 1 jar unsweetened applesauce
- 10-ounce bag frozen corn
- 10-ounce bag frozen green beans
- 1 box Garden Burgers
- Popcorn (kernels or low-fat popped popcorn)
- Small bags chopped walnuts, cashews, almonds, sesame seeds
- Small bag ground flaxseed
- Small bag pine nuts
- 1 jar natural peanut butter or other nut butter (almond, cashew)
- Large box oat bran hot cereal, steel-cut oats, or rolled oats
- 2 boxes whole grain crackers
- 2 pounds whole wheat pasta
- 1 pound brown rice
- 1 box frozen whole grain waffles
- 1 package whole grain English muffins
- 1-pound bag whole grain tortilla chips
- 1-pound bag dried pearl barley
- 2 bags rice cakes
- 1 bag whole wheat tortillas, 8-inch diameter (tortillas freeze well)
- 1 pound whole grain pastry flour
- 1 quart low-fat frozen dessert (sorbet, frozen yogurt, low-fat ice cream)
- 1 tub trans fat–free margarine
- V8 or tomato juice (preferably low sodium)
- Canned chopped tomatoes
- Marinara sauce
- Green tea

Omelets, and Smoked Turkey Hash), midmorning snacks have been omitted and lunch calories reduced.

- You can drink diet soda and coffee or tea (hot or iced) in moderate amounts. Limit yourself to two cups of coffee (with 2 tablespoons of milk or cream per cup) and two 12-ounce servings of diet soda a day. Fittante recommends drinking eight 8-ounce glasses of water daily, along with green tea, which is a good source of antioxidants.

Do you use diabetic exchanges or count carbs? Here's how each meal breaks down.

DRESS FOR SUCCESS

On this plan, you can use any low-fat dressing you like, but Ann Fittante, MS, RD, of the Joslin Diabetes Center in Seattle recommends using dressings made with olive, canola, or flax oil. Unlike many bottled low-fat brands, these dressings are 100 percent healthy fats, with no artery-clogging trans fats.

Flax oil is light and nutty tasting, so it's perfect for salad dressing. Plus, it's a rich source of omega-3 fatty acids, which have proven health benefits. Here's the recipe for Flaxseed Vinaigrette.

4 tablespoons flax oil

2 tablespoons balsamic or red wine vinegar

1 medium clove crushed garlic

Pinch of salt

Freshly ground pepper, rosemary, thyme, and other fresh or dried herbs to taste

In a small bowl, whisk together the oil, vinegar, garlic, salt, and spices. Each tablespoon contains about 70 calories and 8 grams of fat. To make a larger batch, use 1 cup flax oil, ½ cup balsamic or red wine vinegar, 3 to 5 cloves of crushed garlic, and spices.

Note: Flax oil is highly vulnerable to heat and light. To keep it fresh and tasty, store it in the refrigerator. Use it in salad dressing or add it to cooked food. For cooking, use canola or olive oil.

- Each serving of bread, starch, fruit, and milk contains 15 grams of carbohydrate (one carbohydrate choice) and approximately 80 calories and can be interchanged within each day's plan.
- Meals are from 30 to 60 grams of carbohydrate, and snacks are 15 to 30 grams of carbohydrate.
- Exchange lists for recipes combine bread/starch, fruit, milk, and vegetables into one "carbohydrate (carb)" category. For example, one serving of Mexican Pork Stew (page 379) contains 244 calories, 24 grams protein, 18 grams carbohydrate, and 10 grams fat. Diet exchanges are three meat, one carb (half a starch, 1½ vegetable).
- Since fiber is not absorbed by the body, you can subtract it from the total amount of carbohydrates listed in each recipe. This can lower the carbohydrate amount significantly. "For example, one serving of Greek-

SNACKS FOR EVERY CRAVING

This meal plan allows three snacks a day—two 80-calorie snacks and one 150-calorie snack. Below, you'll find snacks that will satisfy, whether you crave sweet, savory, salty, or crunchy.

FREEBIES (25 CALORIES OR LESS)

Enjoy the following items any time of day.

Raw vegetables

Green salad with vinegar or lemon juice

6 ounces low-sodium tomato or vegetable juice

Low-sodium bouillon or broth

Tea, hot or iced (green tea is preferred, but any kind is fine)

Seltzer with lemon or lime

80-CALORIE SNACKS

1 serving fresh fruit: 1 medium apple, banana, orange, pear, or peach; 2 kiwis; 1 large plum; 5 medium apricots; 1 cup grapes, cherries, berries, cubed melon, papaya, or applesauce; ½ grapefruit; ½ small mango; 3 figs; 4 dates

½ cup canned fruit (rinse off light or heavy syrup)

Fruit smoothie (blend 6 ounces milk, ½ cup berries, and ice)

1 cup Strawberry-Watermelon Slush (page 409)

⅓ cup Garlicky Spinach Dip (page 327) and raw veggies

1½ cups Grilled Vegetables (page 352)

2 tablespoons raw veggies with dip or hummus

½ cup Spicy Roasted Chickpeas (page 323)

1 cup vegetable soup

3 cups air-popped popcorn

1 slice whole grain toast or bread

2 large rice or popcorn cakes

Style Lentil Soup (page 335) contains 55 grams of carbohydrate and 26 grams of fiber, so the carb count is actually 29 grams for one serving," says Fittante.

A PLAN WITH WIGGLE ROOM

Fittante has found that her patients are more likely to follow a healthier way of eating if there's a bit of wiggle room, so she built that flexibility right in.

For example, feel free to interchange meals. "Most of the breakfasts are 225 calories; most lunches, 425 calories; and most dinners, 550 calories," says Fittante. "So, with a few exceptions, you can choose to

1 cup fat-free milk or soy milk

½ cup fat-free plain yogurt or low-fat cottage cheese

1 ounce string cheese

Hard-cooked egg

Chocolate Chipper (page 405)

Nutty Brownie (page 403)

3 graham cracker squares or small gingersnaps

150-CALORIE SNACKS

Fruit

2 servings fruit (see previous list)

1 serving fruit with 1 cup fat-free, plain yogurt

1 serving cut-up fruit with 2 table-spoons nuts and a dollop of low-fat vanilla yogurt

Fruit smoothie (blend 1 serving fresh or frozen fruit, 8 ounces milk or soy milk, and ice cubes)

2 cups Strawberry-Watermelon Slush (page 409)

1 serving Sunny Waldorf Salad (page 346)

1 serving Spinach-Orange Salad with Sesame (page 347) and 1 rice cake

½ cup cottage cheese with 1 serving cut-up fruit

Veggies

8 Stuffed Mushrooms (page 326)

1 serving Zucchini Bites (page 325)

⅔ cup Garlicky Spinach Dip (page 327) with raw veggies

3 servings Grilled Vegetables (page 352)

2 servings Big Broiled Balsamic Mushrooms (page 353) with ½ serving crackers

Beans and Grains

½ serving hummus (page 324) and ½ serving crackers

3 servings (¾ cup) Spicy Roasted Chickpeas (page 323)

continued

eat the same breakfast each day, or pick one or two of your favorites. That goes for lunch and dinner meals."

Here's what else you'll want to know.

- Fruits, including berries and nuts, can be interchanged. However, don't exchange a fruit for a nut or vice versa.
- Vegetables can be interchanged. If the vegetables contain no added fat, have as much as you want.
- Any low-fat, low-calorie salad dressing (25 calories or less per table-spoon) can be substituted for the dressings suggested.
- Lean meats can be interchanged. For example, if a meal calls for tuna and you dislike it, choose another meat like turkey, ham, or lean roast beef.

SNACKS FOR EVERY CRAVING *(CONT.)*

1 serving Mediterranean Chickpea Salad (page 348) with ½ serving crackers

⅔ cup Edamame Salad (page 219)

1½ cups edamame, unshelled (green soybeans)

1 serving Barley with Spring Greens (page 351)

Cereals

1 cup cooked oatmeal, oat bran, or Multigrain Cereal (page 319)

Breads and Crackers

1 slice whole grain toast with 2 teaspoons nut butter

1 slice raisin toast with 1 teaspoon trans fat–free margarine

½ English muffin with 1 tablespoon apple butter

1 serving whole grain crackers

2 rice cakes with 2 teaspoons nut butter

½ ounce whole grain crackers with 1 teaspoon nut butter

1 serving whole grain crackers with 1 ounce string cheese

4 breadsticks

1 serving Shrimp in Mustard-Horseradish Sauce (page 321) with 3 to 4 whole grain crackers

1 hard-cooked egg with 1 slice dry toast

Crunchies

4 cups popcorn popped in oil

6 cups air-popped popcorn

1 serving whole grain tortilla chips with salsa

1 ounce nuts

- You're a vegetarian? No problem! Substitute any of the following for 2 ounces of meat: one egg, ½ cup beans, 4 ounces tofu, 1½ ounces low-fat cheese (i.e., goat, feta, reduced-fat Cheddar), ½ cup whole grain (like quinoa or barley), ¾ ounce nuts, or 1 tablespoon nut butter.

- "Low-fat yogurt" refers to any plain or flavored yogurt that's 150 calories or less per 6- to 8-ounce serving.

- "Frozen dessert" refers to any low-fat frozen yogurt, ice cream, sorbet, or sherbet that is 120 calories or less per ½-cup serving.

- Feel free to dress up "naked foods" (such as fruit or plain low-fat yogurt) with 1 teaspoon of honey, jam, maple syrup, or molasses (16 calories) or with artificial sweeteners.

A NOTE ABOUT ALCOHOL

The American Diabetes Association says that people with diabetes can have alcohol in moderation—one drink a day for women, two drinks a

Sweets

1 Blueberry-Yogurt Muffin (page 320) or 1-ounce low-fat muffin

6 to 8 ounces low-fat flavored yogurt

½ cup low-fat pudding

½ cup low-fat frozen yogurt or low-fat ice cream

1 frozen fruit pop

4 graham crackers (made without hydrogenated fat)

4 to 6 gingersnaps (made without hydrogenated fat)

1/12 angel food cake with ½ cup sliced strawberries

1½ Nutty Brownies (page 403)

1 Chocolate Chipper (page 405) and 6 ounces 1% milk

1 Peanut Butter Cookie (page 401) and 6 ounces 1% milk

1 serving Chocolate Soufflé Cake (page 410)

1 serving Sumptuous Strawberries in Spiced Phyllo (page 408)

1 serving Raspberry-Almond Tart (page 406)

1 serving Zucchini–Chocolate Chip Snack Cake (page 404)

1 serving Chocolate Hazelnut Flourless Cake (page 402)

EXTRAS

To fit alcohol into the meal plan, skip a snack and include an alcoholic beverage with your meal.

4 ounces wine (80 calories)

6 ounces wine (100 calories)

1½ ounces hard liquor (100 calories)

12 ounces beer (150 calories)

day for men. Alcohol should be consumed with food since it can cause low blood sugar in some people who take medications for diabetes. "But if you want a glass of wine or a beer at dinner, you'll need to omit something during the day to accommodate the extra calories in alcohol," says Fittante. Here's a cheat sheet.

- One 6-ounce glass of wine contains 100 calories; substitute for two fats.
- One 12-ounce beer contains 150 calories; substitute for one starch and one fat.
- A shot of hard liquor (1½ ounces gin, rum, vodka, or whiskey) contains 105 calories; substitute for two fats).

Follow the plan faithfully, and at the end of 28 days, you'll probably be slimmer, healthier, and calmer. So what are you waiting for? Get ready . . . get set . . . get healthy!

WEEK 1 DAY 1

Breakfast

1 serving Multigrain Cereal (page 319) mixed with 1 tablespoon chopped walnuts

Snack

1 small pear

8 baby carrots

Lunch

1 serving Greek-Style Lentil Soup (page 335)

1–2 cups spinach salad with ½ ounce crumbled feta cheese, dressed with 2 tablespoons low-fat dressing

Snack

1 small apple

Dinner

1½ cups whole wheat pasta with marinara sauce and 1 tablespoon Parmesan or Romano cheese

1 cup broccoli sautéed with garlic and onions in 1 teaspoon olive oil

Snack

½ cup pudding made with fat-free milk

Note: Freeze 1½ cups lentil soup in a container for Day 4's lunch.

WALK THIS WAY

Week 1 walking goals: Rookies—aim for 15 minutes a day. Walking veterans—aim for 30 minutes or more a day.

TAKE A TRANQUILITY BREAK

Tonight, take a 15- or 20-minute shower by candlelight. Use a scented bath gel you've purchased especially for this first day of your lifestyle makeover.

Daily Analysis

Calories: 1,567

Carbohydrate: 241 grams

Fiber: 56 grams

Protein: 56 grams

Fat: 42 grams

Cholesterol: 136 milligrams

Saturated fat: 9 grams

Sodium: 1,823 milligrams

Exchanges

Carbs: 15 (8 bread/starch, 4 fruit, 1 milk, 6 vegetable)

Meats: 3

Fats: 4

WEEK 1 DAY 2

Breakfast

1 slice whole grain toast spread with
1 teaspoon all-natural almond butter

1 cup 1% milk

Snack

3 cups air-popped popcorn

Lunch

Tuna sandwich: ½ cup tuna and
2 teaspoons low-fat mayonnaise
spread on 2 slices whole grain
bread, topped with lettuce and
tomato

1 cup raw sugar snap peas or other raw
vegetable dipped in 2 tablespoons
low-fat dressing

Snack

1 orange

Dinner

3 ounces baked chicken

1 small baked potato with 2 tablespoons low-fat sour cream

1–2 cups salad with 1 tablespoon low-fat dressing

1 cup steamed green beans

6 ounces wine or extra 80-calorie snack

Snack

¼ cup applesauce mixed with ½ cup low-fat plain or vanilla yogurt
and cinnamon

Note: Cook an extra 3 ounces of chicken for tomorrow's lunch.

Daily Analysis

Calories: 1,554
Carbohydrate: 200 grams
Fiber: 27 grams
Protein: 79 grams
Fat: 40 grams

Saturated fat: 11 grams
Cholesterol: 131
   milligrams
Sodium: 2,224 milligrams

Exchanges

Carbs: 12 (6 bread/starch,
   2 fruit, 2 milk, 6 vegetable)
Meats: 5
Fats: 4
1 alcohol

WEEK 1 DAY 3

Breakfast

Breakfast smoothie: Blend 1 cup 1% milk or plain yogurt, 1 small banana, 1 tablespoon ground flaxseed, and ½ cup frozen berries until smooth.

Snack

Sliced raw vegetables and 1 ounce string cheese

Lunch

1 Chicken Salad Roll-Up (page 345)

1 cup honeydew melon

Snack

½ serving hummus (page 324) or 3 tablespoons prepared hummus and raw vegetables

Dinner

1 vegetable patty (like a Garden Burger) spread with 1 teaspoon relish and 1 tablespoon ketchup and topped with lettuce, tomato, and onion (if desired)

1 whole grain roll

2 cups tossed salad with ¼ avocado and 2 tablespoons low-fat dressing

1 cup 1% milk

Snack

½ cup low-fat frozen dessert

Note: Save the remainder of the hummus for Friday's lunch.

WALK THIS WAY

To improve your walking posture, wear a hat and/or sunglasses so you won't be tempted to tilt your head down to avoid sun glare.

TAKE A TRANQUILITY BREAK

Pick up a guidebook on flowers, trees, or birds, and take notice of your natural surroundings.

Daily Analysis

Calories: 1,557

Carbohydrate: 220 grams

Fiber: 31 grams

Protein: 83 grams

Fat: 44 grams

Saturated fat: 13 grams

Cholesterol: 107 milligrams

Sodium: 2,290 milligrams

Exchanges

Carbs: 13 (5 bread/starch, 3 fruit, 3 milk, 6 vegetable)

Meats: 5

Fats: 5

WEEK 1 DAY 4

Breakfast

6 ounces low-fat plain or vanilla yogurt mixed with 2 tablespoons granola, 1 tablespoon ground flaxseed, and 1 teaspoon sunflower seeds

Snack

2 large rice cakes

¼ avocado or 1 ounce string cheese

Lunch

1½ cups leftover Greek-Style Lentil Soup

Small whole grain roll dipped in 1 teaspoon olive oil

Small salad sprinkled with 1 tablespoon chopped walnuts and dressed with 1 tablespoon low-fat dressing

Snack

1 orange

Dinner

1 serving Breaded Baked Cod with Tartar Sauce (page 383)

¾ cup roasted yams

1 cup Swiss chard sautéed in garlic and 1 teaspoon olive oil

1 cup 1% milk

Snack

Fruit smoothie: Blend ¾ cup 1% milk, ½ cup berries, and a few ice cubes until smooth.

WALK THIS WAY

Create backup plans. Map out short, medium, and long walks near home, work, and your child's school so you can put in some walking time on even the busiest days.

TAKE A TRANQUILITY BREAK

This takes just 60 seconds, but it's a powerful exercise. Visualize yourself as your favorite tree. Imagine your feet rooted to the earth, grounding and supporting you. Know that you are stronger and more resilient than you give yourself credit for.

Daily Analysis

Calories: 1,499
Carbohydrate: 199 grams
Fiber: 30 grams
Protein: 87 grams
Fat: 44 grams
Saturated fat: 9 grams
Cholesterol: 196 milligrams
Sodium: 2,385 milligrams

Exchanges

Carbs: 13 (8 bread/starch, 2 fruit, 2 milk, 3 vegetable)
Meats: 4
Fats: 5

WEEK 1 DAY 5

Breakfast

1 cup cooked oat bran cereal mixed
with 1 tablespoon ground flaxseed
and 1 tablespoon chopped almonds

½ banana

Snack

6 ounces low-fat plain or vanilla
yogurt with 1 teaspoon honey

Lunch

1 medium whole grain pita stuffed
with 1 serving hummus (page 324) or
6 tablespoons prepared hummus.
Add fresh lettuce, sliced tomatoes,
and chopped cucumbers.

6 ounces low-sodium vegetable or
tomato juice

Snack

3 cups air-popped popcorn

Dinner

1 serving Not Your Mother's Meat Loaf
(page 372)

½ cup mashed potatoes with 1 teaspoon trans fat–free margarine

½ cup corn

Green salad with 1 tablespoon low-fat dressing

Snack

Cottage cheese parfait: Layer ½ cup cottage cheese (sweetened
with artificial sweetener and cinnamon, if you like) with ½ cup
blueberries; sprinkle with 1 teaspoon nuts

WALK THIS WAY

*Invest in smarter socks.
Surprise—synthetic
fabrics trump 100 percent
cotton because they wick
away sweat to keep feet
dry and blister-free.*

TAKE A TRANQUILITY BREAK

*Make a "gratitude list."
Take 5 minutes and write
down everything you can
think of that you're
grateful for: your
children, tinted
moisturizer, your lilac
tree that gives you
fragrant bouquets for
your kitchen table each
spring, your faith—
anything and everything.*

Daily Analysis

Calories: 1,544
Carbohydrate: 226 grams
Fiber: 36 grams
Protein: 94 grams
Fat: 39 grams

Saturated fat: 8 grams
Cholesterol: 104
   milligrams
Sodium: 2,294
   milligrams

Exchanges

Carbs: 15 (10 bread/starch,
   3 fruit, 1 milk, 4 vegetable)
Meats: 4
Fats: 3

WEEK 1 DAY 6

Breakfast

1 serving Puffy Frittata with Ham and Green Pepper (page 313)

1 slice whole grain toast spread with 1 teaspoon apple butter

Lunch

1 cup low-sodium vegetable soup

½ serving Not Your Mother's Meat Loaf (page 372) on 2 slices whole grain bread, topped with 1 teaspoon each low-fat mayonnaise and ketchup

Snack

1 peach

Dinner

Pasta sauté: Sauté garlic and onion in ½ tablespoon olive oil. Add 2 cups kale, collards, and/or bok choy and sauté for another 5–10 minutes. Sprinkle with basil and oregano; add 1 tablespoon pine nuts, 2 tablespoons sun-dried tomatoes, and ¼ cup Parmesan or Romano cheese. Serve over 1 cup cooked whole wheat pasta.

Tomato and cucumber salad tossed with 1 tablespoon low-fat dressing or red wine vinegar.

Snack

1 sliced apple dipped in 2 tablespoons low-fat plain or vanilla yogurt

> **TAKE A TRANQUILITY BREAK**
>
> *Set the alarm 10 minutes ahead. Those 600 seconds are yours to spend as you will. Enjoy your first cup of coffee. Look in on a sleeping child or snoring partner. Read a few pages of your newest paperback.*

Daily Analysis

Calories: 1,547
Carbohydrate: 223 grams
Fiber: 32 grams
Protein: 76 grams

Fat: 53 grams
Saturated fat: 16 grams
Cholesterol: 526 milligrams
Sodium: 3,071 milligrams

Exchanges

Carbs: 12 (6 bread/starch, 4 fruit, 6 vegetable)
Meats: 6
Fats: 4

WEEK 1 DAY 7

Breakfast

1 serving Whole Grain Crepes with Banana and Kiwifruit (page 315)

Snack

1 Chocolate Chipper (page 405)

Green tea

Lunch

1½ cups chili made with beans and lean ground meat

2 ounces cornbread

1 cup green salad with 1 tablespoon low-fat dressing

Snack

6 ounces low-fat plain or vanilla yogurt mixed with 1 teaspoon honey and sprinkled with cinnamon and nutmeg

Note: Save a 1-ounce piece of cornbread for tomorrow's lunch.

Dinner

1 serving Grilled Flank Steak with Chile-Tomato Salsa (page 374)

¾ cup brown rice

1 cup steamed asparagus and carrots mixed with 1 teaspoon olive oil and chopped garlic

Snack

1 cup Strawberry-Watermelon Slush (page 409)

WALK THIS WAY

Check your shoes for uneven heel wear or tops that look like your feet have pushed them to one side—signs that it's time to invest in new walking footwear.

TAKE A TRANQUILITY BREAK

Say no. Just say no.

Daily Analysis

Calories: 1,561
Carbohydrate: 232 grams
Fiber: 29 grams
Protein: 78 grams
Fat: 35 grams

Saturated fat: 11 grams
Cholesterol: 163 milligrams
Sodium: 2,354 milligrams

Exchanges

Carbs: 11.5 (7 bread/starch, 2 fruit, 1 milk, 5 vegetable)
Meats: 6
Fats: 5

WEEK 2 DAY 1

Breakfast

1 egg, prepared any style with cooking spray

1 whole grain English muffin spread with 2 teaspoons apple butter

Snack

1 cup frozen grapes

Lunch

1 cup low-sodium tomato soup made with fat-free milk

Large salad with 2 ounces grilled chicken and ⅛ avocado, dressed with 1 tablespoon low-fat dressing

1 ounce leftover cornbread

Snack

2 rice cakes spread with 2 teaspoons all-natural peanut butter

Dinner

3 ounces Grilled Salmon with Mint-Cilantro Yogurt (page 385)

1 serving Quinoa with Peppers and Beans (page 354)

1 cup steamed spinach with lemon juice

1 cup 1% milk

Snack

½ cup sliced fruit topped with 2 tablespoons low-fat sour cream or low-fat plain or vanilla yogurt

WALK THIS WAY

Week 2 walking goals: Rookies—aim for 20 minutes a day. Walking veterans—aim for 40 minutes or more a day.

TAKE A TRANQUILITY BREAK

Swing on the swings at your neighborhood playground or park. Can anyone stay stressed with the wind in her hair?

Daily Analysis

Calories: 1,593
Carbohydrate: 216 grams
Fiber: 30 grams
Protein: 99 grams

Fat: 45 grams
Saturated fat: 11 grams
Cholesterol: 203 milligrams
Sodium: 2,847 milligrams

Exchanges

Carbs: 14 (8 bread/starch, 3 fruit, 2 milk, 4 vegetable)
Meats: 6
Fats: 4

WEEK 2 DAY 2

Breakfast

1 slice whole grain toast spread with 1 teaspoon trans fat–free margarine and 1 teaspoon jam

1 cup 1% milk

Snack

Egg salad "sandwich": Mash 1 hard-cooked egg; add 2 teaspoons low-fat mayonnaise. Spread on tomato slices.

Lunch

Turkey sandwich: 2 ounces turkey on 2 slices whole grain bread spread with 1 tablespoon low-fat mayonnaise or mustard and topped with spinach, tomato, and onion (if desired)

²⁄₃ cup Edamame Salad (page 219)

8 baby carrots

Snack

1 Chocolate Chipper (page 405)

Herbal tea

Dinner

3 ounces Sautéed Tuna Steaks with Garlic Sauce (page 384)

1 serving Barley with Spring Greens (page 351)

1 cup 1% milk

Snack

1 cup berries topped with 2 tablespoons low-fat plain or vanilla yogurt

> **WALK THIS WAY**
> *Buy a pedometer and wear it during your daily routine. Challenge yourself to increase your mileage by 100 steps today.*
>
> **TAKE A TRANQUILITY BREAK**
> *After work today, turn out the lights. Light a fragrant candle. Lose yourself in the flickering flame.*

Daily Analysis

Calories: 1,401
Carbohydrate: 170 grams
Fiber: 30 grams
Protein: 81 grams
Fat: 47 grams
Saturated fat: 10 grams
Cholesterol: 308 milligrams
Sodium: 1,900 milligrams

Exchanges

Carbs: 10 (6 bread/starch, 1 fruit, 2 milk, 5 vegetable)
Meats: 6
Fats: 5

WEEK 2 DAY 3

Breakfast

1 serving Multigrain Cereal (page 319)

1 hard-cooked egg

Snack

½ cup low-fat cottage cheese

Raw vegetables

Lunch

Bean and beef burrito: Cook 2 ounces lean ground beef and fill 1 large whole wheat tortilla. Top with ¼ cup pinto beans, chopped onion and tomato salsa, ⅛ avocado (if desired), and 2 tablespoons low-fat sour cream.

1 apple

Snack

½ cup canned peaches (drained)

Dinner

⅓ cup Garlicky Spinach Dip (page 327) with raw vegetables

2 servings Chicken Pesto Pizza (page 331)

Snack

1 Chocolate Chipper (page 405)

¾ cup 1% milk

Note: Save 1 serving of pizza for Day 5's lunch.

WALK THIS WAY

Start climbing. Hill walking burns up to 60 percent more calories—and it's great for firming your butt. No hills in your area? Hop on a treadmill with an incline setting.

TAKE A TRANQUILITY BREAK

Smile at two people while you're driving today. Make a connection, even though you're both insulated by the glass and metal of your vehicles.

Daily Analysis

Calories: 1,484

Carbohydrate: 189 grams

Fiber: 24 grams

Protein: 80 grams

Fat: 50 grams

Saturated fat: 15 grams

Cholesterol: 322 milligrams

Sodium: 1,566 milligrams

Exchanges

Carbs: 13 (8 bread/starch, 3 fruit, 1 milk, 3 vegetable)

Meats: 6

Fats: 4

WEEK 2 DAY 4

Breakfast

Egg sandwich: Prepare 1 egg, any style, with cooking spray; top with 1 ounce low-fat cheese and place between 2 slices whole grain toast or in a whole grain English muffin.

Snack

1 apple

Lunch

1 cup low-sodium vegetable or chicken noodle soup

Large salad: Mix 1½ cups greens, ½ cup chopped vegetables, ¼ cup canned chickpeas, ¼ cup canned kidney beans, ½ cup chopped apple or grapes, ⅛ avocado, and bean sprouts. Dress with 2 tablespoons low-fat dressing.

1 serving whole grain crackers or 1 small whole grain roll

Snack

6–8 ounces low-fat plain or vanilla yogurt

Dinner

1 Italian-Style Beef Burger (page 375) spread with 2 teaspoons mustard and 1 tablespoon ketchup and topped with lettuce, tomato, and onion (if desired)

1 whole grain roll

2 cups tossed salad with 2 tablespoons low-fat dressing

1 cup 1% milk

Snack

1 serving whole grain tortilla chips and salsa

Daily Analysis

Calories: 1,567
Carbohydrate: 194 grams
Fiber: 26 grams
Protein: 95 grams
Fat: 53 grams
Saturated fat: 17 grams
Cholesterol: 367 milligrams
Sodium: 3,149 milligrams

Exchanges

Carbs: 14 (7 bread/starch, 3 fruit, 2 milk, 6 vegetable)
Meats: 6
Fats: 3

WEEK 2 DAY 5

Breakfast

1 whole grain waffle topped with ¾ cup sliced strawberries and a dollop of low-fat plain or vanilla yogurt

Snack

1 ounce roasted cashews

Lunch

1 slice leftover Chicken Pesto Pizza

Tossed salad with 2 tablespoons low-fat dressing

6–8 ounces low-fat plain or vanilla yogurt

Snack

1 orange

Dinner

3 ounces baked pork chop

1 medium baked potato with 2 tablespoons low-fat sour cream

1 cup steamed green beans

½ cup steamed carrots

1 cup applesauce

Snack

2 Chocolate Chippers (page 405)

Herbal tea

WALK THIS WAY

Reduce the impact. Choose an asphalt- or tar-paved road over a concrete sidewalk—the road's actually softer. If the road edge slants to the curb, reverse your walking direction every few days to avoid injuries caused by the uneven surface.

TAKE A TRANQUILITY BREAK

Tonight, go outside, find a spot with an unobstructed view of a patch of sky, and take it in. When was the last time you felt awed by the universe?

Daily Analysis

Calories: 1,506
Carbohydrate: 216 grams
Fiber: 25 grams
Protein: 63 grams

Fat: 50 grams
Saturated fat: 13 grams
Cholesterol: 125 milligrams
Sodium: 925 milligrams

Exchanges

Carbs: 14 (7 bread/starch, 5 fruit, 1 milk, 4 vegetable)
Meats: 4
Fats: 5

WEEK 2 DAY 6

Breakfast

1 cup steel-cut oats mixed with
1 tablespoon ground flaxseed,
1 tablespoon walnuts, and
1 teaspoon honey or brown sugar

Snack

3 cups air-popped popcorn

Lunch

Healthy nachos: Place ½ cup canned beans (kidney, black, red, or pinto) on 1½ servings whole grain tortilla chips. Top with chopped tomatoes and onions and 1 ounce grated low-fat extra-sharp Cheddar cheese. Bake or microwave until cheese melts. Top with salsa, ⅛ avocado, and a dollop of low-fat sour cream.

Snack

1 banana

Dinner

1 serving New American Fried Chicken (page 363)
1 serving Spicy Oven Fries (page 322)
Leafy green tossed salad with 2 tablespoons low-fat dressing
1 cup 1% milk

Snack

½ cup low-fat frozen dessert

WALK THIS WAY
Start slowly. Five minutes of easy striding can help you log more miles by warming up your muscles. Finish with 5 minutes of a pleasant, easy cooldown, and you'll be ready to do it all again tomorrow.

TAKE A TRANQUILITY BREAK
Take a 20-minute nap. Refuse to feel guilty.

Daily Analysis

Calories: 1,549
Carbohydrate: 209 grams
Fiber: 27 grams
Protein: 71 grams
Fat: 53 grams
Saturated fat: 14 grams
Cholesterol: 135 milligrams
Sodium: 1,356 milligrams

Exchanges

Carbs: 13 (9 bread/starch, 2 fruit, 1 milk, 3 vegetable)
Meats: 4
Fats: 5

WEEK 2 DAY 7

Breakfast

1 Berry-Good Smoothie (page 318) with 1 tablespoon ground flaxseed

Snack

2 large rice cakes spread with 2 teaspoons natural almond butter

Lunch

1 serving Adzuki Beans with Miso Dressing (page 356) or 1 cup baked beans

2 cups spinach salad with 1 ounce crumbled feta cheese and 2 tablespoons low-fat dressing

Snack

1 pear

Dinner

1 serving Roast Swordfish with Herbed Crust (page 388)

Medium baked sweet potato with 1 teaspoon trans fat–free margarine

½ cup steamed cauliflower

Large salad sprinkled with 1 tablespoon sunflower seeds and dressed with 1 tablespoon low-fat dressing

1 cup 1% milk

Snack

3 cups air-popped popcorn

WALK THIS WAY

Paper inspiration: On separate pieces of paper, jot down five reasons you're getting fit, and store the notes in a pretty container. Read one the next time your motivation lags.

TAKE A TRANQUILITY BREAK

If worries have you tossing and turning, place a small lidded dish or box by your bed. Tonight before bed, symbolically "place" your worries in the container to deal with tomorrow.

Daily Analysis

Calories: 1,565
Carbohydrate: 216 grams
Fiber: 34 grams
Protein: 79 grams

Fat: 48 grams
Saturated fat: 10 grams
Cholesterol: 97 milligrams
Sodium: 1,515 milligrams

Exchanges

Carbs: 14 (7 bread/starch, 3 fruit, 2 milk, 5 vegetable)
Meats: 4
Fats: 4

WEEK 3 DAY 1

Breakfast

1 Blueberry-Yogurt Muffin (page 320)

1 cup 1% milk

Snack

1¼ cups cubed watermelon

Lunch

1 cup low-sodium vegetable soup

Tuna sandwich: ½ cup tuna and
2 teaspoons low-fat mayonnaise
spread on a whole grain roll

Raw vegetables dipped in low-fat
dressing

Snack

1 ounce whole grain tortilla chips and salsa

Dinner

1 serving Tuscan Bean Stew (page 334)

Large salad with 2 tablespoons low-fat dressing

Snack

6 ounces low-fat plain or vanilla yogurt with ½ cup blueberries

---

WALK THIS WAY

*Week 3 walking goals:
Rookies—aim for 25
minutes a day. Walking
veterans—aim for 50
minutes or more a day.*

TAKE A TRANQUILITY BREAK

*Volunteer one night to
charity. Be reminded of
the good fortune you
have in your life by
helping others.*

Daily Analysis

Calories: 1,555

Carbohydrate: 243 grams

Fiber: 33 grams

Protein: 86 grams

Fat: 36 grams

Saturated fat: 8 grams

Cholesterol: 93
milligrams

Sodium: 2,852
milligrams

Exchanges

Carbs: 14 (8 bread/starch,
2 fruit, 2 milk, 6 vegetable)

Meats: 5

Fats: 3

WEEK 3 DAY 2

Breakfast

1 serving Berry-Good Smoothie (page 318) with 1 tablespoon ground flaxseed

Snack

1 Blueberry-Yogurt Muffin (page 320)

Lunch

Nut-butter sandwich: Spread 1 tablespoon all-natural peanut butter or other nut butter and ½ tablespoon blackstrap molasses (or ½ tablespoon jam) on 2 slices whole grain bread

Carrot and celery sticks

Snack

1 banana

Dinner

1 serving Pork Chops with Apple Cider, Walnuts, and Prunes (page 377)

1 medium baked potato with 2 tablespoons low-fat sour cream

1 cup steamed green beans

Salad with 1 tablespoon low-fat dressing

½ cup low-fat frozen dessert

Snack

½ cup unshelled edamame or 1 ounce soy nuts

WALK THIS WAY

Build bone, burn more fat: Hop on and off curbs; zigzag between pavement, dirt, and grass; and charge up the hills.

TAKE A TRANQUILITY BREAK

Have a picnic—outside in warmer weather, inside if it's cold. (Spread a checked tablecloth on the living room or family room floor!) Make it as simple or elaborate as you like.

Daily Analysis

Calories: 1,571
Carbohydrate: 253 grams
Fiber: 35 grams
Protein: 58 grams
Fat: 45 grams

Saturated fat: 10 grams
Cholesterol: 86 milligrams
Sodium: 1,280 milligrams

Exchanges

Carbs: 14 (8 bread/starch, 3 fruit, 2 milk, 4 vegetable)
Meats: 4
Fats: 4

WEEK 3 DAY 3

Breakfast

1 serving high-fiber dry cereal
  sprinkled with 2 tablespoons
  ground flaxseed

1 cup 1% milk

Snack

3 small gingersnaps

Lunch

1 cup low-sodium clam or fish
  chowder made with 1% milk

1 serving whole grain crackers

1 plum

Snack

½ cup low-fat cottage cheese with 1 serving cut-up fruit

Dinner

1 serving Chicken and Mushroom Pasta Casserole (page 397)

1 cup steamed carrots

Salad with 1 tablespoon chopped almonds and 1 tablespoon low-fat
  dressing

½ cup low-fat frozen dessert

Snack

½ cup applesauce sprinkled with cinnamon

WALK THIS WAY

*Pick up the pace. Burn
50 percent more calories
simply by upping your
speed from 3 to 4 miles
per hour. To get there,
first do 30-second bursts
of fast walking at
2-minute intervals.*

TAKE A TRANQUILITY BREAK

*Burn incense when you
pay your bills.*

Daily Analysis

Calories: 1,465
Carbohydrate: 240 grams
Fiber: 34 grams
Protein: 69 grams
Fat: 32 grams

Saturated fat: 11 grams
Cholesterol: 77
  milligrams
Sodium: 2,979
  milligrams

Exchanges

Carbs: 14 (6 bread/starch,
  3 fruit, 4 milk, 3 vegetable)
Meats: 5
Fats: 3

WEEK 3 DAY 4

Breakfast

1 whole grain waffle topped with ¾ cup sliced strawberries and a dollop of low-fat plain or vanilla yogurt

Snack

1 rice cake and 1 teaspoon almond butter

Lunch

Pizza English muffin: Layer a whole grain English muffin with 3 tablespoons tomato sauce; then 2 ounces part-skim mozzarella, diced onions, garlic, peppers, and mushrooms. Sprinkle with oregano, basil, and red-pepper flakes. Broil until the cheese melts.

Tossed salad with 1 tablespoon low-fat dressing

Snack

1 mango

Dinner

1 serving Country-Style Potato and Green Bean Soup with Ham (page 340)

Chef salad: Mix 1 ounce sliced turkey, 1 ounce sliced roast beef, and ½ cup black beans into a bed of lettuce, tomato, peppers, celery, carrots, and onions. Dress with 2 tablespoons low-fat dressing.

1 cup 1% milk

Snack

Tea

1 slice raisin toast spread with 1 teaspoon trans fat–free margarine and sprinkle of sugar and cinnamon

WALK THIS WAY

Hit the beach. Walking on sand—by the sea or simply in a sand volleyball court—boosts calorie burn 20 to 50 percent and wakes up leg muscles you never knew you had.

TAKE A TRANQUILITY BREAK

Buy yourself an Etch A Sketch and give yourself a daily artistic challenge.

Daily Analysis

Calories: 1,533
Carbohydrate: 214 grams
Fiber: 36 grams
Protein: 82 grams

Fat: 45 grams
Saturated fat: 15 grams
Cholesterol: 118 milligrams
Sodium: 2,188 milligrams

Exchanges

Carbs: 14 (8 bread/starch, 3 fruit, 1 milk, 6 vegetable)
Meats: 5
Fats: 4

WEEK 3 DAY 5

Breakfast

Bean burrito: Spread 1 whole grain tortilla with ¼ cup beans, 2 tablespoons salsa, ½ ounce low-fat Cheddar cheese, and a dollop of low-fat sour cream.

Snack

1 banana

Lunch

1 serving leftover Country-Style Potato and Green Bean Soup with Ham

1 serving whole grain crackers with ½ ounce low-fat Cheddar cheese

Snack

1 ounce cashews

Dinner

Sole with Stir-Fried Vegetables (page 386)

1 cup brown rice

¼ cup low-fat plain or vanilla yogurt mixed with ½ cup canned peaches (drained)

Snack

3 cups air-popped popcorn sprinkled with chili powder

WALK THIS WAY

A wonderful night for a moonwalk. Dress in reflective clothing, grab your flashlight and a friend, and head out for a late-night stroll. Enjoy the night noises and the stars—and stay on the sidewalk for safety.

TAKE A TRANQUILITY BREAK

Detail your car. Clean out your closet. Transforming chaos into order can be very calming.

Daily Analysis

Calories: 1,546
Carbohydrate: 219 grams
Fiber: 30 grams
Protein: 76 grams

Fat: 44 grams
Saturated fat: 15 grams
Cholesterol: 124 milligrams
Sodium: 1,913 milligrams

Exchanges

Carbs: 13 (8 bread/starch, 3 fruit, 1 milk, 3 vegetable)
Meats: 7
Fats: 3

WEEK 3 DAY 6

Breakfast

½ grapefruit

1 serving Asparagus and Goat Cheese Omelet (page 314)

1 slice whole grain toast spread with 1 teaspoon jam

Lunch

1 cup low-sodium navy bean soup

Roast beef sandwich: 2 ounces roast beef on 2 slices whole grain bread spread with 1 tablespoon low-fat mayonnaise and topped with lettuce, tomato, and onion

Snack

1 serving fresh fruit or other 80-calorie snack

Dinner

1 serving Eggplant Parmesan (page 394)

1 cup polenta or whole wheat pasta

Tossed salad with 1 tablespoon low-fat dressing

1 cup 1% milk

Snack

1¼ cups cubed watermelon

WALK THIS WAY

Sprint! Today, walk only half your normal time (13 minutes for rookies, 25 for veterans)—but do it at a faster pace than usual.

TAKE A TRANQUILITY BREAK

Visit a local museum. If you think it's not your thing, think again— walking amid beautiful artwork can be rejuvenating.

Daily Analysis

Calories: 1,540
Carbohydrate: 182 grams
Fiber: 27 grams
Protein: 80 grams
Fat: 59 grams
Saturated fat: 21 grams
Cholesterol: 534 milligrams
Sodium: 3,580 milligrams

Exchanges

Carbs: 12 (7 bread/starch, 3 fruit, 1 milk, 3 vegetable)
Meats: 5
Fats: 5

WEEK 3 DAY 7

Breakfast

1 egg, any style, prepared with cooking spray

1 slice whole grain toast

½ cup home-fried potatoes cooked in 2 teaspoons olive oil and flavored with chopped garlic and onion

Lunch

Tuna salad: Mix 1 tablespoon low-fat mayonnaise and 2 tablespoons diced celery and carrots into ½ cup tuna. Arrange on a bed of greens.

½ whole wheat pita

1 cup fruit salad

1 cup 1% milk

Snack

3 graham cracker squares

Dinner

2 ounces grilled chicken

1 serving Indian-Spiced Potatoes and Spinach (page 350)

Tossed salad with 1 tablespoon low-fat dressing

1 cup 1% milk

Snack

2 cups Strawberry-Watermelon Slush (page 409)

WALK THIS WAY

Bring your iPod. Up-tempo music can keep you strutting faster, longer.

TAKE A TRANQUILITY BREAK

Color with your children or grandchildren. Don't have either? Buy a box of Crayolas and a coloring book for yourself.

Daily Analysis

Calories: 1,445
Carbohydrate: 202 grams
Fiber: 31 grams
Protein: 85 grams

Fat: 37 grams
Saturated fat: 9 grams
Cholesterol: 302 milligrams
Sodium: 2,103 milligrams

Exchanges

Carbs: 14 (6 bread/starch, 4 fruit, 2 milk, 6 vegetable)
Meats: 4
Fats: 4

WEEK 4 DAY 1

Breakfast

1 cup cooked oatmeal mixed with
   1 tablespoon walnuts, 1 tablespoon
   ground flaxseed, and 2 teaspoons
   blackstrap molasses or jam

Snack

6–8 ounces low-fat plain or vanilla
   yogurt

Lunch

2 ounces grilled salmon on a bed of
   greens with 1 tablespoon low-fat
   dressing

1 whole grain roll or 1 serving of crackers

1 apple

Snack

1 orange

Dinner

1 serving Spicy Meatballs with Coconut Milk (page 371), served over
   1 cup whole wheat noodles or brown rice

1 cup steamed broccoli and yellow squash

Snack

1 cup 1% milk

3 small gingersnaps

WALK THIS WAY

*Week 4 walking goals:
Rookies—aim for 30
minutes a day. Walking
veterans—aim for 60
minutes or more a day.*

TAKE A TRANQUILITY BREAK

*Meditate on this thought
today: "Progress, not
perfection." To be a
perfectionist is to be
chronically dissatisfied.*

Daily Analysis

Calories: 1,488
Carbohydrate: 209
   grams
Fiber: 26 grams
Protein: 80 grams

Fat: 41 grams
Saturated fat: 15 grams
Cholesterol: 165
   milligrams
Sodium: 1,104 milligrams

Exchanges

Carbs: 14 (7 bread/starch,
   4 fruit, 2 milk, 4 vegetable)
Meats: 5
Fats: 3

WEEK 4 DAY 2

Breakfast

Breakfast smoothie: Blend 1 cup 1% milk or plain yogurt, 1 small banana, 1 tablespoon ground flaxseed, and ½ cup frozen berries until smooth.

Snack

1 rice cake spread with 1 teaspoon all-natural nut butter

Lunch

1 cup low-sodium split pea soup with ½ serving whole grain crackers

Large salad with 1 sliced hard-cooked egg and 2 tablespoons low-fat dressing

1 cup 1% milk

Snack

1 small pear

Dinner

1 serving Shrimp and Crab Cakes (page 387)

Spinach salad with 1 tablespoon low-fat dressing

½ cup coleslaw made with low-fat mayonnaise

1 slice whole grain bread

Snack

½ cup low-fat frozen dessert

WALK THIS WAY

Put on some weight. Walking with hand weights can strain your shoulders. A better way to burn more calories: Invest in a weighted vest for walkers; it will distribute weight equally.

TAKE A TRANQUILITY BREAK

Find a seasonal way to play today. If it's summertime, run through your sprinkler. If it's fall, rake up a pile of leaves and jump in them. In the winter, build a mini snowman and put him on your front stoop. You get the idea.

Daily Analysis

Calories: 1,578
Carbohydrate: 222 grams
Fiber: 30 grams
Protein: 79 grams
Fat: 48 grams

Saturated fat: 11 grams
Cholesterol: 372 milligrams
Sodium: 2,801 milligrams

Exchanges

Carbs: 14 (7 bread/starch, 4 fruit, 2 milk, 5 vegetable)
Meats: 4
Fats: 4

WEEK 4 DAY 3

Breakfast

1 serving Multigrain Cereal (page 319)

1 cup 1% milk

Snack

½ cup sliced pineapple

Lunch

Stuffed baked potato: Scoop out the flesh of a large baked potato. Mix with 1 ounce chicken, ½ cup vegetables (onions, broccoli, mushrooms) sautéed in cooking spray, 1 ounce sharp cheese or ½ cup cottage cheese, and 2 tablespoons salsa or low-fat sour cream. Spoon back into shell.

Snack

¾ cup Spicy Roasted Chickpeas (page 323)

Dinner

1 serving Mexican Lasagna (page 396)

Salad with 1 tablespoon low-fat dressing

1 cup fruit salad topped with 1 tablespoon chopped almonds and 2 tablespoons low-fat plain or vanilla yogurt

Snack

3 cups air-popped popcorn

WALK THIS WAY

Get wet on purpose. A good rain jacket will let you walk in the rain and stay dry—no more inclement-weather excuses!

TAKE A TRANQUILITY BREAK

Go fly a kite. Literally.

Daily Analysis

Calories: 1,463
Carbohydrate: 227 grams
Fiber: 33 grams
Protein: 72 grams
Fat: 35 grams

Saturated fat: 12 grams
Cholesterol: 105 milligrams
Sodium: 1,340 milligrams

Exchanges

Carbs: 14 (9 bread/starch, 3 fruit, 1 milk, 4 vegetable)
Meats: 5
Fats: 4

WEEK 4 DAY 4

Breakfast

Bean burrito: Fill the bottom of
1 whole grain tortilla with ½ cup
beans and 2 tablespoons salsa.
Sauté 2 egg whites, onions,
peppers, and mushrooms; add to
tortilla. Fold tortilla; top with
2 tablespoons low-fat plain yogurt
or low-fat sour cream.

Lunch

1 cup low-sodium minestrone soup

Turkey sandwich: 2 ounces turkey on
2 slices rye bread spread with
2 teaspoons mustard or low-fat
mayonnaise and topped with
lettuce, tomato, and onion (if
desired)

Snack

1½ cups edamame or other 80-calorie
snack

Dinner

1 serving Sizzling Beef Kebabs (page 373), served over ⅔ cup brown
rice pilaf

1 serving Avocado, Grapefruit, and Papaya Salad (page 349)

Snack

6–8 ounces low-fat plain or vanilla yogurt

WALK THIS WAY

*Breathe away stress.
During your warmup,
focus on taking air in
through your nose—
filling your belly and
then your rib cage and
chest—and then out
through your mouth.*

TAKE A TRANQUILITY BREAK

*Being playful is a great
way to calm your mind.
While you wait in the
checkout line at the
store, ponder a playful
question: "What if people
could read minds?" or
"What if men could give
birth?"*

Daily Analysis

Calories: 1,464
Carbohydrate: 203
    grams
Fiber: 49 grams
Protein: 88 grams

Fat: 40 grams
Saturated fat: 9 grams
Cholesterol: 89
    milligrams
Sodium: 1,731 milligrams

Exchanges

Carbs: 12 (8 bread/starch,
    1 fruit, 1 milk, 6 vegetable)
Meats: 5
Fats: 4

WEEK 4 DAY 5

Breakfast

- 1 slice whole grain toast spread with 1 teaspoon all-natural cashew butter and 1 teaspoon honey
- 6–8 ounces low-fat plain or vanilla yogurt

Snack

- ½ cup Spicy Roasted Chickpeas (page 323)

Lunch

- Hamburger on a whole grain roll spread with 1 teaspoon each mustard, ketchup, and relish and topped with lettuce, tomato, and onion (if desired)
- Tossed salad with ½ tablespoon low-fat dressing

Snack

- 3 medium fresh apricots or other 80-calorie snack

Dinner

- Orange Roughy Veracruz (page 390)
- 1 medium potato
- 1 serving Mustard-Crusted Brussels Sprouts (page 352)
- 1 cup 1% milk

Snack

- 1 small slice angel food cake topped with ½ cup strawberries and 2 tablespoons low-fat plain or vanilla yogurt

Daily Analysis

Calories: 1,564
Carbohydrate: 215 grams
Fiber: 28 grams
Protein: 88 grams
Fat: 45 grams

Saturated fat: 12 grams
Cholesterol: 117 milligrams
Sodium: 2,698 milligrams

Exchanges

Carbs: 13 (7 bread/starch, 2 fruit, 2 milk, 5 vegetable)
Meats: 5
Fats: 3

WEEK 4 DAY 6

Breakfast

Egg sandwich: Top a whole grain English muffin with 1 egg, prepared any style with cooking spray, and 1 slice lean ham or Canadian bacon

Snack

½ grapefruit

Lunch

2½ cups vegetable primavera: Sauté 1½ cups broccoli, carrots, onions, eggplant, and mushrooms in 1 tablespoon olive oil. Spread over 1 cup whole wheat penne pasta; sprinkle with 2 tablespoons Parmesan or Romano cheese

Snack

½ serving RyKrisp crackers spread with ¼ cup cottage cheese and sliced tomatoes

Dinner

1 serving Flounder Florentine (page 389)

Baked sweet potato with 2 teaspoons trans fat–free margarine or sour cream

½ cup carrots, roasted or steamed without fat

1 cup 1% milk

Snack

½ cup low-fat pudding

WALK THIS WAY

Waltz. Changing the rhythm of your walk boosts your energy. Instead of the usual two-count step, count in threes to a waltz rhythm. Silently chant Yes I can to keep time.

TAKE A TRANQUILITY BREAK

Go to the drugstore and select a card for someone who needs one. Write a short but loving message inside and mail it— today.

Daily Analysis

Calories: 1,546
Carbohydrate: 218 grams
Fiber: 31 grams
Protein: 84 grams
Fat: 41 grams

Saturated fat: 13 grams
Cholesterol: 322 milligrams
Sodium: 2,044 milligrams

Exchanges

Carbs: 12 (8 bread/starch, 1 fruit, 2 milk, 4 vegetable)
Meats: 6
Fats: 4

WEEK 4 DAY 7

Breakfast

1 serving Smoked Turkey Hash (page 318)

1 egg, prepared any style with cooking spray

1 slice whole grain toast

Lunch

1 serving Santa Fe Stuffed Sandwich (page 343)

1 serving Spinach-Orange Salad with Sesame (page 347)

Snack

½ ounce pistachios

Dinner

1 serving Chicken Tetrazzini (page 362)

2 servings Grilled Vegetables (page 352)

1 cup 1% milk

Snack

6 ounces low-fat plain or vanilla yogurt topped with ½ cup sliced strawberries

---

WALK THIS WAY

For a double dose of feel-good vibes, lend your feet to a good cause. Signing up for a charity walk will help you stick with your program—and give you the glow that comes from helping others.

TAKE A TRANQUILITY BREAK

Learn by heart a poem you've always loved.

Daily Analysis

Calories: 1,541
Carbohydrate: 189 grams
Fiber: 38 grams
Protein: 111 grams
Fat: 42 grams

Saturated fat: 11 grams
Cholesterol: 408 milligrams
Sodium: 2,492 milligrams

Exchanges

Carbs: 12 (4 bread/starch, 2 fruit, 2 milk, 10 vegetable)
Meats: 7
Fats: 3

7

SOLUTIONS FOR SPECIFIC BLOOD SUGAR PROBLEMS

CHAPTER 20

METABOLIC SYNDROME: YOUR ODDS ARE ONE IN FOUR

What if a single killer was responsible for the health conditions you fear most, including heart attack and stroke, infertility and diabetes, even Alzheimer's disease and cancer? What if you could easily fight back by dusting off your sneakers and grabbing an apple instead of a fast-food apple pie?

WOULDN'T YOUR DOCTOR TELL YOU?

The disease is real. Metabolic syndrome—out-of-whack blood sugar and high insulin levels brought on by too little exercise and too much belly fat—affects at least 51 million adults and children in America, the Centers for Disease Control and Prevention estimates. But the number could be as high as 140 million adults and another 10 million kids— virtually every overweight grown-up and child—because metabolic syndrome is tied directly to excess body fat and inactivity (stress and lack of sleep make it even worse). As Americans grow heavier and even less active, rates of metabolic syndrome are expected to rise. "This condition underlies some of the deadliest, most costly diseases we face," says Daniel Einhorn, MD, medical director of the Scripps Whittier

Institute for Diabetes in La Jolla, California. "Genetics plays a role, but 90 percent is the result of too many pounds and not enough exercise."

While experts call it one of the 21st century's biggest health crises, few of us are hearing about it from our family doctors. Yet.

It's a ticking time bomb, the toxic result of our crazy-busy, grab-a-snack, no-time-for-exercise, chained-to-the-computer lifestyles. "The health consequences may take 15 or 20 years to develop," says metabolic syndrome researcher C. Ronald Kahn, MD, president of the Joslin Diabetes Center in Boston. "Once, metabolic syndrome was a disease of old age. Today, it's starting at age 15 or 20 or 30 . . . and even in preteens. We're setting ourselves up for some very dramatic, widespread health impacts for people in the prime of life."

SHADOW EPIDEMIC OR SCANDAL?

There's a dangerous, double silence around metabolic syndrome. You can't see or feel it, and unless you're under the care of a cardiologist (heart doctors were among the first to realize its significance), an infertility specialist, or an especially astute family doctor, you may not hear about it from your physician anytime soon.

In the first place, there's no simple blood test and no symptoms. You must piece together a string of early warning signs, including an increasingly snug waistband on your favorite jeans, slightly high blood pressure, and slightly low levels of "good" HDL cholesterol.

Second, there's no drug to fix it. Pharmaceutical researchers are looking hard at several drugs with "magic bullet" potential—pills like the diabetes drugs rosiglitazone and metformin that might tame insulin levels early enough to prevent or at least significantly cut the risk for many major diseases at once. But for now, with no drug to tout, drugmakers seem unwilling to launch the kind of multi-million-dollar "health awareness campaign" for metabolic syndrome that's raised public consciousness about high cholesterol, asthma, and arthritis.

Another reason most docs are in the dark: Insulin resistance—the core problem in metabolic syndrome—first became an official medical diagnosis with a code number doctors could enter on insurance forms in 2002. "Even with a diagnosis code, there aren't any treatments yet that insurance companies will pay for; most don't cover weight loss or exercise," notes Yehuda Handelsman, medical director of the Metabolic Institute of America in Tarzana, California.

Metabolic syndrome is so new that experts can't even agree on a good name. Nobody's quite happy with the four in current use: metabolic syndrome, dysmetabolic syndrome, insulin resistance syndrome, and syndrome X.

RISK-CHECK QUIZ:
DO YOU HAVE METABOLIC SYNDROME?

There is no simple test for metabolic syndrome. Instead, experts look for a pattern of seemingly insignificant health problems that, when pieced together like a jigsaw puzzle, show that this killer condition is silently at work.

"These are all small signals that together can indicate a problem," says researcher Marie-Pierre St-Onge, PhD, assistant professor in the Division of Physiology and Metabolism at the University of Alabama at Birmingham. "Start by taking your waist measurement. If it's high, go to your doctor or to a blood pressure screening for a blood pressure check. If that's even slightly elevated, go ahead and get your cholesterol and triglycerides checked."

If you have three or more of these "little" health problems, you most likely have metabolic syndrome.

- A waist measurement of more than 35 inches if you're a woman, 40 inches if you're a man
- Blood pressure of 130/85 millimeters of mercury (mmHg) or higher
- Triglyceride levels of 150 milligrams per deciliter (mg/dl) or higher
- Low HDL levels—less than 50 mg/dl if you're a woman, less than 40 mg/dl if you're a man
- Fasting glucose level of 100 mg/dl or higher
- If you're at higher-than-normal genetic risk for metabolic syndrome (because you have a parent, sibling, aunt, or uncle with diabetes or are of Asian descent), your risk rises with a waist measurement of 31 to 35 inches if you're a woman, 35 to 37 inches if you're a man, the American Heart Association announced in late 2005.

For now, detecting metabolic syndrome requires looking for the right clues. "The important thing is that you or your doctor already have the information you need—your waist measurement, health history, family history, blood lipid test results. and blood pressure numbers—to figure out if you've got metabolic syndrome," Dr. Einhorn says. "But you'll probably have to ask your doctor to review them with you."

Individually, the early warnings seem almost insignificant—something to worry about someday when you're not so busy; maybe you hope they'll go away on their own. But here's why you should pay attention now: "If you've got the risk factors, you're in the danger zone already," Dr. Einhorn says. "Your insulin levels are already high, already doing damage."

The fix? Another do-it-yourself project. So far, the only steps proven to help everyone overcome metabolic syndrome are weight loss and regular exercise. Stress reduction and a good night's sleep will help, too.

WHEN CLEVER GENES WORK TOO WELL

In prehistoric times, insulin resistance may have been a famine survival tool, a genetic trick that kept blood sugar from being absorbed too quickly by hungry muscle cells and made it available for the brain and reproductive system. But when ancient genes collide with 21st-century lifestyles, the trick becomes a killer.

Normally, tiny amounts of insulin are enough to prompt muscle and liver cells to absorb sugar, their preferred fuel, after a meal. Insulin activates receptors on the cell's surface, sending a signal: "Hey, dinner's here! Come and get it!" The cell dispatches molecular pickup trucks called GLUT4 transporters to the surface to haul in the glucose.

But if you're overweight and inactive, as two out of three Americans now are, body fat interferes. "Fat is the culprit," says Sonia Caprio, MD, associate professor of endocrinology and pediatrics at Yale University School of Medicine. "As you become obese, even in children, immune fighters called macrophages surround fat tissue and release inflammatory compounds—chemical messengers like interleukin-6 and C-reactive protein—into the bloodstream. These interfere with insulin receptors on muscle and liver cells. And the receptors cannot signal properly."

The result: Insulin receptors are jammed, cells can't absorb glucose, and blood sugar levels rise. In desperation (because muscle and liver cells need sugar), tiny islet cells in your pancreas churn out more and more insulin to force hungry cells to take up the sugar. "It works," Dr. Einhorn says. "Lots of insulin forces cells to absorb the sugar. In fact, it works so well that your blood sugar levels can stay normal, or only slightly elevated, for decades." But, unseen and unfelt, insulin levels will be at dangerous levels, round the clock, for years.

Sitting around makes things worse. "Muscle contractions from physical activity can make cells absorb blood sugar regardless of insulin levels or insulin resistance," Caprio says. "If you don't get exercise, you're relying even more on insulin and insulin receptors to get sugar into cells."

A sedentary life full of stress and late nights is even worse: New research from Harvard and Duke Universities suggests that both lack of sleep and high anxiety exacerbate metabolic syndrome, perhaps by upping levels of stress hormones.

Smoking can also raise risk. In a new study of 3,649 men, risk for metabolic syndrome was 17 percent higher for those who smoked up to 20 cigarettes daily and 66 percent higher for those with a pack-and-a-half-a-day habit.

SMART SOLUTIONS: SIX WAYS TO PREVENT OR REVERSE METABOLIC SYNDROME

The best prescription for avoiding, or taming, metabolic syndrome isn't a drug at all—it's a healthy lifestyle, Dr. Einhorn says. Here's what works.

Trim a few pounds. Losing only 5 to 7 percent of your body weight is enough to boost insulin sensitivity. If you weigh 175 now, that's a loss of just 9 to 12 pounds.

Eat smarter carbs. In one recent study, insulin-resistant volunteers lost 15 pounds apiece, but only those who ate a healthy diet became less insulin resistant. On their plates: fruit, veggies, and grains that rank at the bottom of the glycemic index (GI), a system that rates foods based on their effect on blood sugar levels. Low-GI items such as beans, whole grains, veggies, and most fruits digest slowly and release sugar steadily into the bloodstream. High-GI items, such as cake and sweetened drinks, boost blood sugar—and insulin—fast.

Add fish and walnuts. Omega-3 fatty acids in salmon, sardines, white albacore tuna, and other fatty cold-water fish (and in walnuts and flaxseed) can raise your HDL while lowering your LDL and triglycerides—protecting you from metabolic syndrome's cardiovascular ravages.

Walk around the block. The benefits of exercise go beyond slimming: Activity quickly cuts blood sugar and insulin levels by forcing blood sugar into muscle cells. As little as 20 minutes of walking every day can help. "Anything is vastly better than nothing when it comes to exercise," Dr. Einhorn says.

Add strength training. Take a class at your local gym or invest in hand weights or resistance bands. Strength training makes cells obey insulin more readily by increasing the number of receptors that ferry blood sugar inside.

Stop smoking. By boosting insulin resistance, smoking raises the risk for heart disease, diabetes, and cancer even higher.

CHAPTER 21

PREDIABETES: MORE THAN A "TOUCH OF SUGAR"

D on't underestimate prediabetes. This "sweet nothing" is a *real* blood sugar problem.

You've got prediabetes if your blood glucose is higher than normal, yet too low to warrant a diagnosis of full-blown type 2 diabetes. Glucose levels in this gray area may seem like no big deal; you can't see or feel the extra sugar, and it's easy to hope it'll just go away by itself. Until recently, nobody seemed to worry much. Doctors downplayed prediabetes as "high-normal blood sugar" or "borderline diabetes," while people with this shadowy condition often shrugged it off as "just a touch of sugar."

Why you *should* pay attention: Prediabetes is the next step in the metabolic breakdown that leads to full-blown diabetes—a phase beyond insulin resistance and metabolic syndrome. While insulin resistance simply makes your cells ignore insulin's signals to absorb blood sugar (prompting your body to pump out more insulin), in prediabetes, a second problem develops: Your body no longer can make enough insulin to force cells to absorb blood sugar.

Prediabetes is reversible. But ignore it, and your odds for developing full-blown diabetes within a decade are nearly 100 percent, warns the American Diabetes Association. Prediabetes also dumps enough extra glucose into your bloodstream to damage blood vessels and nerves, setting the stage for horrific diabetic complications including blindness, kidney failure, infections and amputation, and puts you in a red alert risk category for fatal heart attacks and stroke, sobering new research reveals.

"By the time most people are diagnosed with type 2 diabetes, they've usually had prediabetes for 10 to 15 years and undiagnosed diabetes for another 5 to 10 years," says Anne Peters, MD, director of the University of Southern California's clinical diabetes programs. "By then, the progression that leads to higher and higher blood sugar levels and more serious complications is pretty far along. That's why it's so important to be tested early."

RISK CHECK: YOUR PREDIABETES ODDS

Your chances for prediabetes rise if you:

- Have heart disease risks. In one European study of 39,000 women and men with cardiovascular risks including high blood pressure, low HDL cholesterol, and high LDL cholesterol, one in four had prediabetes.
- Are overweight or obese. If your body mass index is higher than 29, your odds for prediabetes are one in four.
- Are of African American, Hispanic, Native American, Asian, or Pacific Islander descent. Your risk may be double that of white Americans.
- Are over age 45. The CDC estimates that 40 percent of middle-aged and older Americans have prediabetes.

- Have a family history of diabetes. Having parents, siblings, or even aunts, uncles, and grandparents with diabetes indicates that at least one diabetes gene may run in your family. New research shows that nearly half of all Americans have at least one gene that raises risk.
- Have a history of gestational diabetes or had a baby weighing more than 9 pounds at birth. Women in this group have a 20 to 50 percent chance of developing prediabetes within 10 years after pregnancy.
- Had a low birth weight. People who weighed less than 5.5 pounds at birth are at 23 percent higher risk; weighing under 5 pounds raises risk by 76 percent.

The good news: If you have prediabetes, you can cut your risk for progressing from prediabetes to full-blown diabetes by 60 percent *without drugs*—and protect your nerves, blood vessels, and organs against high blood sugar's assault. In the landmark Diabetes Prevention Program study of 3,234 Americans with prediabetes, those who lost just 7 percent of their body weight (about 10 pounds if you now weigh 150), exercised for half an hour 5 days a week, and followed a diet high in fiber and low in saturated fat cut their risk significantly. In fact, this simple plan—a mirror image of the *Sugar Solution* eating plan—was more effective at stopping the progression of prediabetes than the diabetes drug metformin, researchers found.

"Every year a person can live free of diabetes means an added year of life free of the suffering, disability, and the medical costs incurred by this disease," says Edward Horton, MD, director of clinical research at Boston's Joslin Diabetes Center and principal investigator of the Joslin arm of the DPP.

FROM BELLY FAT TO BETA CELLS

An estimated 41 million Americans probably have prediabetes, twice as many as in the year 2001, the Centers for Disease Control and Prevention estimates.

You've got prediabetes if your blood sugar is between 100 and 125 milligrams of glucose per deciliter of blood (mg/dl) on a fasting blood sugar test (in which you don't eat for 8 to 12 hours before a blood sample is drawn) or between 140 and 199 mg/dl on a glucose tolerance test. This longer check, considered a more accurate and sensitive measure of prediabetes, involves fasting and then drinking a glucose-rich beverage. A blood sample drawn 2 hours later helps your doctor check how well your body handles blood sugar after a meal.

"I call this the Rodney Dangerfield of human diseases. It doesn't get any respect," says John Buse, MD, PhD, CDE (certified diabetes educator), associate professor of medicine at the University of North Carolina School of Medicine in Chapel Hill, and director of the university's Diabetes Care Center. That's because even doctors underestimate the importance of prediabetes.

The trouble begins with insulin resistance and metabolic syndrome, early blood sugar control problems linked to inactivity and overeating. "Overweight, a high-fat diet, and visceral fat all intertwine to produce insulin resistance," says Dr. Buse. "People who are insulin resistant are storing excess dietary fat in all kinds of inappropriate places, such as in muscle cells and in the liver, which makes it harder for their body to use sugar as fuel."

Insulin levels rise higher and higher as your body tries to force cells to absorb blood sugar. Then prediabetes adds a new twist: After years of overwork, the insulin-producing beta cells in your pancreas begin to give out, and blood sugar begins to rise. Beta cell burnout is even more dangerous than insulin resistance for one simple reason: It's irreversible.

Genetics plays a key role in how soon beta cells cry uncle. And America's obesity epidemic means that beta cell burnout—once a problem for senior citizens—is happening earlier and earlier. In one recent study of overweight kids, researchers from the Keck School of Medicine of the University of Southern California found signs of it among preteens.

A high-sugar diet may hurt beta cells. Fat counts, too. Lab studies at the University of California, San Diego, School of Medicine recently found that a high-fat diet suppresses an enzyme, called GnT-4a glycosyltransferase, that helps beta cells sense blood sugar levels and make the right amount of insulin. "This molecular trigger begins the chain of events leading from hyperglycemia to insulin resistance and type 2 diabetes," says lead researcher Jamey Marth, PhD, professor of cellular and molecular medicine at UCSD and investigator with the Howard Hughes Medical Institute. "This finding suggests new approaches to the prevention and treatment of diabetes."

Undercover Complications

Until recently, experts thought high blood sugar wasn't a problem at prediabetic levels. Now, there's chilling proof that all the major complications of diabetes begin brewing during prediabetes. Among them:

A 1.5-fold increase in cardiovascular disease and a higher risk

THE SUGAR SURVIVORS: Maureen Marinelli

In 1998, Maureen Marinelli was diagnosed with impaired glucose tolerance, a symptomless condition in which blood sugar rises higher than normal—enough to put you at risk of serious complications but not quite high enough to fit current definitions of type 2 diabetes.

Her lifestyle was one big risk factor. A US Postal Service employee and official for the letter carriers union in Boston, Marinelli, 49, spent her days embroiled in hardball politics and delicate contract negotiations. At home, she was a single mother raising a teenage son.

"It's an understatement to say that my life was stressful," she says. "I ate on the run; my idea of a good lunch was a quarter-pound cheeseburger, fries, and a large soda. I weighed 189 and had high cholesterol, high blood pressure, and reflux from all the stress." Too often, late-night stress relief was a pack of cupcakes or a bag of barbecue potato chips. And she barely had time for her passion, tap dancing.

With the help of a nutrition- and-lifestyle counselor, Marinelli lost 18 pounds. She now eats more fruits, veggies, and whole grains and tap-dances two or three times a week. As a result, she expects to keep her risk of diabetes and heart disease in the normal range for life.

"I feel good about what I'm doing," she says. "I have more energy. I'm protecting my health. I'm no saint, but now when I go to the drive-thru, I get a small cheeseburger and a diet soda."

for fatal heart attack and stroke. As we explored in Chapter 20, the high insulin levels, high blood pressure, inflammation, extra risk of blood clots, and out-of-whack blood fats of metabolic syndrome raise heart attack and stroke risk. The risk rises still higher when blood sugar goes up. Why? Researchers believe that extra sugar stiffens blood vessels, makes particles of "bad" LDL cholesterol stickier and more likely to form plaques in artery walls, creates a flood of cell-damaging free radicals, and suppresses levels of heart-healthy HDL cholesterol while it raises levels of risky triglycerides.

Vision-threatening damage to tiny capillaries in your eyes. About 8 percent of people with prediabetes had signs of diabetic retinopathy in a recent NIH study. "Changes in the eye may be starting earlier and at lower glucose levels than we previously thought," notes researcher Richard Hamman, MD, DrPH, professor and chair of the department of preventive medicine and biometrics at the University of Colorado School of Medicine.

Nerve damage. Researchers for the University of Michigan Health System reported recently that 30 to 50 percent of their patients who complain of tingling, burning, or numbness in the hands and feet also have prediabetes.

Kidney damage. High blood pressure, high cholesterol, and high blood sugar may combine in early diabetes to produce early signs of kidney damage, report scientists from the National Institutes of Health and Harvard Medical School. In a 7-year study of 2,398 women and men, they found that those with prediabetes were 65 percent more likely to develop kidney disease than those without it.

Stop Prediabetes Today

In 2001, an overjoyed Tommy G. Thompson—then US Secretary of Health and Human Services—made a surprising announcement: In a landmark study of over 3,000 people with prediabetes, those who lost a little weight, walked briskly for a half hour 5 days a week, and ate a healthy diet low in saturated fat yet high in fiber cut their odds for developing type 2 diabetes by 58 to 71 percent. In contrast, study volunteers who took a drug, metformin (Glucophage), saw diabetes risk drop by just 30 percent. "In view of the rapidly rising rates of obesity and diabetes in America, this good news couldn't come at a better time," said Thompson.

Since then, researchers have continued to study volunteers who participated in the Diabetes Prevention Program. A new analysis of DPP data by University of Michigan statisticians suggests that a healthy lifestyle can delay the development of diabetes by 11 years. Meanwhile, in a similar study conducted in Finland, researchers have found that people who lost weight and exercised still had a significantly lower risk for diabetes 10 years later.

SMART SOLUTIONS
The *Sugar Solution* Plan for Fighting Prediabetes

Don't wait! Experts say the easy steps below can reverse high-normal blood sugar.

Get tested. Have your blood sugar tested now and again in 6 months to a year to see if there's been a change.

Lose weight. In the Finnish study, even extremely overweight people lowered their risk of diabetes by 70 percent when they lost just 5 percent of their total weight—even if they didn't exercise.

Trim the fat. Aim for less than 30 percent of total daily calories from fat and less than 10 percent from saturated fat, the kind in meat and full-fat dairy products.

Eat smarter carbs. This means carbohydrate foods such as fruits, vegetables, and whole grain cereals and breads that are rich in vitamins, minerals, and especially fiber, which studies show may help lower blood sugar by slowing the digestive process and, hence, how fast glucose enters the bloodstream.

Go for seven to nine. *Prevention* recommends nine servings of fruits and vegetables a day. Try to make at least half of your grain choices (including breads, rice, and pasta) whole grain to raise your fiber intake still higher.

Walk on your lunch break. DPP study volunteers walked for just 150 minutes a week—a half hour 5 days a week.

Be accountable. In the DPP and the Finnish study, volunteers kept a daily record of what and how much they ate, along with their diet's fat content—and it proved key in helping them achieve their dietary goals.

CHAPTER 22

DIABETES: THE NEW AMERICAN EPIDEMIC

Don Werkstell's motto is "check, check, and recheck." A former Department of Homeland Security inspector, he made sure that cargo flying in and out of terminal A at Dallas–Fort Worth Airport posed no threats. Diagnosed with type 2 diabetes in 2004, he now applies the same "check and check again" philosophy to his own blood sugar.

"I have to know what my numbers are. It's the only way to keep my blood sugar low and avoid all the complications of diabetes," says Werkstell. "I check my blood sugar all the time and guide my exercise and food choices by it. And every few months, I get a long-term test called an A1c. Diabetes runs in my family. I've seen what can happen if you don't take care of yourself."

Most of the 21 million Americans with type 2 diabetes aren't as "in control" as Werkstell. Despite government-sponsored health campaigns and newspaper and TV headlines, most of us are still in diabetes denial.

- One-third of all Americans with diabetes don't know they have it.
- Among those who do, most are still in danger. In mid-2005, a stunning new survey of 157,000 diabetic women and men revealed that while 85 percent think they're keeping the lid on high blood sugar, two out of three actually have dangerously high levels that can lead

to kidney failure, blindness, amputation, deadly heart attacks, and stroke. The survey was commissioned by the American Academy of Clinical Endocrinologists.

- When Harvard Medical School researchers recently checked up on diabetes care at 30 of the nation's top university medical centers, they uncovered shocking neglect. Half the time, people with diabetes were sent home without the medicines they needed to lower dangerously rising blood sugar—leaving them at unnecessary risk for complications.

What's gone wrong? People with diabetes—and their doctors—underestimate the urgent need to keep blood sugar tightly controlled via diet, exercise, stress reduction, regular blood sugar checks, and medication if necessary.

In fact, a new University of California, Los Angeles, study underscores the power of diet for people with diabetes. In this small, controlled 3-week study, 6 of 13 overweight or obese men with type 2 diabetes finished *diabetes-free,* with normal blood sugar levels. How? With meals that were low in fat (12 to 15 percent of calories), moderate in protein (12 to 25 percent), and high in carbs (65 to 70 percent). Participants also walked for 45 to 60 minutes a day. But eating low-fat foods and no refined carbs—absolutely no toaster pastries or brownies—was critical to their success, says researcher Christian Roberts, PhD, the author of the study. He predicts that sticking to the diet long-term may undo heart damage associated with diabetes.

But if you've had diabetes for a few years, diet may not be enough.

"Every time you see your doctor about your diabetes, you should discuss how well your treatment plan is working and whether it needs to be changed," says Kenneth J. Snow, MD, acting chief of the Adult Diabetes Division at the Joslin Diabetes Center in Boston. "You can't judge your diabetes by the number of pills you take. You should gauge it by your blood sugar—and by how well your treatment plan mix of diet, exercise, and medication is working to keep it low."

Cutting-edge diabetes treatment calls for aggressive care, particularly for the millions of people whose diabetes developed earlier in life, says Anne Peters, MD, director of the University of Southern California's clinical diabetes program and author of *Conquering Diabetes: A Cutting-Edge, Comprehensive Program for Prevention and Treatment*. "If your doctor seems behind the curve, ask what's going on. This is especially important if you're in your thirties, forties, fifties, or even your sixties. If your diabetes is diagnosed when you're younger or if you plan on living a long life, there's less room for error. High blood sugar is more dangerous when it goes on for years and years."

If your blood sugar is higher than your target goals, your doctor should be talking about a revised treatment plan, Dr. Peters says. If he or she doesn't bring it up, you should.

DIABETES 101

You've got type 2 diabetes if your blood sugar is over 125 milligrams of glucose per deciliter of blood (mg/dl) on a fasting blood sugar test, or over 190 mg/dl on an oral glucose tolerance test (in which you fast, then consume a sugary beverage and take a blood test 2 hours later). If your blood sugar has soared to these levels, it means that nearly every aspect of your body's blood sugar control system has been damaged at a cellular level.

Diabetes is the last stop in a decades-long series of breakdowns in that system. Here's how the progression from normal blood sugar to diabetes unfolds: Thanks to a powerful combination of genetics, overweight, inactivity, abdominal fat, and stress, cells throughout your body first become insulin resistant—ignoring this vital hormone's signals to absorb blood sugar. To compensate, beta cells in your pancreas crank out extra insulin. Finally, beta cells wear out. Insulin production drops; blood sugar rises. At first, sugar levels are only slightly higher than normal, a condition called prediabetes. But finally, as more beta cells cease functioning, your blood sugar rises to officially diabetic levels.

Many people discover their diabetes only after years of undetected high blood sugar has led to outward symptoms. Fatigue, thirst, getting up frequently at night to use the bathroom, frequent infections and slow-healing wounds, sexual difficulties (such as vaginal dryness and erection problems), and digestion trouble (diarrhea, vomiting, and slow digestion, all due to nerve damage) are all warning signs of type

2 diabetes. (If you have any of these problems, call your doctor and schedule a blood sugar test!)

Once diagnosed, you're in a whole new world. Suddenly, you must learn to operate a blood sugar meter—and find room for it in your purse and in your busy schedule. Meals morph into arithmetic problems if you're trying to control blood sugar by counting carbohydrate grams or exchanges. And the pills! You might take one, two, or even 10 to 15 medications to lower your blood sugar and protect against diabetes-related heart risks such as high blood pressure and high cholesterol. You need to worry about your feet (even the smallest bump or cut could lead to a major infection), your eyes (high blood sugar can lead to vision problems), your kidneys (excess blood sugar can lead to kidney failure), and more. Small wonder, then, that people with diabetes report feeling more stressed and depressed.

The Sugar Solution's glucose-lowering strategy can help you feel in control again. Here's what to do.

SMART SOLUTIONS: A 3-STEP BLOOD SUGAR CONTROL PLAN
Step 1: Eat Right, Exercise . . . and Relax!

Luscious fruits, fresh veggies, whole grains, good fats, lean meats, and a minimum of refined carbohydrates: The foundations of the *Sugar Solution* eating plan can help you tame high blood sugar quickly, effectively, and deliciously. The meals suggested in this book even contain exchange-list information for people with diabetes who use that type of system to stay on track with healthy eating.

"Start with the fundamentals," says endocrinologist Richard Hellman, MD, a clinical professor of medicine at the University of Missouri/Kansas City School of Medicine and medical director of the Heart of America Diabetes Research Foundation. "The foundation of good diabetes care is always a healthy diet and regular exercise. Often, if you see your blood sugar levels slipping on daily checks, it's because of that. Even if you need more medication, your diet still helps because it can help prevent weight gain, supplies important nutrients, and will still have an impact on your blood sugar. Exercise helps muscle cells become more insulin-sensitive."

THE SUGAR SURVIVORS: Maggie Lopez

Maggie Lopez of Port Orange, Florida, had symptoms of type 2 diabetes—and, with her Hispanic heritage and ample waistline, a host of risk factors. "I was tired and thirsty all the time, and I always seemed to have to visit the bathroom," says the operations supervisor of a call center.

Because she was still in her thirties, Lopez, now 42, never suspected diabetes. But her doctor did and ordered a blood test. The diagnosis: type 2. The treatment: weight loss and healthy eating.

Lopez received a crash course in healthy living. She cut down on bread, rice, and other starches and chose healthy meals when she ate at restaurants. She also began walking 30 minutes each day after work.

That was 5 years ago. Today, Lopez is 32 pounds lighter and feels better than she has since high school. She takes an oral diabetes medication, rosiglitazone maleate (Avandia), and monitors her blood sugar at least twice a day.

Motivated by his wife, Lopez's 5-foot-7-inch, 270-pound husband, Salvador, had his blood sugar tested and was also diagnosed with type 2. "He's lost about 50 pounds since he was diagnosed and feels great," says Lopez. And her daughter, 19-year-old Elizabeth, is also more careful about what she eats. Says Lopez, "Being diagnosed has been a blessing in disguise."

Here's how to tailor the plan to fit your needs:

Talk with a registered dietitian or certified diabetes educator. Many insurance plans, including Medicare, cover at least one visit. These food specialists can help you customize the carbohydrate levels and portion sizes to meet your body size and unique blood sugar processing "style." They can also help you make the plan fit your lifestyle.

Fit exercise into your day, your way. In Chapter 14, you'll find several walking programs, plus lots of ways to identify activities that match your personality. We urge you to include 10 to 15 minutes of strengthening exercises each day (or two or three longer sessions each week) to build muscle mass that burns more blood sugar, around the clock. Why not keep dumbbells and/or resistance bands near the TV, so you can fit in your strengthening routine while you watch your favorite shows?

Take advantage of the spa effect. Cutting stress reduced blood sugar significantly in one Duke University study of 108 people with type 2 diabetes. Those who took a stress-reduction class lowered their A1c levels by as much as 1 point. Learning to say *ahhh* not only gives you a blood sugar advantage but also makes you feel great. Lead researcher Richard Surwit, PhD, suggests these stress-less techniques: yoga, mindfulness-based stress reduction, a relaxing hobby, and progressive relaxation. Cutting back on caffeine can also help; the jolt in coffee and even tea can raise stress hormones and blood sugar levels.

Step 2: Check Your Blood Sugar Every Day, and Your A1c Level Two to Four Times a Year

To stay healthy and avoid complications, you need tight blood sugar control. How do you know if your diet, exercise, and medication plan is really working? By testing your blood sugar every day with your blood sugar meter—and seeing your doctor several times a year for an A1c test, which reveals your average blood sugar for the past 2 to 3 months.

"Daily checks and A1c tests look at blood sugar in two very different ways," says Francine Kaufman, MD, former president of the American Diabetes Association, head of the Center for Diabetes and Endocrinology at Childrens Hospital Los Angeles, and author of *Diabesity: The Obesity-Diabetes Epidemic That Threatens America—And What We Must Do to Stop It*. "A daily test is a snapshot. Taken with a blood sugar meter, it tells you what your level is at one moment. It's very useful for finding out how high your blood sugar is at key times of day—first thing in the morning before you eat, before a meal, after exercise—or to see how well your body handles the natural rise in blood sugar after you eat."

In contrast, Dr. Kaufman says, the A1c is like a full-length movie. It tells you what's happened, on average, to your blood sugar over the past 2 to 3 months.

"With results of both tests, you can see if there's a disconnect between your diabetes management plan and your real blood sugar levels," Dr. Kaufman explains. "What if your daily checks look good, but your A1c is high? You may discover that the meter you use for daily checks isn't working right or that there's a time of day when your sugar's much higher than you ever realized. You may need to alter your medication dosage, adjust the size of your meals or your food choices, work on lowering stress, or resolve to exercise more. If you weren't getting A1c checks every few months, you'd never know there was a problem."

An A1c test measures the amount of sugar attached to hemoglobin in your bloodstream. Found inside red blood cells, hemoglobin carries oxygen from your lungs to cells throughout your body. But it also links up with sugars such as blood glucose along the way. Like Christmas cookies rolled in sweet sprinkles, hemoglobin picks up more and more sugar if there's an excess in your blood. Research confirms that every one-point rise in your A1c level significantly raises your risk for heart attack; stroke; and damage to eyes, kidneys, and nerves. An A1c above 7 percent raises heart attack risk 25 percent, ups stroke risk 30 percent, triples your chances of nerve damage in legs and feet, and raises odds

OUCHLESS TESTING

If blood sugar checks hurt, these strategies could help.

- Adjust your blood sugar meter so that the lancet penetrates as little skin as possible.
- Use a fresh lancet for each test. Reused lancets grow dull and hurt. (Medicare and private insurance usually cover the cost of lancets, so there's no need to save money by reusing them again and again.)
- Try taking your blood sample from your palm or the side of your finger instead of your finger pads. Some meters can also test on your thigh or upper arm.
- Be patient. Checking your blood sugar may soon be as simple as slicing an onion. A new study from India reveals that tears may be just as effective as blood samples at tracking blood sugar levels. The discovery will allow researchers to develop a new kind of test strip that could measure blood sugar levels simply by being placed near the corner of the eye.

for nerve damage in the eyes by up to 50 percent. Every one-point drop in your A1c cuts your risk for complications by up to 41 percent.

But daily tests are important, too. "The A1c cannot give you the quick results you need to see if a new sugar control strategy is working," Dr. Kaufman says. "You need to know right away if your medication is effective, whether a new food raises your levels too high, or how physical activity impacts your blood sugar. Everyone's body is different. Daily tests let you see just how your body is reacting, so that you can fine-tune your plan." Here's how to get the most from this testing strategy.

Daily Blood Sugar Check(s)

When to check: Work with your doctor. If you've just been diagnosed or are starting a new medication, you may need to test three to six times a day. If your treatment is working well, you may need fewer checks. Smart tip: If you test just once or twice a day, check at different times on different days. That will give you a more complete idea of how your sugar levels rise and fall.

Shoot for these numbers: For a fasting test (such as first thing in the morning) or before a meal: 90–130 mg/dl; 2 hours after a meal: less than 180 mg/dl.

Best test equipment: A glucose monitor that's less than 2 or 3 years old or an older meter that's been calibrated with your doctor's help. "After a while, meters wear out," says Karmeen Kulkarni, MS, RD, CDE, president of the ADA's health care and education program and a certified diabetes educator at St. Mark's Hospital in Salt Lake City. "New meters have some great features—you can store your previous readings, then download them into your computer, for example."

Cost: Meters may cost as little as $10 for a very basic model to more than $300 for a sleek version that doubles as a personal digital assistant (PDA). Supplies, such as lancets for drawing blood and test strips, cost extra. Money-saving tip: Check with your insurance company to see which meters they cover or how much they'll kick in. Some insurers also cover the cost of test strips.

Smart test tip: Write your results down. If you don't use a meter that automatically records your readings, keep a blood sugar log of the date, time of day, and whether it's a fasting reading or after a meal. Add

HIGH STAKES

A growing stack of research confirms that keeping your A1c level in a healthy range (experts recommend a reading of 6.5 to 7 percent for people with diabetes, lower if possible) is a powerful, effective strategy for sidestepping a host of serious, scary complications. This test measures average blood sugar for the last 2 to 3 months. Here's how a high A1c threatens your health.

Heart trouble. In a recent British study of 10,232 women and men with type 2 diabetes, University of Cambridge researchers found that every one-point increase in HBA1c levels raised heart disease risk 24 percent for men and 28 percent for women. Other research shows that it doubles heart failure risk.

Brain attacks. The same study found that stroke risk rose 30 percent when HBA1c levels rose above 7 and tripled at levels above 10.

Amputation. Tulane University scientists found in a recent study of 4,526 women and men that an HBA1c over 7 triples the risk for peripheral vascular disease—the nerve damage responsible for foot and leg amputations among people with diabetes.

Blindness. In a study of 11,247 women and men, researchers from the International Diabetes Institute in Australia found that the odds for retinopathy—damage to the tiny blood vessels inside the retina—rose 25 percent when A1c levels were over 7.5 percent for up to 4 years, and 50 percent when A1c remained high more than 8 years.

Kidney damage and failure. The higher your A1c, the greater the odds for kidney failure, say Israeli researchers who found that high blood sugar, high blood pressure, and high cholesterol levels all raise kidney risk for people with diabetes.

The bright side. You're in control. University of Oxford scientists say that reducing your A1c (by tightening your blood sugar control) cuts all of these risks dramatically. A one-point drop in your A1c level will reduce heart attack risk 14 percent, lower heart failure risk 16 percent, cut stroke risk 21 percent, cut risk for amputation due to peripheral vascular disease by 41 percent, and reduce risk for blindness or kidney failure by 35 percent.

comments about factors that could have influenced your reading, such as a stressful experience, a just-completed exercise routine, or a new food (or a splurge). Take your records to every diabetes checkup so your doctor can review them with you.

A1c Test

When to check: Every 2 to 3 months if your blood sugar is high. If it's been under tight control for a long time (at least a year), your doctor may OK twice-yearly A1c checks.

Shoot for this number: An A1c reading of 6.5 to 7. "Normal A1c levels for people without diabetes are 6 percent or lower," says diabetes specialist Jaime A. Davidson, MD, of the Dallas-based Endocrine and Diabetes Associates of Texas. "The closer to normal, the better, but be reasonable. If your A1c is high and you bring it down even somewhat, you've reduced your risk for complications."

Best test equipment: The kind at your doctor's office or a commercial lab. Home A1c tests are available for about $25, but experts recommend lab tests. You get more consistent results, your doctor reads the report, and she can help chart your progress.

Cost: Forty dollars at a private lab. Insurance may cover most or all of the cost.

Smart test tip: Many doctors test A1c levels just once a year. Ask about more frequent checks, Davidson suggests, especially if you've started a new medicine or have difficulty keeping your daily blood sugar under control.

Step 3: Update Your Attitude about Diabetes Medications

"Most people with type 2 diabetes will need more medications as time goes by—and it's not their fault," says Kenneth J. Snow, MD, acting chief of the Adult Diabetes Division at Boston's Joslin Diabetes Center. "It's just the natural progression of diabetes. But doctors don't always explain this, and people are very surprised and troubled when it happens."

It's important to understand that diabetes *does* progress. With type 2 diabetes, insulin-producing cells in your pancreas dwindle; as insulin levels fall, blood sugar continues to rise. When British scientists tracked this process in a group of 4,075 women and men with newly diagnosed type 2 diabetes, they found that 75 percent needed several drugs to control blood sugar after 9 years. Just 9 percent kept their blood sugar within a safe range with diet and exercise alone. The researchers concluded that in less than 10 years after diagnosis, most people with type 2 will need insulin shots to keep blood sugar low.

Diet, exercise, and stress reduction are fundamentals of good diabetes care. But when you need more help, ask for it. "Every time you see your doctor about your diabetes, you should discuss how well your treatment plan is working and whether it needs to be changed," Dr. Snow says. Don't wait for your doctor to suggest an adjustment. In a 12-year study of 570 diabetics, researchers at Kaiser Permanente Northwest found that doctors often delayed for months or years before upgrading the treatment plans of diabetes patients with high blood sugar.

CHAPTER 23

POLYCYSTIC OVARY SYNDROME: THE HIDDEN FERTILITY ROBBER

Stubborn extra pounds. Erratic menstrual cycles. Acne. Infertility. And a big hair problem: It's thinning up on top yet growing luxuriantly on your face and body. Like the pieces of a strange puzzle, the warning signs and symptoms of polycystic ovary syndrome (PCOS) don't seem to add up to a single medical problem.

For most of the 20th century, doctors treated the individual symptoms of PCOS as unrelated medical problems. That changed in 1976, when researchers stumbled upon a pair of common denominators—high insulin levels and insulin resistance—that have changed the way PCOS is diagnosed and treated. "High insulin isn't the only factor in PCOS, but it is very important," says infertility specialist Sandra Carson, MD, a reproductive endocrinologist and PCOS researcher at Baylor College of Medicine in Houston. "It may act on the ovaries to increase male hormones. The end result is that you stop ovulating, gain weight, develop acne, and can even have abnormal face and body hair." Over the long term, it also raises your risk for diabetes, heart disease, and several forms of cancer.

Serious stuff. Yet most PCOS is never diagnosed or treated—despite the fact that it's the most widespread hormonal problem faced by American women, affecting up to 13 million. "One in 10 reproductive-age women in the United States suffers from PCOS, but up to three-fourths are unaware they have it," says endocrinologist Rhoda H. Cobin, MD, a clinical professor of medicine at Mount Sinai School of Medicine in New York City and past president of the American Association of Clinical Endocrinologists. "It is important to alert these women to the serious health complications associated with PCOS. Early detection and careful management can prevent many from occurring."

And it's no longer a problem for grown women only. The childhood obesity epidemic has led to another emerging health problem: an increase in the number of *young* girls developing PCOS, the American Association of Clinical Endocrinologists recently warned. Early weight gain can prompt early menstrual periods, raising risk for PCOS and ovulation problems. "PCOS usually was diagnosed in women in their twenties and thirties. This unfolding epidemic is putting girls as young as 11 years old at risk for serious health complications," says John Nestler, MD, chair of the division of endocrinology and metabolism in the Virginia Commonwealth University School of Medicine. Adolescent girls with PCOS are also at significant risk for metabolic syndrome and type 2 diabetes.

THE BLOOD SUGAR CONNECTION

The PCOS threat is far-reaching. Among women with PCOS, 80 percent are insulin resistant, 33 percent have prediabetes, and 10 percent will develop type 2 diabetes before the age of 40, say researchers from the University of Chicago. PCOS can be a killer, raising your lifetime risk for diabetes 7 to 10 times higher than normal, doubling your odds for a heart attack or stroke, and leaving you more vulnerable to cancers of the breast and uterine lining, among others.

New research reveals the following risks.

Heart-threatening inflammation: In a study of 210 women, nearly 40 percent of those with PCOS had danger-zone levels of an inflammatory compound called C-reactive protein, compared with less than 10 percent of women without PCOS, report scientists from Israel's Rambam Medical Center in Haifa. C-reactive protein raises risk for clogged arteries, blood clots, and high blood pressure.

Clogged arteries: University of Pittsburgh cardiologists who scanned the neck arteries of 267 young women (ages 30 to 44) found a tenfold higher risk for dangerous plaque in artery walls of study volunteers with PCOS. Clogged carotid arteries are a potent marker for heart disease risk.

Metabolic syndrome: PCOS doubles your risk for metabolic syndrome, a cluster of heart-threatening health problems including high blood pressure, high triglycerides, and low levels of heart-protecting HDL cholesterol, say Virginia Commonwealth University endocrinologists who discovered the risk after screening 161 women with PCOS. "Women with PCOS should automatically be screened for the metabolic syndrome to prevent the risk of early onset cardiovascular disease," says lead study author John Nestler, MD.

Sleep apnea: University of Chicago researchers who checked 40 women with PCOS found that 75 percent were at high risk for sleep apnea. These women also had higher levels of insulin, a risk factor for diabetes.

Cancer: PCOS can triple your risk for cancer of the endometrium, the lining of the uterus. Research also suggests that PCOS could raise your risk for breast cancer three to four times above normal.

THE MANY FACES OF PCOS

Some women with PCOS have warning signs that start with adolescence, such as irregular menstrual periods. Others have no obvious symptoms—until infertility or miscarriage makes their hopes for motherhood difficult to attain. PCOS can cause a host of problems, including those listed here.

Menstrual trouble: You may have irregular bleeding (including lengthy bleeding episodes, scant or heavy periods, or spotting), infrequent periods (cycles are often more than 6 weeks apart), or amenorrhea—no periods at all.

Chronic pelvic pain: Polycystic ovaries, sometimes three times bigger than normal, can lead to the feeling of pelvic fullness and pelvic pain during intercourse.

Bloating and fluid retention: Due to a complex interplay of hormones affecting fluid balance, many women with PCOS experience persistent premenstrual syndrome.

Abnormal growth of facial and body hair: Known as hirsutism, this growth commonly appears where women don't want it—the face, neck, chest, abdomen, thumbs, toes, and sideburns.

Loss of scalp hair: Thinning is usually most evident at the top of the head rather than as a receding hairline.

Oily skin, acne, and dandruff: Elevated androgen levels can cause the skin to produce excess sebum, a waxy goo that can clog the pores and cause pimples, blackheads, and inflammation. It can also make the skin on the scalp flaky, producing dandruff.

Skin problems: A woman with PCOS can develop skin tags—benign, hormonally induced growths that resemble grains of puffed rice—on her neck, eyelids, armpits, upper chest, and groin. Or she may develop acanthosis nigricans—dark patches of skin that appear under her breasts or on her neck, armpits, elbows, knees, hands, or groin. These dark patches are a hallmark of high insulin levels and may fade as insulin sensitivity improves.

Infertility: If you've tried to conceive for 6 to 12 months without success and have any of the other symptoms listed here, talk with your doctor.

Obesity: The extra pounds associated with PCOS often settle in the abdomen, giving a woman with the condition a distinctive apple-shaped figure. It's now known that "apples" have a higher risk of heart disease and type 2 diabetes than "pears"—women who carry their weight in their hips and thighs.

Diagnosis, Please

If you think you might have PCOS, take our quiz on page 288. Then see your doctor. She will first rule out other health problems that can cause PCOS-like symptoms, including hypothyroidism (when your thyroid gland produces too little thyroid hormone), hyperprolactinemia (when your pituitary gland makes too much prolactin, a hormone that regulates ovulation), and ovarian or adrenal tumors.

"Women with PCOS often have three major clinical problems: periods, weight, and skin. If all three exist, there is over a 95 percent chance that the diagnosis is PCOS," says Samuel S. Thatcher, MD, PhD, director of the Center for Applied Reproductive Science in Johnson City, Tennessee, and author of *PCOS: The Hidden Epidemic*. If PCOS seems to be a possibility, your doctor should also perform these screening tests, which can help assess your diabetes and heart risk and provide information abut your fertility.

- A fasting comprehensive biochemical panel (a battery of blood tests used to evaluate liver and kidney function by measuring proteins and enzymes) and lipid panel (to check LDL, HDL, total cholesterol, and triglycerides)
- A 2-hour glucose tolerance test (GTT) with insulin levels

MEDICAL BREAKTHROUGHS

The link between PCOS and insulin has opened new doors for women hoping to overcome the syndrome and have children and lead healthier lives. On the cutting edge: Scientists are studying the effects of several insulin-sensitizing diabetes drugs on women with PCOS. Here's what they're learning.

Rosiglitazone may help fertility. In a recent Stanford University study of 42 women with PCOS, half of those who took the diabetes drug rosiglitazone for 12 weeks ovulated and saw insulin resistance and insulin levels drop.

Metformin could help alleviate cardiovascular risks. Italian researchers found that when 30 women with PCOS took the diabetes medicine metformin for 6 months, their cardiovascular health improved. Levels of "bad" LDL cholesterol fell, levels of "good" HDL rose, and arteries were more flexible. Meanwhile, American researchers at several universities are tracking whether 678 women with PCOS who take metformin plus the ovulation-inducing fertility drug Clomid will be able to get pregnant.

- Measurement of the ratio of luteinizing hormone to follicle-stimulating hormone (LH:FSH), an indicator of the health of the ovaries. Most premenopausal women have a ratio close to 1:1. Levels of LH higher than FSH suggest PCOS; some doctors believe that an LH:FSH greater than 2:1 or 3:1 indicates PCOS.
- Tests for hormones that can affect fertility, including dehydroepi-

---

RISK CHECK: QUIZ—COULD YOU HAVE PCOS?

Only a doctor can diagnose PCOS. However, the following quiz, from the Polycystic Ovarian Syndrome Association (PCOSA), can help you determine whether you should be evaluated for the condition.

Section 1: Menstrual Irregularities

When not on birth control pills, do you have or have you ever had any of the following problems? Place a check mark next to each applicable item. Score one point for each item unless otherwise indicated.

- ☐ Eight or fewer periods per year
- ☐ No periods for an extended period of time (4 or more months)
- ☐ Irregular bleeding that starts and stops intermittently
- ☐ Fertility problems (two points if you have seen a fertility specialist or been treated with fertility

drugs to induce ovulation)

Section 2: Skin Problems

Place a check mark next to each applicable item. Score one point for each item unless otherwise indicated.

- ☐ Adult acne or severe adolescent acne
- ☐ Excess facial or body hair, especially on upper lip, chin, neck, chest, and/or abdomen
- ☐ Skin tags
- ☐ Balding or thinning hair
- ☐ Dark or discolored patches of skin on your neck or groin, under arms, or in skin folds (two points)

Section 3: Weight and Insulin-Based Problems

Place a check mark next to each applicable item. Score one point for each item unless otherwise indicated.

- ☐ Excess weight or difficulty

androsterone sulfate (DHEA), sex hormone binding globulin (SHBG), androstenedione, and testosterone

SMART SOLUTIONS: A PCOS SYMPTOM-RELIEF PLAN

You may not need to lose weight if you have PCOS; 40 to 50 percent of all women who have it remain at a normal weight. But if you are over-

(continued on page 291)

maintaining weight (two points if your excess weight is centered around your middle)

☐ Sudden unexplained weight gain

☐ Shaking, lack of concentration, uncontrollable hunger, and/or mood swings 2 or more hours after a meal

☐ Score two points if you have a family history of type 2 diabetes, heart disease, or hypertension

Section 4: Related Problems

Although there is little or no documented research, many women with PCOS have experienced the following problems. Place a check mark next to each applicable item. Score one point for each item.

☐ Migraines

☐ Depression and/or anxiety

☐ Rapid pulse and/or irregular heartbeat

☐ Pregnancy complications such as gestational diabetes or excess amniotic fluid

Scoring

0–4 points: Although PCOS is possible, it's unlikely.

5–9 points: If you are concerned about your health and score in this range, you may want to talk with your doctor about the possibility of PCOS, as well as other disorders.

10–14 points: Most women diagnosed with PCOS score in this range. Talk with your doctor about the possibility that you have PCOS.

15–20 points: A score this high warrants urgent consultation with a doctor regarding PCOS or other endocrine-related disorders.

"Just 2 months!" recalls Jeannine Scott with a laugh as she nurses her 4-month-old daughter, Ava. "My husband and I spent a year trying to conceive. I joined a study and was pregnant in 2 months. I feel so blessed."

Scott, who was in her late twenties when daughter Ava was born, was the first success story to emerge from a nationwide study of 678 women with polycystic ovary syndrome (PCOS). The goal: babies—and new insights into possible links between PCOS, the fastest-growing infertility problem in the United States, and metabolic syndrome.

The researchers still are weighing the data to see how one of three experimental treatment strategies for PCOS-related infertility—the ovulation-stimulating drug Clomid, a diabetes medicine called Metformin, or a combination of the two—gave women in the study an edge when it came to conceiving and carrying healthy babies to term.

For Scott, PCOS was a surprise diagnosis: She didn't have the usual symptoms such as weight gain, acne, or problems with unwanted hair growth. It was only after a year of trouble conceiving that tests revealed she had cysts on her ovaries—a sign of PCOS for some, but not all, women with this condition. (Some women with cysts do not have PCOS, and new research shows that women without cysts can have the condition as well.)

Enrollment in the study meant frequent blood tests, which revealed her pregnancy within about 2 weeks of conception, Scott says. (At that point, the medications were stopped.) She's thrilled with her little girl: "Her hair is brown just like her father's, and her eyes are blue like mine," she says.

weight, losing even 5 to 10 percent of your body weight can reduce insulin resistance and androgen levels and improve menstrual regularity and the appearance of your skin. In fact, some women see improvements within days of reducing calorie intake.

Paring pounds can be tough for women with PCOS, probably because of high insulin levels that may promote fat storage and discourage fat burning in your body. At many PCOS clinics, dietitians recommend a low-glycemic eating plan that relies on healthy fats, lean protein, and "good carbs" (fruits, veggies, and whole grains)—like the *Sugar Solution* plan—to keep blood sugar lower and steadier. Research is beginning to suggest that low-glycemic eating may give people with insulin resistance a weight-loss edge by dialing back insulin levels so the body can burn a little more fat. (Of course, you still have to follow a reduced-calorie diet; good carbs aren't a magic bullet!) "While weight loss can be difficult for women with PCOS, studies show that it can help correct the very insulin insensitivity that's making it difficult," says Dr. Thatcher.

Eating lower-GI meals and snacks can help you avoid blood sugar spikes that prompt your pancreas to release a flood of insulin. Keeping insulin lower may, researchers suspect, also lower testosterone levels in your body. Glycemic index (GI) researchers at the University of Sydney in Australia even believe that following a low-GI meal plan could lower insulin and testosterone levels enough to ease PCOS-related metabolic problems, including menstrual cycle irregularities, tiredness, body-hair overgrowth, acne, and mood swings.

CHAPTER 24

PREGNANCY DIABETES: RISKS FOR BABIES AND MOMS

Inside the womb, a growing baby demands more and more fuel for healthy growth and development. Behind the scenes, a "silent partner" makes sure she gets it: Unseen and unfelt, pregnancy itself quietly reprograms your blood sugar control system to deliver extra energy to a rapidly developing child.

The process is elegant, ancient, and unstoppable. Hormones secreted by your placenta make your own body increasingly insulin resistant (a process that stops with childbirth). Your blood sugar rises— providing your baby with extra energy to grow on.

But for at least 6 percent of pregnant women, this recipe for prenatal "baby food" goes awry. Blood sugar soars too high, leading to gestational diabetes. It's a threat for mom and baby alike, raising a woman's risk for preterm birth, difficult labor, Caesarean section, urinary tract infections, dangerous pregnancy high blood pressure (called pre-eclampsia), and type 2 diabetes after pregnancy. For babies, gestational diabetes increases the odds for higher birth weight and injury during delivery, as well as perilous low blood sugar, jaundice, and breathing problems after birth.

"It's important to detect and treat gestational diabetes as early in the pregnancy as possible," says Russell K. Laros Jr., MD, professor of obstetrics and gynecology and reproductive sciences at the University of California, San Francisco, and a specialist in high-risk pregnancies.

Equally important: Doing all you can to lower your risk for gestational diabetes *before* you become pregnant. Some risk factors are outside your control, including your age (being over 25), ethnicity (Hispanic, African American, Native American, or Pacific Islander heritage), and genetics (family history of type 2 diabetes). Yet a growing

RISK CHECK: IS GESTATIONAL DIABETES IN YOUR FUTURE?

Answer the questions below to determine your odds for gestational diabetes.

1. Are you a member of a high-risk ethnic group (Hispanic, African American, Native American, or Pacific Islander)?
   ☐ Yes   ☐ No

2. Are you overweight or obese?
   ☐ Yes   ☐ No

3. Are you related to anyone who has diabetes now or had diabetes in their lifetime?
   ☐ Yes   ☐ No

4. Are you older than 25?
   ☐ Yes   ☐ No

5. Did you have gestational diabetes with a past pregnancy?
   ☐ Yes   ☐ No

6. Have you had a stillbirth or a very large baby with a past pregnancy?
   ☐ Yes   ☐ No

7. Do you have a history of abnormal glucose tolerance?
   ☐ Yes   ☐ No

Scoring

- If you answered yes to two or more of these questions, you are at high risk for gestational diabetes.
- If you answered yes to only one of these questions, you are at average risk for gestational diabetes.
- If you answered no to all of these questions, you are at low risk for gestational diabetes.

stack of research shows that controlling three factors before conception—what you eat, how much you move, and the number on your bathroom scale—can significantly lower your odds for developing diabetes during pregnancy.

TAKE CONTROL OF YOUR HEALTH—AND YOUR BABY'S

Extra weight, inactivity, and a high-fat, high-sugar diet mute your body's response to insulin, the hormone that escorts blood sugar into cells. If you are not pregnant, this insulin resistance can persist, undetected, for years without progressing to full-blown diabetes.

But pregnancy changes all the rules. Suddenly, your body is storing new "mommy fat" on your hips and torso. At the same time, your placenta is pumping hormones including human placental lactogen, progesterone, leptin, and tumor necrosis factor alpha into your bloodstream, reducing your body's sensitivity to insulin. If you were already insulin resistant when you became pregnant, these changes can push your blood sugar up to dangerous diabetic levels.

Your prepregnancy weight is a strong predictor of gestational diabetes risk. If you're lean, your odds are about 3 percent; if you're overweight, they double. An obese woman's risk is three to four times higher than normal, say Harvard School of Public Health researchers who followed the health of 14,613 nurses for 5 years as part of the landmark Nurses Health Study.

Your weight can also dictate just how dangerous gestational diabetes will be. Among 624 Canadian women who all had pregnancy diabetes, those who weighed the most prior to pregnancy were three times more likely to have a Caesarean section and four times more likely to develop preeclampsia.

Meanwhile, overweight is putting more and more women at risk for gestational diabetes. When researchers at the University at Buffalo in New York reviewed the health records of 79,000 women who became pregnant between 1999 and 2003, they found that the number who were overweight at conception rose 11 percent in just 5 years—and the number who were obese rose 8 percent.

"Obese patients who become pregnant are at increased risk of

WHY WAIT? TEST EARLY FOR LOWER BLOOD SUGAR

New research suggests testing for gestational diabetes just 2 months earlier than usual—at 16 weeks rather than the standard 24 to 28 weeks—can cut complications dramatically. Yet early tests aren't the norm for most high-risk moms-to-be, a big group comprising more than half of all pregnant women.

Gynecologists have long thought that the standard blood sugar test yielded accurate diabetes results only in the 24th week of pregnancy or later. But when Duke University researchers screened 255 women for gestational diabetes during their 16th week of pregnancy, then rechecked at 24 weeks, they found that early tests were 99.4 percent accurate. "Screening at 16 weeks is a better predictor of gestational diabetes," says Gerard Nahum, MD, associate clinical professor in Duke University Medical Center's department of obstetrics and gynecology and lead author of the Duke testing study. "It's more sensitive than screening later and allows us to focus earlier on women who are at greatest risk. It's also a more

practical screening technique because blood samples drawn during early pregnancy for other tests can also be used for this purpose."

Earlier testing could cut the number of spontaneous premature births related to GD *in half*, say Spanish researchers who tracked 235 women with an early diagnosis of GD and another 189 diagnosed in the sixth month of pregnancy, between 24 and 28 weeks.

The check for gestational diabetes: a simple oral glucose tolerance test, in which you fast for 8 to 12 hours, then have a fasting blood sugar check. Next, you drink a sugary beverage containing 100 grams of glucose and have your blood sugar measured over the next 3 hours. You've got gestational diabetes if you have any two of these results: fasting blood sugar over 95 mg/dl; blood sugar of 180 mg/dl 1 hour after drinking the sugary beverage; 155 mg/dl after 2 hours; 140 mg/dl after 3 hours.

developing gestational diabetes, as well as pregnancy-related hypertension, preeclampsia, neonatal death, and labor complications," says John Yeh, MD, lead author and chair of the department of gynecology/obstetrics at the university's medical school.

BLOOD SUGAR'S DANGERS FOR MOMS AND BABIES

Among the ways gestational diabetes can threaten a woman's health during pregnancy:

- Nearly double the risk for preeclampsia. Pregnancy-related high blood pressure can lead to fatal seizures for mothers-to-be and to premature delivery, low birth weight, and even stillbirth. When obstetricians at St Luke's–Roosevelt Hospital Center, University Hospital of Columbia University in New York, tracked the records of 1,664 women with gestational diabetes, they found that one in 10 also had preeclampsia.
- Twice the likelihood of Caesarean section. Up to 30 percent of all women with gestational diabetes have Caesarean sections, compared with 17 percent of women without pregnancy diabetes, according to the federal government's Agency for Healthcare Research and Quality.
- A 42 percent higher risk for unplanned preterm birth. Researchers from the Kaiser Permanente health systems in Oakland, California, discovered this risk when they examined the birth records and blood sugar levels of 46,230 women.
- An almost total guarantee you'll develop full-blown type 2 diabetes later. About 10 percent of women with gestational diabetes progress to diabetes within a year or so of giving birth; 70 percent are diabetic within a decade. After 28 years, 92 percent will have diabetes, say researchers from Helsinki University Hospital in Finland.

For babies, the risks include:

- High birth weight—9 pounds and up. This can lead to the baby suffering a fractured collarbone or injury to nerves in the neck during delivery.

- Low blood sugar after birth. In the womb, your baby's pancreas churns out extra insulin to help control extra blood sugar from your body. After birth, when your baby no longer receives blood sugar from you, the extra insulin can push her blood sugar low enough to cause seizures and nervous system damage.
- A two- to sixfold higher risk for preterm birth and admission to the neonatal intensive care unit, report University of Toronto researchers who tracked the offspring of 624 pregnant women with blood sugar problems. Babies can have jaundice and breathing problems, too.

SMART SOLUTIONS TO PREVENT GESTATIONAL DIABETES

If you're planning a pregnancy, here's how you can use the *Sugar Solution* plan to defeat gestational diabetes before it starts. (Note: If you're already pregnant, see your doctor. The *Sugar Solution* isn't designed to meet the special nutritional and caloric needs of pregnant women.)

Go low-glycemic for less insulin resistance. Eating foods that keep blood sugar lower and steadier—such as steel-cut oats, barley, and whole grain breads instead of instant oatmeal, white rice, and white bread—improved insulin sensitivity twice as much as following a low-fat diet in a University of Minnesota study of 39 overweight women and men, ages 18 to 40. Their food choices and menu plans were very similar to the *Sugar Solution* eating plan: lots of fresh produce, whole grains, and good fats (even dessert!) in place of refined carbohydrates and saturated fats.

Lace up your sneakers, haul out your bicycle. Exercise tunes up your body's insulin sensitivity. Getting 4 hours of activity per week prior to pregnancy cut gestational diabetes risk 76 percent in a study of 909 women conducted by researchers from Seattle's Swedish Medical Center.

Already pregnant? Ask your doctor about the best gentle exercise routine for you. University of Buffalo researchers who followed 12,799 pregnant women found that overweight women who performed any amount and type of weekly exercise cut their risk for gestational diabetes in half. To exercise safely during pregnancy, first check with your doctor to be sure it's right for you. Keep workouts to less than 45 minutes so your body temperature stays within safe levels. Sip water before, during, and after your workout. And think gentle, not marathon. This is not the time to increase your fitness level. A half-hour stroll around the shopping mall, a neighborhood walk, and a slow half-hour swim each week may be all you need.

Give yourself the relaxation advantage. Get enough sleep, and take time to pursue serenity. Plenty of research finds connections between being well rested and a lower risk for insulin resistance and diabetes. Shaking off stress can be even more effective: Stress hormones can unleash extra blood sugar, trigger junk food binges, and pack extra calories onto your midsection as fat (a risk factor for insulin resistance).

Another reason to learn the art of *ahhh* now: Prenatal researchers

---

IF YOU ALREADY HAVE TYPE 2 DIABETES. . .

The American Diabetes Association recommends that women with type 1 and type 2 diabetes have their blood sugar under tight control for at least 3 to 6 months before trying to conceive. Why? Having high blood sugar in the early weeks and months of pregnancy—when a baby's organ systems are forming—raises the risk for birth defects two to five times higher than normal.

A new study from Boston's Joslin Diabetes Center helps explain the risk: Excess sugar may deprive a growing embryo of oxygen during early development in the very first weeks of pregnancy—before you even realize you're pregnant. Low oxygen may shut off development by triggering the production of cell-damaging free radicals, says lead researcher Mary R. Loeken, PhD, a scientist in Joslin's Section on Developmental and Stem Cell Biology and an assistant professor of medicine at Harvard Medical School. "High sugar levels and low oxygen may also create an environment in which genes involved in neural tube and heart development aren't switched on," she says.

---

have found profound links between a pregnant mom's stress levels and her child's later health status. In one study of 74 ten-year-olds, researchers from Bristol University in England found that cortisol levels in saliva samples were highest among kids whose moms had been the most anxious late in pregnancy.

Stop smoking. It's bad for your health, bad for your baby's—and it raises your risk for gestational diabetes by 50 percent.

Schedule a fasting blood sugar check 6 to 12 weeks after you give birth. Once you've had gestational diabetes, your risk for type 2 diabetes will remain significantly higher for the rest of your life (as will your risk for developing gestational diabetes during any subsequent pregnancies). Your doctor should test your blood sugar within 3 months of delivery, then recheck annually to catch diabetes early.

SMART SOLUTIONS FOR MOMS-TO-BE WITH HIGH BLOOD SUGAR

If you have type 2 diabetes before pregnancy or develop diabetes during pregnancy, these expert tips can help control blood sugar and cut complications risk.

Buy a blood sugar meter and test, test, test. Like a person with type 2 diabetes, women with gestational diabetes must test blood sugar frequently—usually upon waking, before meals, and 1 to 2 hours after each meal—to be sure it's staying within a safe range for mom and baby. Your doctor will tell you what your blood sugar goals should be. In general, the targets for women with gestational diabetes are:

- Less than 105 milligrams of glucose per deciliter of blood (mg/dl) when you wake up in the morning
- Less than 155 mg/dl an hour after a meal
- Less than 130 mg/dl 2 hours after eating

Keep a blood sugar log where you can write down your results and also note your meals, exercise, and any unusual stresses you've experienced that could affect your blood sugar level.

Be prepared for insulin therapy. Up to 39 percent of women with gestational diabetes will also need insulin shots to help control high blood sugar during pregnancy. Insulin is safe and effective and won't cross the placenta to reach your baby. Meanwhile, research suggests that a type of diabetes medication called a sulfonylurea may also work—and it's a pill, not a shot. But more research is needed.

CHAPTER 25

CHILDHOOD DIABETES: KIDS IN CRISIS

A seventh grader suddenly grows moody. He can't stay awake in class. He's usually an A student, but his grades are slipping. He's overweight and has odd brownish patches on the skin beneath his arms. Diagnosis: type 2 diabetes.

A 4-year-old girl stands 42 inches tall and weighs 92 pounds—too tall and too heavy for standard childhood height and weight charts. Born prematurely, she had been fed extra portions at breakfast, lunch, and dinner by her worried parents in the hope that she would grow and be healthy. But the plan went awry. Diagnosis: type 2 diabetes, with blood sugar and insulin levels twice the norm.

Every day, across the nation and the world, the parents of overweight and inactive children and teens are hearing surprising news from their pediatricians and family doctors: *Your child has type 2 diabetes.* Once an adults-only disease, this blood sugar crisis is becoming a crisis of childhood. Since 1994, the number of kids diagnosed with type 2 has increased six- to tenfold. And now pediatricians are beginning to see troubling diabetic complications as well: blood sugar–related damage to the retinas in the eyes of preteens; high blood pressure; high cholesterol; and, in girls as young as 11, even early signs of reproductive trouble, including irregular menstrual periods and ovulation problems related to blood sugar control problems.

"When type 2 diabetes strikes an older adult, it may take 10 to 20 years before the major long-term complications like heart disease, stroke, and blindness develop. But now that more people in their thirties, twenties, and even teens are getting the disease, we will see these complications in younger and younger people," says C. Ronald Kahn, MD, president of Boston's Joslin Diabetes Center. "With the staggering increase of type 2 diabetes in younger people around the globe, my greatest nightmare is that in about 15 or 20 years, we will face an epidemic of diabetes and its complications that will be a huge burden for mankind, governments, and the health care system."

AN EPIDEMIC OF SODA, FRIES, AND VIDEO GAMES

Until a decade ago, almost all diabetes in kids was type 1, a genetic disease in which blood sugar soars because the immune system destroys insulin-producing cells in the pancreas. Type 2 was called adult-onset diabetes because nearly all its victims were over age 30—and most were elderly. "Ten years ago, we saw maybe one or two kids a year with type 2," says Francine Kaufman, MD, a diabetes specialist at Childrens Hospital Los Angeles and past president of the American Diabetes Association. Now, in children's hospitals and pediatric clinics, up to 46 percent of all new diabetes cases are type 2. Some are in children as young as age 4, she says.

Future shock: The Centers for Disease Control and Prevention (CDC) recently estimated that one in three kids born in 2001 will develop type 2 diabetes sometime during his or her life. Among African American, Hispanic, Asian, and Native American children, the odds are closer to one in two, says K. M. Venkat Narayan, chief of the CDC's diabetes epidemiology section. "The fact that the diabetes epidemic has been raging was well known to us. But looking at the risk in these terms was very shocking," he says.

Meanwhile, one in eight elementary-school-age kids may have metabolic syndrome, a precursor to diabetes, say researchers from the University of North Carolina at Chapel Hill. In their study of 3,203 kids, 42 percent had low levels of "good" HDL cholesterol (a hallmark of

RISK CHECK: IS YOUR CHILD HEADED FOR TYPE 2 DIABETES?

Schedule a blood sugar test (ask for a fasting plasma glucose test) every 2 years beginning at age 10 if your child is overweight and has two or more of these diabetes risk factors. For kids under 10, talk with your doctor.

- A family history of type 2 diabetes in first- and second-degree relatives
- Member of an at-risk race/ethnic group: Native American, African American, Latino, Asian American, South Pacific Islander
- Signs of insulin resistance or conditions associated with insulin resistance, such as acanthosis

nigricans, high blood pressure, high cholesterol, high triglycerides, or polycystic ovary syndrome

If your child is overweight, schedule a doctor's appointment if you see any of these warning signs that she may already have type 2 diabetes.

- Frequent urination
- Excessive thirst
- Extreme hunger
- Unexplained weight loss
- Increased fatigue
- Irritability
- Blurry vision

metabolic syndrome), and 9 percent had high triglycerides, another sign. Sixteen percent had high insulin levels, and nearly 8 percent had high blood pressure. Five percent had prediabetes, in which blood sugar is already creeping toward diabetic levels.

OVERWEIGHT BLUES

There's no invading virus or sinister bacteria to blame for this epidemic, no vaccine to ward it off or quick-fix pill to cure it. Type 2 diabetes is a lifestyle disease—a body-fat disease—caused by too much TV, too little activity, and too much high-calorie junk food that raises blood sugar and pads little tummies with extra fat. Its rise mirrors the huge upswing in childhood obesity that's left 30 percent of American kids overweight and another 15 percent obese.

"At least 80 percent of type 2 diabetic kids are overweight," says Judith Fradkin, MD, an endocrinologist at the National Institute of Diabetes and Digestive and Kidney Diseases in Washington, DC. While some kids have a genetic predisposition to type 2 diabetes, it's almost always extra pounds and inactivity that push their bodies over the edge.

"People used to think that body fat was just a place to store excess

---

SOLVE THE OVERWEIGHT QUESTION

Is your child just a little plump—or carrying dangerous excess weight? This pediatrician-recommended strategy will help you know for sure. You need a tape measure, an accurate scale, and a computer with Internet access.

Step 1: Chart her body mass index (BMI). Measure your child's height (in stocking feet) and weight, and write down both numbers. Then plug them into the CDC's BMI calculator at http://www.cdc.gov/ nccdphp/dnpa/bmi/calc-bmi.htm. You'll get a number (usually between 16 and 30) that reflects her weight in relation to her height.

Step 2: Is her BMI healthy? Healthy BMIs for children and even teens rise and fall with age. They're also different for girls and boys. To assess your child's BMI, plot it into

the CDC's new growth charts for girls and boys ages 2 to 20. You'll need a computer with Internet access for this step. The CDC BMI charts for children can be found at this Web address: www.cdc.gov/ nccdphp/dnpa/growthcharts/ training/modules/module1/text/ module1print.pdf.

Step 3: Talk with your doctor. Discuss what you've found before you assume there's a problem. Ask her to look at your child's growth pattern (some kids put on extra weight in the weeks or months before a growth spurt) and take into account his body type and any circumstances that could make BMI extra high or extra low (such as youth sports). Ask that your child's weight continue to be assessed as he grows.

---

calories," Fradkin says. "But as it turns out, fat tissue is biologically active, making hormones and signaling molecules that travel to other parts of the body, telling them to be resistant to the action of insulin."

Nutrition researchers lay part of the blame on the uptick in consumption of sweetened beverages among kids—many of whom can buy them from soda machines conveniently placed in their school cafeterias. In one recent eye-opening study, overweight kids who consumed the most sugar, especially in sweet drinks, showed signs of a decline in the function of their insulin-producing beta cells—a chilling precursor to type 2 diabetes.

The rest of the story? Kids are moving less than ever. Instead, they're watching TV, sitting at computers, or playing video games for an estimated 6.5 hours per day. Many elementary schools no longer offer recess, in an effort to pack more instructional time into the day. Just one in three junior high schools even requires physical education, according to the CDC. In 1969, nearly half of all kids who lived within a mile of school walked or biked to class. Today, fewer than 16 percent do. The rest ride in buses or cars. Some parents even drive their kids the short distance to the bus stop.

DEADLY LEGACY

Kids with type 2 face adult-size complications. When Canadian researchers followed 51 Native Americans, ages 18 to 33, who had developed type 2 before age 17, they found three on dialysis for kidney failure, one who was blind at age 26, one with a toe amputated, and two dead of heart attacks; 21 of 56 pregnancies had ended in miscarriage or stillbirth.

"Our worst fears are being realized," says David Ludwig, MD, director of the Optimal Weight for Life (OWL) Clinic, a program for prediabetic kids at Children's Hospital Boston. "We're getting the first reports of people who were diagnosed as teenagers and have had diabetes for 10 years. They're now in their late twenties and are developing kidney failure, and some have required amputations. And they're dying at a higher-than-expected rate."

Perhaps the gravest and most overlooked danger: Because of high blood sugar and insulin levels, 20-year-olds with diabetes have cardiovascular diseases once found only in older, out-of-shape adults, such as high blood pressure, high cholesterol, and plaque-choked artery walls. This boosts their risk of early heart attacks and stroke. "It's unprecedented—an impending catastrophe," Dr. Ludwig says.

SMART SOLUTIONS: THE FAMILY PLAN THAT STOPS TYPE 2 DIABETES

Bottom line: Type 2 diabetes doesn't have to happen to your child. It can be prevented or at least delayed with the same steps proven to keep at-risk adults diabetes free. All it takes is a family commitment to healthy eating and activity. "The kids who do best in our obesity treatment program are the ones whose parents are not just supportive but are also participating in the same healthful lifestyle program," Dr. Ludwig notes.

Here's what else you can do to help prevent type 2 diabetes in your child.

Goal #1: Eat Healthy

Base meals on fruits, veggies, hearty whole grains, lean protein, fish rich in omega-3 fats (such as wild salmon), low-fat dairy, and moderate amounts of heart-healthful monounsaturated fat from olive and canola oils, suggests Jan P. Hangen, RD, nutrition team leader at the OWL Clinic. (You can use the meal plans and recipes in this book.)

Drink more low-fat milk, less soda. Harvard Medical School researchers discovered that overweight young adults with the highest dairy consumption were 66 percent less likely to develop metabolic syndrome than those with the lowest dairy consumption. Aim for two or three daily servings of milk, yogurt, and low-fat cheese.

Soda, juice, and other sugar-filled drinks are making our children fat, warn nutritionists at Cornell University. They recently followed 30 children, ages 6 to 13, for 2 months and found that those who drank more than 16 ounces of sweetened drinks per day gained an average of

2½ pounds. That's because children don't eat less to compensate for the extra liquid calories.

Serve dinner at home whenever possible. Meals prepared in your own kitchen usually have less fat and fewer calories, and you can control portion sizes better. Reconsider the drive-thru, too. In a recent University of Minnesota study that tracked 3,031 young adults for 15 years, those who ate fast food two or more times weekly were 10 pounds heavier and twice as likely to be insulin-resistant, compared with those who averaged less than one drive-thru dinner weekly. When you do go out to dinner, ask the restaurant to serve half your child's dinner and wrap the other half for later. Even kiddie portions can be oversize.

Goal #2: Move

At a minimum, children should get moderate to vigorous activity for an hour a day most days of the week, the CDC recommends. So should you. So why not get active together? Exercising as a family is the most effective—and fun—way to ensure that both your child and you get the activity your bodies need. Go to the driving range, swim at your community pool, challenge your child to miniature golf, learn to in-line skate together, or just take long walks. You're not only building healthier bodies and habits, but you're showing your kid that the best things in life aren't found on the TV screen or inside a french fry container.

Limit TV to 1 to 2 hours a day, maximum. Not only are children completely inactive while watching TV (burning even fewer calories than they would reading or playing Monopoly), but they're a captive audience for an endless stream of junk food ads.

Instead, make after school your child's playtime. Have plenty of indoor exercise instigators on hand for rainy days, such as jump ropes, a mat printed with a hopscotch board, mini basketball sets, hula hoops, and music kids can dance to. And make physical activity a social occasion. Set up active playdates for elementary schoolers. Children age 12 and older may prefer a structured exercise class or a team sport so they can be active with their friends.

Get infants active, too. Let your baby spend more time on the floor, rolling over and crawling for toys you put just beyond his grasp.

Goal #3: Reward the Effort

Children need to be rewarded for adopting healthier habits, not for pounds lost. "The biggest mistake parents make is offering children food-related rewards in exchange for weight loss," says Hangen. "Reaching a healthy weight is not an event, it's a process—one that takes a long time and requires making some permanent lifestyle changes."

The next time your child begs for candy after dinner in exchange for eating all his peas and carrots, try offering yourself as a reward instead. Together, you can put on a puppet show, build an amazing castle out of blocks, play dress-up—whatever activity your child would enjoy. "We're all so short on time, yet it's the most precious commodity in the world," says Hangen.

Parents help by cheering success and letting kids know it's okay to mess up once in a while, says Hangen. "Whenever there is a self-esteem issue—about body weight or health—there's some guilt and shame hiding underneath. You need to get kids away from their fear long enough to think they can change," she says. "Humor and empathy are key. After all, they're still kids."

And once in a while, go for a chocolate bar or ice cream or spend a night together watching *Harry Potter* videos on the couch.

8

100-PLUS MOUTHWATERING RECIPES

BREAKFASTS

PUFFY FRITTATA WITH HAM AND GREEN PEPPER

2 tablespoons butter

1 small onion, chopped

1 green bell pepper, chopped

½ teaspoon salt

½ teaspoon ground black pepper

8 slices (6 ounces) ham, chopped

8 large eggs, at room temperature

¼ cup water

½ cup (2 ounces) shredded Cheddar
cheese (optional)

Melt 1 tablespoon of the butter in a 12" nonstick skillet over low heat. Add the onion, bell pepper, ¼ teaspoon of the salt, and ¼ teaspoon of the pepper. Cook, stirring occasionally, until crisp-tender, for 3 to 4 minutes. Stir in the ham and cook for 1 minute, stirring occasionally. Transfer to a plate.

Separate the eggs, placing the yolks in a medium bowl and the whites in a large bowl. Lightly beat the yolks with the water and the remaining ¼ teaspoon salt and ¼ teaspoon pepper. Beat the egg whites until they form stiff, but not dry, peaks. Fold the yolks into the whites.

Melt the remaining 1 tablespoon butter in the skillet over low heat. Pour in the eggs and spread them evenly with a rubber spatula. Scatter the ham mixture and cheese (if using) over the top, cover, and cook until the eggs are set, for 25 to 30 minutes. Slide the frittata onto a plate and serve immediately (puffiness will subside in 5 to 7 minutes).

Makes 4 servings

Per serving: 290 calories, 22 g protein, 8 g carbohydrates, 19 g fat, 448 mg cholesterol, 467 mg sodium, 2 g dietary fiber
Diet Exchanges: 1 vegetable, 3 meat, 2½ fat
Carb Choices: ½

ASPARAGUS AND GOAT CHEESE OMELETS

16 asparagus spears (10 ounces), trimmed and cut into ½" lengths

8 large eggs

¼ cup 1% milk

¼ cup chopped fresh basil

½ teaspoon salt

½ teaspoon ground black pepper

4 teaspoons butter

1 clove garlic, minced

½ cup (3 ounces) crumbled goat cheese

Preheat the oven to 250°F. Coat a large baking sheet with cooking spray.

Cook the asparagus in boiling water over high heat until crisp-tender, for 2 to 5 minutes. Drain in a colander and pat dry on paper towels.

To make one omelet at a time: Break 2 of the eggs into a small bowl. Add 3 tablespoons of the milk and lightly beat with a fork. Stir in 1 tablespoon of the basil, ⅛ teaspoon of the salt, and ⅛ teaspoon of the pepper. Melt 1 teaspoon of the butter in an 8" nonstick skillet over medium heat.

Add one-fourth of the garlic and cook until soft, for 2 minutes. Add in one-fourth of the asparagus, then pour in the egg mixture. Cook until the eggs are almost set, for 4 minutes, lifting the edge occasionally to let the raw eggs flow under. Spoon 2 tablespoons of the cheese along the center. Fold the omelet in half, remove to the prepared baking sheet, and place in the oven to keep warm.

Prepare 3 more omelets in the same manner.

Makes 4

Per serving: 292 calories, 20 g protein, 7 g carbohydrates, 20 g fat, 450 mg cholesterol, 570 mg sodium, 1 g dietary fiber
Diet Exchanges: 1 vegetable, 3 meat, 3 fat
Carb Choices: ½

WHOLE GRAIN CREPES WITH BANANA AND KIWIFRUIT

CREPES

1 cup whole grain pastry flour

¼ teaspoon salt

1 egg

1 cup + 3 tablespoons unsweetened
soy milk or whole milk

1½ teaspoons vanilla extract

2 teaspoons butter

FILLING

½ cup (4 ounces) plain yogurt

1 banana, cut into 24 diagonal slices

2 kiwifruits, peeled, halved
lengthwise, and sliced

2 teaspoons lime juice (optional)

½ teaspoon ground cinnamon

To make the crepes: In a large bowl, combine the flour and salt.

In a small bowl, beat the egg, then stir in the milk and vanilla. Pour into the flour and mix well.

Melt ½ teaspoon of the butter in an 8" nonstick skillet over medium heat. Pour 3 tablespoons of the batter into the skillet and tilt the skillet to coat the bottom in a thin layer (if the batter seems too thick, add 1 to 2 tablespoons water). Cook the first side until nicely browned, for 2 minutes. Using a spatula, turn the crepe and cook the second side for 1 to 2 minutes (the second side will look spotty). Slide the crepe onto a plate and cover with foil to keep warm. Continue in the same manner, rebuttering the pan after every second crepe.

To make the filling and assemble: Place a crepe on a serving plate, attractive side down, and spread with 1 tablespoon of the yogurt. Arrange 2 banana slices and a quarter of a kiwifruit in strips one-third of the way from one edge. Sprinkle with ¼ teaspoon of the lime juice (if using) and a pinch of the cinnamon and roll up. Continue assembling.

Makes 4 servings (eight 6" to 7" crepes)

Per serving: 205 calories, 8 g protein, 34 g carbohydrates, 6 g fat, 62 mg cholesterol, 198 mg sodium, 6 g dietary fiber

Diet Exchanges: 1 fruit, 1 bread, 1fat

Carb Choices: 2

WHOLE GRAIN PANCAKES WITH BERRY CREAM SYRUP

PANCAKES

¾ cup whole grain pastry flour

¼ cup buckwheat flour

1½ teaspoons baking powder

½ teaspoon baking soda

⅛ teaspoon salt

1 cup buttermilk

1 large egg, at room temperature, separated

3 tablespoons + 2 teaspoons melted butter

8 drops liquid stevia

SYRUP

¼ cup red or black raspberry fruit spread

2 tablespoons heavy cream

3–4 teaspoons orange juice or apple cider (optional)

To make the pancakes: In a large bowl, combine the pastry flour, buckwheat flour, baking powder, baking soda, and salt.

In a glass measuring cup, mix the buttermilk, egg yolk, 3 tablespoons of the butter, and the stevia. Stir into the flour mixture until well combined. In a small bowl, whip the egg white until it forms stiff, but not dry, peaks. Fold into the batter. (It will be light but not fluid.)

Heat a nonstick griddle over medium-low heat and add half of the remaining butter. For each pancake, spoon ¼ cup of the batter onto the griddle, making 4 cakes at a time, each about 4" in diameter. Cook until the edges begin to look dry, for about 3 minutes. Flip the cakes and cook the second side for 2 to 3 minutes. Continue in the same manner until all the butter and batter are used. Serve hot with the syrup.

To make the syrup: In a small bowl, combine the fruit spread, cream, and enough juice or cider (if using) to make a syrup. (Without the juice or cider, the topping will have the consistency of a spread.)

Makes 4 servings (eight 4" pancakes)

Per serving: 295 calories, 7 g protein, 31 g carbohydrates, 15 g fat, 93 mg cholesterol, 564 mg sodium, 2 g dietary fiber

Diet Exchanges: ½ milk, 1½ bread, 3 fat

Carb Choices: 2

FLORENTINE OMELETTE

2 cups liquid egg substitute

1 teaspoon Italian seasoning

¼ teaspoon salt

8 ounces mushrooms, sliced

1 onion, chopped

1 red bell pepper, chopped

1 clove garlic, minced

2 ounces (1 packed cup) spinach leaves, chopped

¾ cup (3 ounces) shredded low-fat mozzarella cheese

In a medium bowl, whisk together the egg substitute, Italian seasoning, salt, and 3 tablespoons water.

Coat a large nonstick skillet with cooking spray. Set over medium-high heat. Add the mushrooms, onion, pepper, and garlic. Cook, stirring often, for 4 to 5 minutes, or until the pepper starts to soften. Add the spinach. Cook for 1 minute, or until the spinach wilts. Transfer to a small bowl and cover.

Wipe the skillet with a paper towel. Coat with cooking spray and set over medium heat. Pour in half of the egg-substitute mixture. Cook for 2 minutes, or until the bottom begins to set. Using a spatula, lift the edges to allow the uncooked mixture to flow to the bottom of the pan. Cook for 2 minutes, or until set. Sprinkle with half of the reserved vegetable mixture and half of the cheese. Cover and cook for 2 minutes, or until the cheese melts. Using a spatula, fold the omelette in half. Invert onto a serving plate.

Coat the skillet with nonstick spray. Repeat with the remaining egg-substitute mixture, vegetable mixture, and cheese to cook another omelette. To serve, cut each omelette in half.

Makes 4 servings

Per serving: 150 calories, 20 g protein, 10 g carbohydrates, 2 g dietary fiber, 4 g total fat, 2 g saturated fat, 12 mg cholesterol, 505 mg sodium

Diet Exchanges: ½ carb (1 ½ vegetable), 2 meat

SMOKED TURKEY HASH

2 teaspoons vegetable oil

1 large onion, coarsely chopped

1 small green bell pepper, coarsely chopped

1 pound cooked red potatoes, cubed

1 smoked turkey drumstick (1 pound), skinned, boned, and cubed

1 egg white, lightly beaten

2 tablespoons chopped parsley

½ teaspoon dried thyme

⅛ teaspoon salt

3 tablespoons fat-free milk

Warm the oil in a 12" nonstick skillet over medium-high heat. Add the onion and pepper. Cook for 3 minutes, or until the pepper starts to soften.

In a large bowl, toss together the potatoes, turkey, egg white, parsley, thyme, and salt. Add to the skillet. Cook, stirring occasionally, for 10 to 12 minutes, or until lightly browned. Pour the milk around the edges. Cook, stirring, for 3 minutes, or until the milk is absorbed.

Makes 4 servings

Per serving: 245 calories, 20 g protein, 24 g carbohydrates, 5 g fat, 68 mg cholesterol, 620 mg sodium, 3 g dietary fiber
Diet Exchanges: 1 bread, 3 meat
Carb Choices: 1

BERRY-GOOD SMOOTHIE

1 cup fresh or thawed frozen blueberries

1 cup (8 ounces) vanilla yogurt

½ cup cran-blueberry juice

In a blender, combine the blueberries, yogurt, and juice. Blend until smooth.

Makes 2 servings

Per serving: 188 calories, 5 g protein, 38 g carbohydrates, 2 g fat, 6 mg cholesterol, 78 mg sodium, 2 g dietary fiber
Diet Exchanges: 1 milk, 1 fruit
Carb Choices: 2½

MULTIGRAIN CEREAL

2   cups rolled oats

2   cups wheat flakes

2   cups malted barley flakes

2   cups rye flakes

1   box (1 pound) dark or golden raisins

1½ cups flaxseeds, ground

¾   cup sesame seeds

In an airtight container, combine the oats, wheat flakes, barley flakes, rye flakes, raisins, flaxseeds, and sesame seeds. Store in the freezer until ready to use.

To cook: For 1 serving, bring 1 cup water to a boil in a small saucepan. Add a pinch of salt. Add ⅓ cup of the cereal, cover, and cook, stirring occasionally, for 25 minutes, or until thickened and creamy.

Note: For 4 servings, use 3 cups water, ¼ teaspoon salt, and 1½ cups cereal. Cook for 25 to 30 minutes.

Makes 36 servings (⅓ cup each)

Per serving: 160 calories, 5 g protein, 29 g carbohydrates, 4 g fat, 0 mg cholesterol, 8 mg sodium, 5 g dietary fiber

Diet Exchanges: 2 bread

Carb Choices: 2

BLUEBERRY-YOGURT MUFFINS

1½ **cups whole wheat flour**

2 **tablespoons toasted wheat germ**

2 **teaspoons baking powder**

½ **teaspoon salt**

2 **eggs or ½ cup fat-free liquid egg substitute**

1 **cup low-fat plain yogurt**

¼ **cup packed brown sugar**

2 **tablespoons canola oil**

1½ **cups fresh or thawed frozen blueberries**

Preheat the oven to 375°F. Coat a 12-cup muffin pan with cooking spray.

In a large bowl, whisk together the flour, wheat germ, baking powder, and salt.

In a small bowl, whisk together the eggs or egg substitute and yogurt. Whisk in the sugar and oil. Add to the flour mixture and stir just until the dry ingredients are moistened. Stir in the blueberries.

Divide the batter among the muffin cups, filling each about two-thirds full. Bake for 20 minutes, or until a wooden pick inserted in the center of a muffin comes out clean. Transfer to a wire rack and cool slightly.

Makes 12 muffins

Per muffin: 125 calories, 4 g protein, 20 g carbohydrates, 4 g fat, 37 mg cholesterol, 171 mg sodium, 2 g dietary fiber
Diet Exchanges: 1 bread, 1 fat
Carb Choices: 1

Note: Store the muffins in a covered container for up to 1 day at room temperature or up to 1 month in the freezer.

SNACKS AND APPETIZERS

SHRIMP IN MUSTARD-HORSERADISH SAUCE

SHRIMP

1½ quarts water

1 thin lemon slice

Salt to taste

20 large shrimp (1 pound), cleaned and deveined

MUSTARD-HORSERADISH SAUCE

4 teaspoons lemon juice

4 teaspoons Dijon mustard

2½ tablespoons olive oil

1 tablespoon prepared horseradish

2 teaspoons sour cream

¼ teaspoon salt

⅛ teaspoon ground black pepper

2 teaspoons finely chopped scallions

To make the shrimp: In a large saucepan, combine the water, lemon slice, and salt. Bring to a boil over high heat. Reduce the heat and cook for 5 minutes. Add the shrimp and cook until opaque and pink, for 2 to 3 minutes. Drain and discard the lemon slice.

To make the sauce: In a large bowl, mix the lemon juice and mustard. Gradually whisk in the oil to make a slightly thickened sauce. Stir in the horseradish, sour cream, salt, and pepper.

Add the shrimp to the sauce and toss to coat. Sprinkle with the scallions. Serve immediately at room temperature or chilled.

Makes 4 servings

Per serving: 123 calories, 7 g protein, 2 g carbohydrates, 10 g fat, 54 mg cholesterol, 330 mg sodium, 0 g dietary fiber
Diet Exchanges: 1 meat, 1½ fat
Carb Choices: 0

SPICY OVEN FRIES

2 medium russet potatoes, scrubbed and cut into long ¼"-thick strips	1 tablespoon roasted garlic and red pepper spice blend
1 tablespoon canola oil	¼ teaspoon salt
	¼ teaspoon ground black pepper

Preheat the oven to 425°F. Coat a 13" x 9" baking pan with cooking spray.

Place the potatoes in a mound in the prepared baking pan and sprinkle with the oil, spice blend, salt, and pepper. Toss to coat well and spread the potatoes into a single layer. Bake, turning the potatoes several times, for 40 minutes, or until crisp and lightly browned.

Makes 4 servings

Per serving: 125 calories, 3 g protein, 18 g carbohydrates, 4 g fat, 0 mg cholesterol, 144 mg sodium, 2 g dietary fiber
Diet Exchanges: 1 bread, 1 fat
Carb Choices: 1

BUFFALO CHICKEN WITH BLUE CHEESE DRESSING

24 chicken drummettes, skin removed	1 cup (8 ounces) fat-free sour cream
4 tablespoons hot sauce	1 scallion, chopped
2 teaspoons vinegar	1 tablespoon white wine vinegar
¼ teaspoon garlic powder	1 teaspoon sugar
⅓ cup (1½ ounces) crumbled blue cheese	2 large ribs celery, cut into sticks

Preheat the oven to 400°F. Line a baking sheet with foil and coat with cooking spray.

In a large bowl, combine the chicken, 2 tablespoons of the hot sauce, 1 teaspoon of the vinegar, and the garlic powder. Toss to coat evenly and arrange on the prepared baking sheet. Bake for 12 to 15 minutes, or until the juices run clear.

Meanwhile, in a medium bowl, combine the blue cheese, sour cream, scallion, vinegar, and sugar. Stir to mix, mashing the cheese with the back of a spoon.

Remove the chicken from the oven. Drizzle with the remaining 2 tablespoons hot sauce and 1 teaspoon vinegar. Toss to mix. Arrange on a serving platter. Drizzle with any sauce left on the foil. Serve with the blue cheese dressing and celery sticks.

Makes 8 servings

Per serving: 95 calories, 9 g protein, 6 g carbohydrates, 0 g dietary fiber, 3 g total fat, 0 g saturated fat, 30 mg cholesterol, 387 mg sodium
Diet Exchanges: ½ carb (½ bread/starch), 1 meat

SPICY ROASTED CHICKPEAS

2 cups canned chickpeas, rinsed and drained	**½ teaspoon ground coriander**
	¼ teaspoon ground red pepper
1½ teaspoons extra-virgin olive oil	**¼ teaspoon ground black pepper**
½ teaspoon ground cumin	

Preheat the oven to 400°F. Coat a nonstick baking sheet with cooking spray.

In a small bowl, toss the chickpeas with the oil, cumin, coriander, red pepper, and black pepper.

Place the chickpeas in a single layer on the prepared baking sheet. Bake for 30 to 40 minutes, or until crisp and golden.

Makes 8 servings

Per serving: 40 calories, 2 g protein, 7 g carbohydrates, 1 g fat, 0 mg cholesterol, 170 mg sodium, 2 g dietary fiber
Diet Exchanges: ½ bread
Carb Choices: ½

VARIATION
Southwestern Roasted Chickpeas: Replace the coriander with chili powder.

HUMMUS PLATTER

4 whole wheat pitas	½ teaspoon salt
1 can (19 ounces) chickpeas, rinsed and drained	½ cup finely chopped red onions
⅓ cup tahini	2 tablespoons chopped fresh parsley
⅓ cup lemon juice	2 red bell peppers, thinly sliced
3 cloves garlic, chopped	1 cucumber, thinly sliced

Preheat the oven to 425°F.

Cut each pita into eight triangles and separate each triangle into two pieces. Spread the triangles, rough side up, on two large baking sheets. Bake for 8 to 10 minutes, or until crisp. (This can be done ahead of time. Cool the triangles completely and store them in a covered container for up to 3 days.)

In a food processor, combine the chickpeas, tahini, lemon juice, garlic, and salt. Pulse for 30 seconds to mix. Process for 2 minutes, or until very smooth, scraping down the sides of the container as necessary.

Transfer to a serving dish. Sprinkle with the onions and parsley. Serve with the pitas, peppers, and cucumber.

Makes 8 servings

Per serving: 205 calories, 7 g protein, 29 g carbohydrates, 8 g fat, 0 mg cholesterol, 439 mg sodium, 6 g dietary fiber
Diet Exchanges: 1 vegetable, 1½ bread, 1 fat
Carb Choices: 2

ZUCCHINI BITES

2 eggs

5 egg whites

4 cups shredded zucchini

1½ cups (6 ounces) shredded fat-free
   mozzarella cheese

1 cup chopped onions

½ cup (2 ounces) grated Parmesan
   cheese

½ cup all-purpose flour

1 tablespoon chopped fresh dill

¼ teaspoon baking powder

Preheat the oven to 350°F. Coat a 9" × 13" nonstick baking dish with cooking
spray.

In a large bowl, beat together the eggs and egg whites. Stir in the zucchini,
mozzarella, onions, Parmesan, flour, dill, and baking powder.

Spoon the mixture into the prepared baking dish. Bake for 30 to 35 minutes,
or until a toothpick inserted in the center comes out clean. Cool in the pan
for 5 minutes. Cut into 24 squares. Serve warm or cold.

Makes 8 servings

Per serving (3 squares): 133 calories, 16 g protein, 11 g carbohydrates, 3 g fat, 58 mg cholesterol,
329 mg sodium, 1 g dietary fiber
Diet Exchanges: 2 vegetable, 2 meat, ½ fat
Carb Choices: 1

VARIATION

Sun-Dried Tomato–Zucchini Bites: Replace the dill with 1 tablespoon chopped fresh
basil. Place 8 dry-packed sun-dried tomatoes in a cup or small bowl. Cover with boiling water and let soak for 15 minutes, or until softened. Finely chop and stir into the
zucchini mixture.

STUFFED MUSHROOMS

16 large mushrooms, cleaned

1 tablespoon olive oil

3 tablespoons dry sherry or
nonalcoholic white wine

¼ cup chopped fresh parsley

1 tablespoon grated Parmesan
cheese

1 tablespoon unseasoned dry
bread crumbs

1 clove garlic, minced

¼ teaspoon dried thyme

¼ teaspoon dried oregano

Salt

Ground black pepper

Preheat the oven to 375°F. Coat a 9" × 13" nonstick baking dish with cooking spray.

Remove and finely chop the mushroom stems. Set the caps aside.

In a cup, combine the oil and sherry or wine. Pour 2 tablespoons into an 8" nonstick skillet, reserving 2 tablespoons. Warm the skillet over medium-low heat. Add the chopped stems and sauté for 6 minutes, or until the mixture is dry.

Add the parsley, cheese, bread crumbs, garlic, thyme, oregano and salt and pepper to taste. Remove from the heat and stir in 1 tablespoon of the remaining sherry mixture until moistened.

Spoon the mushroom mixture into the reserved caps. Place in a single layer in the prepared baking dish. Bake for 15 to 20 minutes, or until the caps are tender and heated through. Halfway through the cooking time, brush the caps with the remaining 1 tablespoon sherry mixture. Serve hot.

Makes 16 caps

Per cap: 19 calories, 0.5 g protein, 1 g carbohydrates, 1 g fat, 0.5 mg cholesterol, 12 mg sodium, 0.5 g dietary fiber
Diet Exchanges: Free
Carb Choices: 0

GARLICKY SPINACH DIP

½ cup (4 ounces) fat-free ricotta cheese

¼ cup (2 ounces) fat-free sour cream

2 tablespoons orange juice

1 package (10 ounces) frozen chopped spinach, thawed and squeezed dry

¼ cup chopped scallions

¼ cup chopped fresh basil

2 tablespoons chopped fresh oregano

2 cloves garlic, minced

⅛ teaspoon ground nutmeg

Dash of hot-pepper sauce

Salt

Ground black pepper

In a food processor fitted with the steel blade, combine the cheese, sour cream, and orange juice. Add the spinach, scallions, basil, oregano, garlic, nutmeg, and hot-pepper sauce. Process until smooth, stopping occasionally to scrape down the sides of the container. Add salt and pepper to taste.

Pour into a medium bowl, cover, and refrigerate for at least 30 minutes, or overnight.

Makes 2 cups

Per tablespoon: 11 calories, 1 g protein, 1 g carbohydrates, 0 g fat, 1 mg cholesterol, 16 mg sodium, 0.5 g dietary fiber
Diet Exchanges: Free
Carb Choices: 0

PIZZAS

CLASSIC TOMATO PIZZA

1 tablespoon cornmeal

1 teaspoon olive oil

3 cloves garlic, minced

6 plum tomatoes, chopped

¼ cup chopped fresh basil

¼ teaspoon salt

1 tube (10 ounces) refrigerated pizza dough

¾ cup (3 ounces) shredded low-fat mozzarella cheese

Preheat the oven to 450°F. Coat a large round pizza pan with cooking spray. Sprinkle with the cornmeal.

In a medium nonstick skillet over medium heat, combine the oil and garlic. Cook, stirring occasionally, for 2 to 3 minutes, or until fragrant. Add the tomatoes, basil, and salt. Cover and cook, stirring occasionally, for 5 minutes, or until the tomatoes are soft. Remove from the heat.

Turn the dough out onto a lightly floured work surface. Roll into a 12" circle and place on the prepared pan. Spread the tomato sauce over the dough to within ¼" of the edge. Sprinkle with the cheese. Bake for 10 to 12 minutes, or until the crust is golden brown.

Makes 8 servings

Per serving: 160 calories, 7 g protein, 26 g carbohydrates, 2 g dietary fiber, 4 g total fat, 1 g saturated fat, 6 mg cholesterol, 280 mg sodium

Diet Exchanges: 2 carbs (2 bread/starch)

ONION-ROSEMARY FOCACCIA

1 tablespoon cornmeal

1 tablespoon olive oil

1 red onion, halved and thinly sliced

2 teaspoons dried rosemary, crushed

¼ teaspoon salt

2 tubes (10 ounces each) refrigerated pizza dough

1 teaspoon dried basil

Preheat the oven to 450°F. Coat a baking sheet with cooking spray. Sprinkle with the cornmeal.

Warm the oil in a medium nonstick skillet over medium heat. Add the onion, rosemary, and salt. Cover and cook, stirring occasionally, for 15 to 20 minutes, or until very soft. Remove from the heat and allow to cool slightly.

Turn the dough out onto a lightly floured work surface. Roll into a 12" x 6" rectangle and place on the prepared baking sheet. Sprinkle with the basil. With your fingertips, press the basil into the dough. Top with the onion mixture. Bake for 12 to 15 minutes, or until the crust is browned.

Makes 10 servings

Per serving: 160 calories, 4 g protein, 33 g carbohydrates, 1 g dietary fiber, 2 g total fat, 0 g saturated fat, 0 mg cholesterol, 179 mg sodium
Diet Exchanges: 2 carbs (2 bread/starch)

RATATOUILLE PIZZA

1 tablespoon cornmeal

½ small onion, chopped

1 small eggplant, peeled and cut into small chunks

1 small zucchini, cut into small chunks

2 cloves garlic, chopped

2 plum tomatoes, chopped

¼ cup chopped fresh basil

1 teaspoon drained capers

¼ teaspoon salt

1 tube (10 ounces) refrigerated pizza dough

1¼ cups (5 ounces) shredded low-fat mozzarella cheese

¼ cup (1 ounce) grated Parmesan cheese

Preheat the oven to 450°F. Coat a large round pizza pan with cooking spray. Sprinkle with the cornmeal.

Coat a medium nonstick skillet with cooking spray and set over medium heat. Add the onion, eggplant, zucchini, and garlic. Cook, stirring occasionally, for 5 to 7 minutes, or until soft. Add the tomatoes, basil, capers, and salt. Cook for 3 minutes, or until the tomatoes are soft. Remove from the heat to cool slightly.

Turn the dough out onto a lightly floured work surface. Roll into a 12" circle and place on the prepared pan. Spread evenly with the ratatouille. Top with the mozzarella and Parmesan. Bake for 10 to 12 minutes, or until the crust is golden brown.

Makes 8 servings

Per serving: 192 calories, 10 g protein, 26 g carbohydrate, 2 g dietary fiber, 5 g total fat, 3 g saturated fat, 12 mg cholesterol, 386 mg sodium

Diet Exchanges: 1½ carbs (1 bread/starch, 1 vegetable), 1 meat

CHICKEN PESTO PIZZA

1 tablespoon cornmeal

1 tube (10 ounces) refrigerated
  pizza dough

⅓ cup low-fat prepared pesto

¼ pound cooked boneless, skinless
  chicken breasts, cut into small
  strips

1 roasted red pepper, cut into small
  strips

½ cup rinsed and drained water-
  packed canned artichoke hearts,
  patted dry and quartered

½ cup (2 ounces) crumbled low-fat
  goat cheese or shredded low-fat
  Jarlsberg cheese

Preheat the oven to 450°F. Coat a large round pizza pan with cooking spray.
Sprinkle with the cornmeal.

Turn the dough out onto a lightly floured work surface. Roll into a 12" circle
and place on the prepared pan. Spread with the pesto, leaving a ¼" border.
Arrange the chicken, peppers, and artichokes over the top. Dot with the goat
cheese or sprinkle with the Jarlsberg. Bake for 10 to 12 minutes, or until the
crust is golden brown.

Makes 8 servings

Per serving: 196 calories, 10 g protein, 26 g carbohydrates, 6 g fat, 18 mg cholesterol, 234 mg
sodium, 2 g dietary fiber
Diet Exchanges: 1 vegetable, 1 bread, 1 meat
Carb Choices: 2

CARAMELIZED PEAR PIZZA

1 tablespoon cornmeal	2 teaspoons butter or margarine
¼ cup dried cranberries	1 large pear, cut into ½" thick slices
2 teaspoons + 3 tablespoons sugar	1 tube (10 ounces) refrigerated pizza dough
¼ teaspoon ground cinnamon	
2 cups (16 ounces) fat-free ricotta cheese	⅓ cup apricot preserves
	2 tablespoons slivered almonds

Preheat the oven to 450°F. Coat a large round pizza pan with cooking spray. Sprinkle with the cornmeal.

Place the cranberries in a glass measuring cup and cover with boiling water. Soak for 3 to 5 minutes, then drain and set aside.

In a small cup, mix 2 teaspoons of the sugar with the cinnamon. In a small bowl, mix the ricotta with 2 tablespoons of the remaining sugar.

Melt the butter or margarine in a medium nonstick skillet set over medium heat. Add the pear and the remaining 1 tablespoon sugar. Cook for 4 minutes, or until the pear is soft. Add the reserved cranberries and remove from the heat.

Turn the dough out onto a lightly floured work surface. Roll into a 12" circle and place on the prepared pan. Spread evenly with the ricotta. Scatter evenly with the pear and cranberries. Dollop the preserves on top and sprinkle with the almonds. Dust with the cinnamon sugar. Bake for 8 to 10 minutes, or until the crust is golden brown.

Makes 8 servings

Per serving: 253 calories, 11 g protein, 47 g carbohydrates, 2 g dietary fiber, 3 g total fat, 1 g saturated fat, 20 mg cholesterol, 206 mg sodium
Diet Exchanges: 3 carbs (3 bread/starch)

SOUPS AND SANDWICHES

LAMB AND BARLEY SOUP

1 tablespoon olive oil

1 pound lamb cubes, cut into bite-size pieces

1 small onion, chopped

2 carrots, chopped

4 ribs celery, chopped

1 clove garlic, minced

4 cans (14½ ounces each) reduced-sodium chicken broth

2 tablespoons tomato paste (optional)

⅔ cup hulled or regular barley

¼ teaspoon dried rosemary, crumbled

½ teaspoon dried oregano

½ teaspoon ground black pepper

Heat the oil in a large soup pot over low heat. Add the lamb and cook, stirring frequently, until browned all over, 3 to 5 minutes. Transfer to a plate. Stir the onion, carrots, celery, and garlic into the pot. Cover and cook, stirring occasionally, until the vegetables begin to soften, about 10 minutes.

Return the lamb to the pot and add the broth. Bring to a simmer and add the tomato paste (if using), barley, rosemary, oregano, and pepper. Partially cover and cook until the barley is tender-chewy, 45 to 55 minutes. Skim the fat from the surface of the soup if necessary.

Makes 8 servings

Per serving: 194 calories, 17 g protein, 17 g carbohydrates, 4 g dietary fiber, 7 g total fat, 2 g saturated fat, 42 mg cholesterol, 160 mg sodium
Diet Exchanges: 1 carb (1 bread/starch), 2 meat

TUSCAN BEAN STEW

2 teaspoons olive oil

1½ cups finely chopped fresh fennel or anise

¼ pound Italian sausage, crumbled

1 tablespoon finely minced garlic

3 cups fat-free chicken broth

3 cups dried small white or navy beans, rinsed and soaked overnight and drained

1 teaspoon dried basil

2 ripe plum tomatoes, chopped

½ cup thinly sliced fresh basil leaves

Heat the oil in a 6-quart pressure cooker over medium heat. Add the fennel or anise and sausage and cover with the lid (do not lock). Cook for 4 minutes, or until the fennel or anise is tender and the sausage is browned. Add the garlic and cook for 1 minute.

Add the broth, beans, and dried basil. Cover with the lid, lock in position, and bring to full pressure over high heat (high pressure on those models with a choice). Reduce the heat slightly to moderate steam (detailed directions will be with your cooker). Cook for 10 minutes.

Switch the pressure indicator to quick release or run cold water over the lid to reduce the pressure. (See the manufacturer's directions for the quick release of steam or temperature cooldown.) Unlock the lid. Puree ⅔ cup of the beans in a blender and return to the pot. Stir in the tomatoes and fresh basil.

Makes 6 servings (about 8 cups)

Per serving: 472 calories, 34 g protein, 69 g carbohydrates, 11 g fat, 13 mg cholesterol, 677 mg sodium, 12 g dietary fiber
Diet Exchanges: ½ vegetable, 2½ bread, 4 meat
Carb Choices: 4½

GREEK-STYLE LENTIL SOUP

1 pound brown lentils, picked over and rinsed

9 cups water

6 cloves garlic, minced

3 large carrots, cut into ¼" pieces

2 large onions, chopped

1 teaspoon dried thyme, crushed

1 teaspoon ground black pepper

½ teaspoon dried rosemary, crushed

1½ cups tomato puree

1 teaspoon salt

¼ teaspoon ground cinnamon

2 tablespoons extra-virgin olive oil

1 tablespoon red wine vinegar

3 tablespoons coarsely chopped fresh marjoram or oregano (optional)

In a large saucepan or Dutch oven, combine the lentils, water, garlic, carrots, onions, thyme, pepper, and rosemary. Bring to a boil over high heat. Reduce the heat to low, cover, and simmer, stirring occasionally, for 35 minutes, or until the lentils are tender. Stir in the tomato puree, salt, and cinnamon and simmer for 20 minutes to blend the flavors. Remove from the heat and stir in the oil, vinegar, and marjoram or oregano (if using).

Makes 6 servings (about 10 cups)

Per serving: 351 calories, 23 g protein, 55 g carbohydrates, 5 g fat, 0 mg cholesterol, 434 mg sodium, 26 g dietary fiber
Diet Exchanges: 1½ vegetable, 2 bread
Carb Choices: 4

CLAM CHOWDER WITH GREENS

¼ pound turkey bacon, chopped

1 tablespoon vegetable oil

1 onion, finely chopped

1 clove garlic, minced

1 small bunch (12 ounces) turnip greens or other greens, coarse stems removed and leaves chopped

2 cans (14½ ounces each) reduced-sodium chicken broth

2 cans (10 ounces each) baby clams, drained and juice reserved

1 cup half-and-half

2–2½ tablespoons potato flour

¼ teaspoon ground black pepper

Cook the turkey bacon in a large saucepan over medium-low heat until crisp. Drain on a paper towel–lined plate.

Add the oil to the pan, then add the onion and garlic. Cook, stirring occasionally, until the onion is translucent, 8 to 10 minutes. Add the greens and cook for 2 minutes.

Stir in the broth and the reserved clam juice. Bring to a simmer over medium heat and cook for 10 minutes. Stir in the half-and-half and heat through. Sprinkle 2 tablespoons potato flour over the soup and stir in.

Add the remaining ½ tablespoon flour for a thicker soup if desired. Stir in the pepper and clams and cook for 1 to 2 minutes. Sprinkle the bacon over each serving.

Makes 6 servings

Per serving: 180 calories, 8 g protein, 12 g carbohydrates, 3 g dietary fiber, 11 g total fat, 4 g saturated fat, 42 mg cholesterol, 563 mg sodium
Diet Exchanges: 1 carb (3 vegetable), 1 meat, 1 fat

SICILIAN SAUSAGE STEW

8 ounces Italian-style turkey sausage (hot, sweet, or a mix of both)

2 cups fat-free chicken broth

1 can (16 ounces) no-salt-added tomatoes

2 large potatoes, cut into ½" cubes

1 small yellow summer squash or zucchini, diced

1 can (15 ounces) kidney beans

1 can (15 ounces) white navy or cannellini beans

½ cup diced onions

1 rib celery, diced

2 tablespoons pitted and sliced imported black olives

2 tablespoons chopped fresh parsley

1 tablespoon chopped fresh oregano

2 cloves garlic, minced

1 teaspoon aniseeds

Salt and ground black pepper

Crumble the sausage into a large saucepan and sauté over medium heat until browned, about 5 minutes. Drain off the fat.

Add the stock and stir to loosen any brown bits stuck to the pan. Add the tomatoes (with juice), potatoes, squash or zucchini, kidney beans (with liquid), white beans (with liquid), onions, celery, olives, parsley, oregano, garlic, and aniseeds. Bring to a boil. Reduce the heat to low; cover, and simmer for 25 minutes, or until the vegetables are tender. Add salt and pepper to taste.

Makes 6 servings

Per serving: 271 calories, 20 g protein, 42 g carbohydrates, 11 g dietary fiber, 5 g total fat, 1 g saturated fat, 0 g cholesterol, 414 mg sodium
Diet Exchanges: 2 carbs (2 bread/starch), 2 meat

TOMATO-BASIL SOUP

2½ teaspoons extra-virgin olive oil

4 shallots, minced

3 cloves garlic, minced

2 pounds tomatoes, chopped

3 cups vegetable broth or water

10 large fresh basil leaves

⅓ cup cooked white rice

Salt and ground black pepper

Heat the oil in a large nonstick skillet over medium heat and sauté 2 of the shallots and 1 clove of the garlic for 2 minutes, or until soft. Add the tomatoes and the remaining 2 shallots and 2 cloves garlic. Cook for 10 minutes, stirring frequently.

Add the stock or water and the basil and rice. Add salt and pepper to taste. Simmer for 15 minutes.

Makes 4 servings

Per serving: 101 calories, 3 g protein, 17 g carbohydrates, 3 g dietary fiber, 4 g total fat, 1 g saturated fat, 0 g cholesterol, 144 mg sodium
Diet Exchanges: 1 carb (3 vegetable), ½ fat

Note: This soup is refreshing and delicious served cold. Simply chill it in the refrigerator and add 1 tablespoon fresh lemon juice before serving.

CRISP TORTILLA WITH AVOCADO, BEANS, AND CHEESE

4　corn tortillas (6" diameter)

1　can (15 ounces) pinto beans, drained, with 2 tablespoons liquid reserved

¼　teaspoon salt

¼　teaspoon onion powder

¼　teaspoon garlic powder

1　avocado, thinly sliced

1　jalapeño chile pepper, seeded and chopped (wear plastic gloves when handling)

¾　cup (4 ounces) shredded Muenster cheese

Preheat the oven to 350°F.

Arrange the tortillas on a baking sheet in a single layer. Bake, turning occasionally, until golden and crisp, 18 to 20 minutes.

Meanwhile, in a small saucepan over low heat, combine the beans, reserved liquid, ⅛ teaspoon of the salt, the onion powder, and the garlic powder. Cook until hot, 2 to 3 minutes.

Arrange the avocado slices over the tortillas. Season with the remaining ⅛ teaspoon salt and top with the jalapeño pepper. Spoon the beans over the top and cover with the cheese. Bake until the cheese melts, 5 to 8 minutes.

Makes 4 servings

Per serving: 347 calories, 17 g protein, 24 g carbohydrates, 8 g dietary fiber, 21 g total fat, 9 g saturated fat, 41 mg cholesterol, 610 mg sodium
Diet Exchanges: 1 carb (1 bread/starch), 2 meat, 3 fat

COUNTRY-STYLE POTATO AND GREEN BEAN SOUP WITH HAM

3 cloves garlic, minced

2 very large or 3 medium russet potatoes, quartered lengthwise and sliced ¼" thick

1 large onion, chopped

4 ounces coarsely cubed ham

1½ cups chicken broth

1½ cups water

1 teaspoon dried marjoram, crushed

¼ teaspoon ground black pepper

12 ounces green beans, halved

3 carrots, sliced

½ cup (3 ounces) reduced-fat sour cream

In a large saucepan or Dutch oven, combine the garlic, potatoes, onion, ham, broth, water, marjoram, and pepper. Bring to a boil over high heat. Reduce the heat to low, cover, and simmer, stirring occasionally, for 15 minutes, or until the potatoes are very tender.

Using a potato masher, mash the potatoes slightly, breaking them up to give the soup a chunky texture.

Add the green beans and carrots. Cover and cook, stirring occasionally, for 10 minutes, or until tender. Add the sour cream and bring to a simmer, stirring constantly, until the soup is slightly thickened and creamy.

Makes 4 servings (about 6 cups)

Per serving: 288 calories, 13 g protein, 41 g carbohydrates, 9 g fat, 26 mg cholesterol, 645 mg sodium, 8 g dietary fiber
Diet Exchanges: 1½ vegetable, 1½ bread, 2 meat
Carb Choices: 3

MEDITERRANEAN MUFFULETTA

2 tablespoons chopped dry-packed sun-dried tomatoes

1 large eggplant (1 pound), cut lengthwise into ¼"-thick slices

1 large yellow squash, cut lengthwise into ¼"-thick slices

1 red onion, sliced crosswise

2 red bell peppers, cut into strips

2 ounces fat-free cream cheese, at room temperature

2 ounces goat cheese, crumbled

2 tablespoons fat-free sour cream

2 teaspoons chopped fresh thyme

1 tablespoon chopped pistachios (optional)

1 loaf crusty multigrain French bread, halved lengthwise through the side

Coat a grill rack with cooking spray. Preheat the grill.

Place the tomatoes in a small bowl. Cover with boiling water and soak for 10 minutes, or until soft. Drain and set aside.

Meanwhile, place the eggplant, squash, onion, and peppers on the prepared grill rack and cook for 6 minutes, turning once, or until lightly browned and softened. Remove from the grill and set aside.

In another small bowl, combine the cream cheese, goat cheese, sour cream, thyme, pistachios (if using), and reserved tomatoes.

Remove the soft insides from the crust of each half of the bread and reserve for another use. Spread the tomato mixture over both halves of the bread. Layer the reserved vegetables on the bottom half, then cover with the top half. Cut into 4 sandwiches.

Makes 4 servings

Per serving: 290 calories, 13 g protein, 47 g carbohydrates, 7 g total fat, 4 g saturated fat, 13 mg cholesterol, 8 g dietary fiber, 508 mg sodium
Diet Exchanges: 2½ carbs (2 bread/starch, 1 vegetable), 2 meat

BARBECUED PORK SANDWICHES

1   **chipotle pepper (see note)**

12 **ounces pork tenderloin, trimmed of all visible fat**

¼   **teaspoon ground red pepper**

⅔   **cup diced onions**

1   **tablespoon minced garlic**

¾   **cup reduced-sodium barbecue sauce**

¼   **cup apple cider**

1   **teaspoon brown sugar**

4   **sandwich buns, toasted**

In a small bowl, cover the chipotle pepper with hot water and soak for 5 minutes. Drain. Remove the stems and seeds (wear plastic gloves when handling). Coarsely chop the pepper and set aside.

Coat a large nonstick skillet with cooking spray and warm over medium-high heat. Sear the pork, turning as necessary, for about 5 minutes, or until browned on all sides. Remove and place on a large piece of triple-layered foil. Season with the red pepper and set aside.

Coat a medium nonstick saucepan with cooking spray and warm over medium heat. Add the onions and cook, stirring occasionally, for 5 minutes. If necessary, add 1 to 2 teaspoons water to prevent sticking. Add the garlic and cook for 1 minute. Add the barbecue sauce, cider, brown sugar, and the reserved chipotle pepper. Bring to a boil and simmer for 10 minutes.

Preheat the oven to 350°F. Pour one-third of the sauce over the pork, then tightly seal the foil over the pork. Bake for 25 minutes, or until very tender.

Using 2 forks, shred the pork. Add to the remaining sauce and cook over medium heat until hot. Serve with the buns.

Makes 4 servings

Per serving: 291 calories, 22 g protein, 37 g carbohydrates, 1 g dietary fiber, 6 g total fat, 2 g saturated fat, 49 mg cholesterol, 235 mg sodium
Diet Exchanges: 2 carbs, (2 bread/starch), 2 meat

Note: Chipotle peppers are mesquite-smoked, dried jalapeño peppers. They are also available canned. Omit the soaking if using a canned pepper.

SANTA FE STUFFED SANDWICHES

1 unsliced round (12 ounces) sourdough or multigrain bread

1 can (19 ounces) black beans, rinsed and drained

2 scallions, sliced

2 tablespoons chopped fresh cilantro or parsley

¼ cup barbecue sauce

½–1 teaspoon hot-pepper sauce

5 large leaves lettuce

1 cup (4 ounces) shredded low-fat Monterey Jack cheese

1 tomato, thinly sliced

2 roasted red peppers

With a serrated knife, slice off the top third of the bread and set aside. Hollow out the bottom, leaving a ½"-thick shell. Reserve the bread pieces for another use.

In a medium bowl, coarsely mash half of the beans. Add the scallions, cilantro or parsley, barbecue sauce, and the remaining beans. Stir to mix. Add ½ teaspoon of the hot-pepper sauce. Taste and add up to ½ teaspoon more, if desired.

Line the hollowed bread with the lettuce. Cover with the bean mixture. Sprinkle with the cheese. Cover with the tomato and peppers. Cover with the reserved bread top and press firmly. Cut into 6 wedges.

Makes 6 servings

Per serving: 261 calories, 15 g protein, 39 g carbohydrates, 5 g fat, 13 mg cholesterol, 729 mg sodium, 7 g dietary fiber

Diet Exchanges: 1½ vegetable, 1½ bread

Carb Choices: 2½

GRILLED VEGETABLE MELTS

BASIL SPREAD

1 cup packed fresh basil leaves

2 tablespoons grated Parmesan
cheese

1 tablespoon toasted walnuts

1 clove garlic

¼ cup (2 ounces) fat-free cream
cheese or sour cream

SANDWICHES

2 zucchini, cut lengthwise into
¼"-thick slices

2 yellow and/or red bell peppers,
quartered

1 red onion, cut crosswise into
¼"-thick slices

¼ teaspoon salt

1½ tablespoons balsamic vinegar

8 slices Italian bread, lightly
toasted

4 slices low-fat Jarlsberg cheese

To make the basil spread: In a food processor, combine the basil, Parmesan, walnuts, and garlic. Process to puree. Add the cream cheese or sour cream. Process to mix. Set aside.

To make the sandwiches: Preheat the grill or broiler. Coat a grill rack or broiler-pan rack with cooking spray.

Arrange the zucchini, peppers, and onion in a single layer on the prepared rack. Coat lightly with cooking spray. Sprinkle with the salt. Grill or broil, turning once, for 10 minutes, or until lightly browned. Place on a plate and drizzle with the vinegar.

Arrange 4 of the bread slices on the rack. Spread with the reserved basil mixture. Top with layers of zucchini, peppers, onion, and cheese. Grill or broil for 1 minute, or until the cheese melts. Top with the remaining bread slices.

Makes 4 servings

Per serving: 311 calories, 20 g protein, 46 g carbohydrates, 6 g total fat, 2 g saturated fat, 13 mg cholesterol, 5 g dietary fiber, 705 mg sodium
Diet Exchanges: 2½ carbs (2 bread/starch, 1½ vegetable), 2 meat

CHICKEN SALAD ROLL-UPS

1 can (8 ounces) mandarin oranges

¼ cup Asian plum sauce

1 tablespoon rice wine vinegar or wine vinegar

1 teaspoon grated fresh ginger

½ pound cold cooked boneless, skinless chicken breast, cut into small strips

1 red bell pepper, chopped

½ cup chopped seeded cucumber

2 scallions, thinly sliced

2½ cups packed chopped romaine lettuce

4 whole wheat tortillas (8" diameter)

Drain the oranges, reserving 2 tablespoons of the juice.

In a large bowl, combine the plum sauce, vinegar, ginger, and reserved orange juice. Add the chicken, pepper, cucumber, scallions, lettuce, and oranges. Toss to coat.

Place the tortillas on a work surface. Divide the salad evenly on top. Roll into cylinders and slice in half diagonally.

Makes 4 servings

Per serving: 331 calories, 22 g protein, 48 g carbohydrates, 6 g fat, 50 mg cholesterol, 416 mg sodium, 6 g dietary fiber
Diet Exchanges: ½ fruit, 1½ bread, 3 meat
Carb Choices: 3

SALADS AND VEGETABLES

SUNNY WALDORF SALAD

¾ cup (6 ounces) low-fat plain yogurt

½ cup orange juice

1½ tablespoons honey

½ teaspoon ground cinnamon

3 apples, cut into ½" chunks

1 large orange, separated into segments

1 rib celery, chopped

½ cup golden raisins

3 tablespoons coarsely chopped cashews

In a large bowl, combine the yogurt, orange juice, honey, and cinnamon. Add the apples, orange, celery, raisins, and cashews. Stir to mix.

Makes 6 servings

Per serving: 162 calories, 3 g protein, 34 g carbohydrates, 3 g fat, 2 mg cholesterol, 57 mg sodium, 4 g dietary fiber
Diet Exchanges: ½ milk, 1½ fruit
Carb Choices: 2

BLT BREAD SALAD

6 plum tomatoes, chopped

2 cloves garlic, minced

⅓ cup chopped fresh basil or 1½ teaspoons dried

3 tablespoons balsamic vinegar

½ teaspoon salt

12 slices turkey bacon, cooked and crumbled

½ small red onion, halved and thinly sliced

8 ounces French bread, cubed (about 6 cups)

8 ounces romaine lettuce leaves, shredded

In a large bowl, combine the tomatoes, garlic, basil, vinegar, and salt. Mash the tomatoes and garlic with a fork until coarsely pureed. Add the bacon, onion, and bread. Toss to coat. Let stand for 10 minutes so the bread absorbs some of the juices. Add the lettuce and toss to mix.

Makes 6 servings

Per serving: 180 calories, 8 g protein, 27 g carbohydrates, 3 g dietary fiber, 5 g total fat, 1 g saturated fat, 16 mg cholesterol, 682 mg sodium
Diet Exchanges: 3 carbs (1½ bread/starch, 1½ vegetable)

SPINACH-ORANGE SALAD WITH SESAME

1 teaspoon sugar	1½ teaspoons toasted sesame oil
½ teaspoon cornstarch	10 ounces baby spinach leaves
⅓ cup orange juice	2 navel oranges, separated into segments
1½ tablespoons rice wine vinegar	
1 teaspoon grated fresh ginger or ¼ teaspoon ground	1 small red onion, thinly sliced
	1 kiwifruit, sliced
1 clove garlic, chopped	

Place the sugar and cornstarch in a small saucepan. Gradually add the orange juice and vinegar, whisking to dissolve the dry ingredients. Add the ginger and garlic. Cook, stirring, over medium-high heat for 2 to 3 minutes, or just until the mixture boils. Remove and whisk in the oil. Allow to cool.

In a large bowl, combine the spinach, orange segments, onion, and kiwifruit. Add the dressing and toss to coat evenly.

Makes 4 servings

Per serving: 113 calories, 4 g protein, 23 g carbohydrates, 2 g fat, 0 mg cholesterol, 60 mg sodium, 6 g dietary fiber
Diet Exchanges: 1½ vegetable, 1 fruit
Carb Choices: 2

MEDITERRANEAN CHICKPEA SALAD

1 can (15 ounces) chickpeas, rinsed and drained

3 plum tomatoes, chopped

2 roasted red peppers, chopped

½ small red onion, quartered and thinly sliced

½ cucumber, peeled, halved, seeded, and chopped

2 tablespoons chopped parsley

2 cloves garlic, chopped

3 tablespoons lemon juice

1½ teaspoons extra-virgin olive oil

1½ teaspoons flax oil

¼ teaspoon salt

In a large bowl, combine the chickpeas, tomatoes, peppers, onion, cucumber, parsley, garlic, lemon juice, olive oil, flax oil, and salt. Toss to coat well. Let stand for at least 15 minutes to allow the flavors to blend.

Makes 8 servings

Per serving: 104 calories, 4 g protein, 18 g carbohydrates, 3 g fat, 0 mg cholesterol, 158 mg sodium, 4 g dietary fiber
Diet Exchanges: ½ vegetable, ½ bread, ½ fat
Carb Choices: 1

CHEESY BAKED CAULIFLOWER

2 teaspoons vegetable oil

1 small onion, chopped

2 cloves garlic, minced

2 tablespoons unbleached or all-purpose flour

¼ teaspoon salt

⅛ teaspoon ground nutmeg

1½ cups 1% milk

½ cup (2 ounces) shredded low-fat Monterey Jack cheese

¼ cup (1 ounce) grated Parmesan cheese

1 pound frozen cauliflower pieces, thawed

1 pound frozen sliced carrots, thawed

⅓ cup crushed low-fat round snack crackers

Preheat the oven to 350°F. Coat a medium baking dish with cooking spray.

Warm the oil in a medium saucepan over medium heat. Add the onion and garlic. Cook, stirring often, for 5 minutes, or until soft. Sprinkle with the flour, salt, and nutmeg. Cook, stirring constantly, for 1 minute. Stir in the milk. Cook, stirring often, for 5 minutes, or until thickened.

Remove from the heat. Stir in the Monterey Jack and Parmesan until melted. Add the cauliflower and carrots and stir to coat. Spoon into the prepared baking dish. Sprinkle with the crackers.

Bake for 15 to 20 minutes, or until heated through and bubbly.

Makes 6 servings

Per serving: 247 calories, 12 g protein, 36 g carbohydrates, 5 g dietary fiber, 7 g total fat, 3 g saturated fat, 12 mg cholesterol, 572 mg sodium
Diet Exchanges: 2 carbs (1 milk, 3 vegetable), 1½ meat

AVOCADO, GRAPEFRUIT, AND PAPAYA SALAD

1 **tablespoon olive oil**

2 **teaspoons lemon or lime juice**

1 **avocado, peeled and sliced**

2 **pink grapefruit, peeled and sectioned**

1 **small ripe papaya, peeled and sliced**

2 **scallions, thinly sliced**

4 **cups mixed baby greens**

1 **tablespoon finely chopped cilantro**

In a medium bowl, whisk together the oil and juice. Add the avocado, grapefruit, papaya, and scallions. Toss gently to combine. Cover and refrigerate for 1 hour. Serve over a bed of the greens, sprinkled with the cilantro.

Makes 4 servings

Per serving: 175 calories, 3 g protein, 20 g carbohydrates, 12 g fat, 0 mg cholesterol, 12 mg sodium, 4 g dietary fiber
Diet Exchanges: 1½ vegetable, ½ fruit
Carb Choices: 1

INDIAN-SPICED POTATOES AND SPINACH

2 medium russet potatoes, scrubbed and cut into ½" chunks

2 tablespoons canola oil

3 large cloves garlic, minced

1 medium onion, chopped

1¾ teaspoons ground cumin

¾ teaspoon ground coriander

½ teaspoon ground turmeric

¼ teaspoon ground ginger

¼ teaspoon salt

¼ teaspoon ground black pepper

⅛ teaspoon ground cinnamon

2 cups frozen cut leaf spinach (from a bag)

2–4 tablespoons water

½ cup (4 ounces) fat-free plain yogurt

Place a steamer basket in a large saucepan with ½ inch of water. Place the potatoes in the steamer and bring to a boil over high heat. Reduce the heat to medium, cover, and cook for 20 minutes, or until the potatoes are very tender. Drain the potatoes and transfer to a bowl. Cover to keep warm. Dry the saucepan.

Heat the oil in the saucepan over medium heat. Add the garlic and onion and cook, stirring frequently, for 5 minutes, or until soft. Add the cumin, coriander, turmeric, ginger, salt, pepper, and cinnamon. Cook, stirring, for 30 seconds.

Add the potatoes and cook, stirring frequently, for 5 minutes, or until crisp and golden. Add the spinach and 2 tablespoons of the water. Cover and cook, tossing gently (add additional water 1 tablespoon at a time, if needed), for 5 minutes, or until heated through.

Place in a serving bowl. Spoon the yogurt on top and serve hot.

Makes 4 servings

Per serving: 195 calories, 8 g protein, 24 g carbohydrates, 7 g fat, 1 mg cholesterol, 350 mg sodium, 6 g dietary fiber
Diet Exchanges: 1 vegetable, 1 bread, 1 meat, 1 fat
Carb Choices: 1½

BARLEY WITH SPRING GREENS

1½ cups chicken or vegetable broth

½ cup pearl barley

1 tablespoon extra-virgin olive oil

1 bunch scallions, thinly sliced

3 cloves garlic, slivered

10 cups loosely packed torn mixed greens, such as escarole, Swiss chard, watercress, and arugula

¼ teaspoon salt

⅛ teaspoon ground black pepper

Bring the broth to a boil in a medium saucepan over high heat. Add the barley and return to a boil. Reduce the heat to low, cover, and simmer for 45 minutes, or until tender.

Meanwhile, heat the oil in a large saucepan or Dutch oven over medium-high heat. Add the scallions and garlic and cook, stirring frequently, for 3 minutes, or until the scallions are wilted.

Add the greens, salt, and pepper. Cook, stirring, for 3 minutes, or until just wilted. Fluff the barley with a fork and stir into the greens.

Makes 4 servings

Per serving: 143 calories, 5 g protein, 24 g carbohydrates, 4 g fat, 0 mg cholesterol, 391 mg sodium, 7 g dietary fiber

Diet Exchanges: 2½ vegetable, ½ bread, 1 meat

Carb Choices: 1½

GRILLED VEGETABLES

2 small zucchini, sliced diagonally ¼" thick

2 small yellow summer squash, sliced diagonally ¼" thick

2 small eggplant, sliced diagonally ¼" thick

1 large red bell pepper, halved lengthwise and seeded

2 medium red onions, sliced crosswise ⅛" thick

1 teaspoon ground black pepper

Pinch of salt

Coat an unheated grill rack with olive oil cooking spray. Preheat the grill.

Arrange the zucchini, squash, eggplant, bell pepper, and onions on the rack and coat lightly with the spray. Place the rack over medium-hot coals, arranging it so the vegetables are 6" from the coals. Grill for 4 to 6 minutes on each side, or until golden brown. Sprinkle with the black pepper and salt.

Note: You can also prepare these vegetables indoors under the broiler. Cook them 4 to 6 inches from the heat for 5 to 8 minutes.

Makes 6 servings

Per serving: 80 calories, 3 g protein, 18 g carbohydrates, 1 g fat, 0 mg cholesterol, 47 mg sodium, 7 g dietary fiber
Diet Exchanges: 3 vegetable
Carb Choices: 1

MUSTARD-CRUSTED BRUSSELS SPROUTS

1 slice rye bread with caraway seeds

2 boxes (10 ounces each) frozen Brussels sprouts

2–3 tablespoons Dijon mustard

1 tablespoon prepared horseradish

2 teaspoons olive oil

Preheat the broiler.

Tear the bread into pieces and place in a food processor. Pulse until finely ground.

In a large saucepan, cook the Brussels sprouts according to package directions. Drain and return to the pan. Stir in the mustard and horseradish. Spoon into an 8" x 8" glass baking dish. Sprinkle with the bread crumbs and drizzle with the oil. Broil 3" from the heat for 3 minutes, or until the crumbs are crisp and golden.

Makes 4 servings

Per serving: 112 calories, 7 g protein, 16 g carbohydrates, 4 g fat, 0 mg cholesterol, 400 mg sodium, 5 g dietary fiber
Diet Exchanges: $1\frac{1}{2}$ vegetable, 1 fat
Carb Choices: 1

BIG BROILED BALSAMIC MUSHROOMS

2 tablespoons balsamic vinegar

2 tablespoons water

2 teaspoons olive oil

$\frac{1}{2}$ teaspoon dried thyme

12 ounces portobello mushrooms, trimmed and thickly sliced

Preheat the broiler. Line a broiler-pan rack with foil.

In a large bowl, whisk together the vinegar, water, oil, and thyme. Add the mushrooms and toss gently to coat. Arrange in a single layer on the rack and broil 3" from the heat for 2 minutes. Turn and broil for 2 minutes longer, or until golden.

Makes 4 servings

Per serving: 49 calories, 2 g protein, 6 g carbohydrates, 3 g fat, 0 mg cholesterol, 5 mg sodium, 1 g dietary fiber
Diet Exchanges: $1\frac{1}{2}$ vegetable
Carb Choices: $\frac{1}{2}$

QUINOA WITH PEPPERS AND BEANS

1 cup quinoa	2 medium red bell peppers, cut into thin strips
2½ cups vegetable broth	
2 tablespoons extra-virgin olive oil	1 large onion, cut into thin wedges
3 cloves garlic, minced	1 can (14–19 ounces) black beans, rinsed and drained
1 tablespoon finely chopped peeled fresh ginger	¼ cup chopped fresh cilantro
¾ teaspoon whole cumin seeds	

Place the quinoa in a fine-mesh strainer and rinse under cold running water until the water runs clear.

Bring 2 cups of the broth to a boil in a medium saucepan over high heat. Add the quinoa and return to a boil. Reduce the heat to low, cover, and simmer for 20 minutes, or until tender.

Meanwhile, heat the oil in a 12" nonstick skillet over medium heat. Add the garlic, ginger, and cumin seeds and cook, stirring, for 2 minutes, or until fragrant. Add the peppers and onion and cook, stirring, for 8 minutes, or until tender. Stir in the beans and the remaining ½ cup broth and cook for 2 minutes.

Fluff the quinoa with a fork and stir in the cilantro. Place in a serving bowl and top with the pepper mixture.

Makes 4 servings

Per serving: 307 calories, 14 g protein, 50 g carbohydrates, 10 g fat, 0 mg cholesterol, 637 mg sodium, 9 g dietary fiber
Diet Exchanges: 1½ vegetable, 2 bread, 2 meat
Carb Choices: 3

MEDITERRANEAN BAKED BEANS

1 cup great Northern beans, picked over and rinsed

1 cup red kidney beans, picked over and rinsed

2 cups chicken broth

1½ cups water

6 cloves garlic, minced

2 tablespoons extra-virgin olive oil

1 large sprig fresh sage or ½ teaspoon dried, crushed

½ teaspoon freshly ground black pepper

Place the great Northern and kidney beans in a large bowl. Add cold water to cover by 2". Cover and let stand overnight.

Preheat the oven to 325°F. Drain the beans and place in an ovenproof Dutch oven. Add the broth, water, garlic, oil, sage, and pepper.

Cover and bake for 1 hour and 45 minutes, or until the beans are very creamy and tender. (Add a little more water during baking, if needed.)

Makes 4 servings

Per serving: 292 calories, 15 g protein, 42 g carbohydrates, 16 g dietary fiber, 8 g total fat, 1 g saturated fat, 0 mg cholesterol, 408 mg sodium

Diet Exchanges: 2 carbs (2 bread/starch), 2 meat

ADZUKI BEANS WITH MISO DRESSING

1¼ cups dried adzuki beans, small red beans, or black beans, picked over and rinsed

¼ teaspoon ground black pepper

2 tablespoons mellow white miso

3 tablespoons orange juice

2 tablespoons lemon juice

2 tablespoons olive oil

½ teaspoon grated fresh ginger

3 scallions, sliced diagonally

2 medium cucumbers, peeled, halved, seeded, and cut into thin diagonal slices

1 small carrot, shredded

¼ cup coarsely chopped walnuts

Place the beans in a large bowl. Add water to cover by 2". Cover and let stand overnight.

Drain the beans and place in a medium saucepan. Add water to cover by 2" and bring to a boil over high heat. Stir in the pepper. Reduce the heat to low, cover, and simmer, stirring, for 30 minutes, or until very tender. Drain the beans, place in a serving bowl, and let stand for 20 minutes.

Meanwhile, in a large bowl, whisk together the miso, orange juice, lemon juice, oil, and ginger. Stir in the scallions, cucumbers, carrot, walnuts, and beans. Let stand for 15 minutes to blend the flavors.

Makes 4 servings

Per serving: 351 calories, 15 g protein, 49 g carbohydrates, 12 g fat, 0 mg cholesterol, 327 mg sodium, 10 g dietary fiber
Diet Exchanges: 3 bread, 3 meat
Carb Choices: 3

GREEN BEANS WITH GINGERED WALNUTS

1 tablespoon canola oil	¾ cup walnut halves
1 teaspoon reduced-sodium soy sauce	1 pound green beans, rinsed and trimmed
¼ teaspoon ground ginger	2 teaspoons lemon juice
¼ teaspoon garlic powder	1 tablespoon olive oil

Preheat the oven to 250°F.

Spread the canola oil in a small baking pan and place the pan in the oven. When the pan is hot, remove it and stir in the soy sauce, ginger, and garlic powder. Add the walnuts and stir to coat. Bake, stirring occasionally, for 25 minutes, or until the nuts are crisp and brown. Remove the pan from the oven. Cool the nuts on a paper towel.

In a medium saucepan, steam the beans for about 5 minutes, or until crisp-tender. In a serving bowl, toss the beans with the lemon juice and oil. Add the walnuts and toss. Serve immediately.

Makes 4 servings

Per serving: 180 calories, 4 g protein, 9 g carbohydrates, 4 g dietary fiber, 15 g total fat, 2 g saturated fat, 0 mg cholesterol, 50 mg sodium
Diet Exchanges: ½ carb (2 vegetable), 3 fat

CHICKEN AND TURKEY
MAIN DISHES

CURRIED CHICKEN WITH COCONUT

2 teaspoons peanut oil or walnut oil

1 teaspoon butter

½ large onion, chopped

2 cloves garlic, minced

¾ cup chopped fennel bulb or celery

½ large green or red bell pepper, chopped

4 boneless, skinless chicken breast halves (6 ounces each), cut into 1" cubes

½ teaspoon salt

¼ teaspoon ground black pepper

1 tablespoon curry powder

⅔ cup canned crushed tomatoes

½ cup chicken broth

3 tablespoons chopped peanuts

3 tablespoons shredded unsweetened coconut

In a large saucepan, heat the oil and butter over medium heat until the butter is melted. Stir in the onion, garlic, fennel or celery, and bell pepper. Cover and cook, stirring occasionally, just until translucent, 8 to 10 minutes.

Stir in the chicken, salt, and black pepper. Cook, stirring frequently, until the chicken has lost most of its pink color, 3 to 5 minutes. Sprinkle with the curry powder and cook, stirring, for 30 seconds. Add the tomatoes and broth and bring to a simmer. Cover, reduce the heat to medium-low, and cook until the chicken is tender, about 30 minutes.

Serve with the nuts and coconut for sprinkling on top.

Makes 8 servings

Per serving: 165 calories, 22 g protein, 12 g carbohydrates, 4 g dietary fiber, 6 g total fat, 2 g saturated fat, 51 mg cholesterol, 292 mg sodium
Diet Exchanges: 3 meat

CHICKEN CUTLETS WITH MOZZARELLA, PEPPERS, AND OLIVES

4 boneless, skinless chicken breast halves (6 ounces each)

1 tablespoon fresh basil or ½ teaspoon dried

4 slices (6 ounces) smoked or regular mozzarella cheese, each ¼" thick

½ teaspoon salt

¼ teaspoon ground black pepper

2 tablespoons olive oil

1 large green or red bell pepper, cut into thin strips

⅓ cup dry white wine or chicken broth

⅓ cup (3 ounces) pitted ripe kalamata olives, quartered lengthwise

Preheat the oven to 350°F.

Make a 3"-long horizontal pocket in each chicken piece (cut through the thicker edge to ½" from the opposite edge). Sprinkle the basil over the cheese slices. Slip a cheese slice into each pocket, folding it as needed to fit. Close the edges and secure with toothpicks. Season with ¼ teaspoon of the salt and the pepper.

Heat the oil in a large ovenproof skillet over medium-low heat. Stir in the bell pepper and season with the remaining ¼ teaspoon salt. Cook, stirring occasionally, until lightly browned and starting to wilt, 4 to 5 minutes. Push the pepper to the edge of the skillet and add the chicken. Cook until lightly browned, 2 to 3 minutes. Turn the chicken and arrange the pepper around it. Add the wine or broth and the olives.

Bake, turning once or twice, until the chicken juices run clear and a meat thermometer registers 170°F, 12 to 15 minutes.

Using a slotted spoon, transfer the chicken to plates and top with the peppers and olives. There should be about 2 tablespoons of juice in the pan. If more, set the skillet over medium heat and cook until the liquid is reduced, 1 to 3 minutes. Spoon over the chicken.

Makes 8 servings

Per serving: 210 calories, 24 g protein, 2 g carbohydrates, 0 g dietary fiber, 10 g total fat, 4 g saturated fat, 66 mg cholesterol, 307 mg sodium

Diet Exchanges: 3 meat, 1 fat

CHICKEN PARMESAN

SAUCE

1 tablespoon olive oil

2 cloves garlic, minced

1¼ cups canned crushed tomatoes

2 tablespoons Italian-style tomato paste

⅛ teaspoon dried oregano

½ teaspoon dried basil

¼ teaspoon salt

⅛ teaspoon ground black pepper

CHICKEN

6 slices light whole wheat bread

2 large eggs

2 tablespoons water

4 boneless, skinless chicken breast halves (6 ounces each), pounded to ¼" thick

¼ teaspoon salt

½ teaspoon ground black pepper

¼ cup soy flour or whole wheat flour

2 teaspoons olive oil

6 ounces shredded part-skim mozzarella cheese

To make the sauce: Heat the oil in a small saucepan over low heat. Stir in the garlic and cook, stirring frequently, for 30 seconds. Add the tomatoes, tomato paste, oregano, and basil. Cook, stirring occasionally, until thick and rich, 12 to 15 minutes. Season with the salt and pepper. Cover and keep warm.

To make the chicken: Preheat the oven to 250°F.

Place the bread on a baking sheet and bake until completely dry, 10 to 12 minutes. Let cool slightly. Transfer the bread to a food processor and grind to make about 1 cup crumbs. Transfer to a large plate.

In a shallow bowl, lightly beat the eggs with the water. Season the chicken with the salt and pepper and coat with the flour. Dip into the egg mixture, then press into the crumbs to coat both sides.

Place the broiler-pan rack 4" to 5" from the heat and preheat the broiler. Heat 1 teaspoon of the oil in a large skillet over medium heat. Add 2 of the coated chicken breasts and cook until golden brown on the first side, 2 to 3 minutes. Turn and cook until the chicken is no longer pink and the juices run clear, 2 to 3 minutes. Transfer to a 13" x 9" baking dish.

Repeat with the remaining 1 teaspoon oil and the remaining chicken. Top with the sauce and sprinkle with the cheese. Broil just until the cheese melts, 1 to 2 minutes.

Makes 6 servings

Per serving: 366 calories, 40 g protein, 16 g carbohydrates, 2 g dietary fiber, 16 g total fat, 5 g saturated fat, 153 mg cholesterol, 572 mg sodium
Diet Exchanges: ½ carb (1 bread/starch, ½ vegetable), 5 meat, 2 fat

CHICKEN TETRAZZINI

2 teaspoons + 1 tablespoon butter	6–8 large mushrooms (8 ounces), sliced
1¼ cups (4½ ounces) whole wheat rotelle or other short pasta	½ cup heavy cream
2¼ cups chicken broth	2 tablespoons cornstarch
¼ cup dry white wine or chicken broth	2 tablespoons + 1¼ teaspoons water
1 bay leaf	¼ teaspoon ground black pepper
4 boneless, skinless chicken breast halves (6 ounces each), cut crosswise into ¼"-wide strips	⅔ cup (3 ounces) grated Parmesan cheese

Place the oven rack in the top position and preheat the oven to 425°F. Coat an 8" x 8" baking dish with 2 teaspoons of the butter.

Cook the pasta according to package directions. Drain well and transfer to a large, warmed bowl.

Meanwhile, in a large saucepan, combine 1½ cups of the broth, the wine or broth, and the bay leaf. Bring to a simmer over medium heat. Add the chicken and cook, stirring once, just until cooked through, for 8 minutes. Using a slotted spoon, transfer the chicken to the pasta bowl. Add the mushrooms to the broth and cook until tender, for 3 to 4 minutes. Add the mushrooms to the pasta bowl. Discard the bay leaf.

Measure the broth left in the pan. If more than 1½ cups, boil it until reduced. If less than 1½ cups, add some of the remaining ¾ cup broth. Add the cream and simmer for 1 minute. Increase the heat to medium-high and bring to a boil.

In a cup, combine the cornstarch and water. Whisk into the broth mixture and cook, whisking until thickened, for 30 to 60 seconds. Season with the pepper and add to the pasta bowl. Toss to mix.

Pour the mixture into the prepared baking dish, spreading it evenly. Sprinkle with the cheese and dot with the remaining 1 tablespoon butter, cut into small pieces. Bake on the top rack until light brown and bubbling, for 15 to 20 minutes.

Makes 12 servings

Per serving: 163 calories, 18 g protein, 9 g carbohydrates, 6 g fat, 46 mg cholesterol, 182 mg sodium, 2 g dietary fiber
Diet Exchanges: 1 bread, 2 meat
Carb Choices: ½

NEW AMERICAN FRIED CHICKEN

½ **cup buttermilk**

½ **cup fresh white bread crumbs**

½ **cup fresh whole wheat bread crumbs**

½ **teaspoon paprika**

1 **teaspoon ground black pepper**

½ **teaspoon dried thyme or sage**

1 **tablespoon minced fresh parsley**
   Pinch of salt (optional)

4 **skinless whole chicken legs**

Preheat the oven to 425°F. Coat a baking rack with cooking spray. Place the rack on a foil-lined baking sheet.

Place the buttermilk in a shallow dish. Place the white and whole wheat bread crumbs in another shallow dish.

In a cup or small bowl, combine the paprika, pepper, thyme or sage, parsley, and salt (if using). Add 1 teaspoon of the mixture to the bread crumbs and the remainder to the buttermilk.

Dip the chicken pieces in the buttermilk, then roll them in the seasoned bread crumbs to coat. Place on the prepared rack and lightly coat with cooking spray.

Bake for 15 minutes. Turn the chicken and coat with cooking spray. Bake for 15 minutes, or until the crust is golden brown and the juices run clear when a joint is pierced with a sharp knife.

Makes 4 servings

Per serving: 226 calories, 28 g protein, 8 g carbohydrates, 9 g fat, 90 mg cholesterol, 178 mg sodium, 0 g dietary fiber
Diet Exchanges: 4 meat
Carb Choices: ½

BAKED CHICKEN THIGHS WITH PEPPERS AND OLIVES

1 teaspoon olive oil

1½ cups sliced onions

1 tablespoon minced garlic

1 green bell pepper, thinly sliced

1 red or yellow bell pepper, thinly sliced

5 pitted black olives, sliced

¼ teaspoon dried thyme

¼ teaspoon dried rosemary

Pinch of red-pepper flakes

1¼ pounds boneless, skinless chicken thighs, trimmed of all visible fat

2 teaspoons lemon juice

⅛ teaspoon ground black pepper

1 tablespoon grated Parmesan cheese

2 cups hot cooked rice

Preheat the oven to 425°F.

Coat a no-stick skillet with cooking spray. Add the oil and warm over medium heat. Add the onions and garlic and sauté for 4 to 5 minutes, or until the onions are nearly tender.

Add the green and red or yellow peppers and sauté for 5 to 6 minutes, or until tender. Add the olives, thyme, rosemary, and red-pepper flakes and sauté for 1 minute.

Coat a shallow 3-quart nonstick baking dish with cooking spray. Arrange the chicken in a single layer in the baking dish. Drizzle with the lemon juice and sprinkle with the black pepper. Spoon the vegetables over the chicken and sprinkle with the cheese.

Bake for 25 to 30 minutes, or until the chicken is cooked through. Serve with the rice.

Makes 4 servings

Per serving: 310 calories, 21 g protein, 35 g carbohydrates, 3 g dietary fiber, 10 g total fat, 4 g saturated fat, 59 mg cholesterol, 111 mg sodium

Diet Exchanges: 2 carbs (2 bread/starch), 2 meat, 1 fat

VARIATION

Baked Chicken Thighs with Tomatoes and Pine Nuts: Omit the bell peppers and replace with 2 medium tomatoes, each cut into 8 wedges. Instead of sautéing, add the tomatoes to the baking dish after the chicken. Replace the olives, thyme, and rosemary with 1 tablespoon toasted pine nuts and 1 tablespoon chopped fresh basil. Sprinkle over the chicken and tomatoes.

GRILLED CHICKEN BREASTS IN SAGE VINAIGRETTE

¼ cup balsamic vinegar

1 tablespoon extra-virgin olive oil

2 teaspoons chopped fresh sage

4 boneless, skinless chicken breast halves (4 ounces each)

Preheat the grill or broiler. In a small bowl, whisk together the vinegar, oil, and sage. Brush over the chicken and let marinate for 15 minutes at room temperature.

Remove the chicken from the marinade. Cook over a medium-hot grill or broil about 5" from the heat for 6 to 8 minutes, or until the chicken is cooked through, turning once and basting occasionally with the marinade.

Makes 4 servings

Per serving: 219 calories, 21 g protein, 6 g carbohydrates, 0 g dietary fiber, 4 g total fat, 3 g saturated fat, 94 mg cholesterol, 41 mg sodium

Diet Exchanges: 3 meat, 1 fat

Note: To make a light sauce for the chicken, double the marinade ingredients. After the chicken has marinated and while it is cooking, pour the marinade into a saucepan over medium-low heat. Bring to a boil, then reduce the heat to low and simmer for 2 minutes, whisking constantly. Drizzle over the chicken or serve alongside.

STUFFED CHICKEN BREASTS

1 zucchini, shredded

1 small onion, chopped

1½ teaspoons dried oregano

½ teaspoon dried thyme

½ cup (4 ounces) low-fat cottage cheese

¼ cup (1 ounce) grated Parmesan cheese

½ cup fresh bread crumbs

¼ teaspoon + ⅛ teaspoon salt

4 boneless, skinless chicken breast halves (4 ounces each), trimmed of all visible fat

Preheat the oven to 450°F. Coat a baking sheet with cooking spray.

Coat a large skillet with cooking spray. Add the zucchini, onion, 1 teaspoon of the oregano, and the thyme. Coat with cooking spray. Cook, stirring occasionally, over medium heat for 5 to 6 minutes, or until any juices from the zucchini have evaporated. Remove from the heat. Add the cottage cheese, Parmesan, bread crumbs, and ¼ teaspoon of the salt. Stir to mix.

Place the chicken on a work surface. Butterfly each piece by making a horizontal cut into the thick end of each breast half to create a flap. Do not cut all the way through. Open the cut portion as you would open a book. Lay a piece of plastic wrap over the chicken and flatten with the flat side of a meat mallet or heavy skillet to about ¼" thickness.

Place one-quarter of the zucchini mixture in the center of each breast half. Roll each into a bundle, tucking in the sides as you roll. Tie each bundle with kitchen string. Place on the prepared baking sheet and coat with cooking spray. Season with the remaining ½ teaspoon oregano and ⅛ teaspoon salt.

Bake for 10 minutes. Reduce the oven temperature to 350°F. Bake for 15 minutes, or until a thermometer inserted in the thickest portion registers 160°F and the juices run clear.

Remove from the oven and let stand for 5 minutes. Remove the string before serving.

Makes 4 servings

Per serving: 262 calories, 35g protein, 17 g carbohydrates, 2 g dietary fiber, 5 g total fat, 2 g saturated fat, 73 mg cholesterol, 638 mg sodium

Diet Exchanges: ½ carb (¼ bread/starch, 1 vegetable), 4 meat

TURKEY BURGERS STUFFED WITH CHILES AND CHEESE

1 large jalapeño chile pepper
(1–1½ ounces)

1½ pounds 7% low-fat ground turkey

4 slices (¾ ounce each) Muenster
cheese

4 pimiento-stuffed green olives
(1 ounce), sliced

¾ teaspoon salt

¼ teaspoon ground black pepper

1 tablespoon vegetable oil

Place the jalapeño pepper in a small, heavy skillet. Cook over very low heat, turning frequently, until the skin has blistered and blackened slightly, 10 to 15 minutes. Remove from the skillet and let cool. Peel off the skin and cut the pepper in half lengthwise, discarding the stem, seeds, and ribs (wear plastic gloves when handling). Coarsely chop.

Divide the turkey into 8 pieces. Gently press or pat to make patties about 4" in diameter. Layer the cheese, jalapeño pepper, and olives on 4 of the patties. Top with the remaining 4 patties and pinch the edges together to seal. Season with the salt and pepper.

Heat the oil in a large nonstick skillet over medium-high heat. Add the patties and cook until browned on the first side, 3 to 4 minutes. Flip and cook until browned, 2 to 3 minutes. Reduce the heat to low and cook until the meat is no longer pink but still juicy, 6 to 8 minutes.

Makes 4 servings

Per serving: 370 calories, 41 g protein, 1 g carbohydrates, 0 g dietary fiber, 21 g total fat, 7 g saturated fat, 143 mg cholesterol, 799 mg sodium
Diet Exchanges: 6 meat, 3 fat

BREADED TURKEY THIGHS WITH MUSTARD SAUCE

¼ cup apple cider vinegar

2 tablespoons Dijon mustard

2 tablespoons brown sugar

1 teaspoon grated fresh ginger

½ teaspoon dried thyme

2 boneless, skinless turkey thighs

½ cup fresh bread crumbs

In a small bowl or cup, combine the vinegar, mustard, brown sugar, ginger and thyme.

Cut each turkey thigh in half. Place the turkey between two sheets of wax paper and pound to equal thickness. Transfer to a shallow bowl and pour on half of the mustard sauce. Cover and marinate for 15 minutes.

Preheat the broiler. Coat a baking rack with cooking spray and place on a foil-lined nonstick baking sheet. Remove the turkey from the marinade, gently shaking off the excess. Discard the marinade. Coat the turkey with the bread crumbs.

Place the turkey on the prepared rack and broil 8" from the heat for 6 to 8 minutes per side, or until the turkey is cooked through and the crumbs are golden.

In a small saucepan over low heat, warm the remaining half of the mustard sauce. Serve with the turkey.

Makes 4 servings

Per serving: 195 calories, 22 g protein, 12 g carbohydrates, 0 g dietary fiber, 7 g total fat, 2 g saturated fat, 63 mg cholesterol, 817 mg sodium

Diet Exchanges: ½ carb (½ bread/starch), 3 meat

SESAME TURKEY CUTLETS

2   **tablespoons hoisin sauce**

2   **tablespoons water**

1   **pound turkey breast cutlets**

Ground black pepper

1   **tablespoon toasted sesame seeds (see note)**

In a small bowl, stir together the hoisin sauce and water; set aside.

Rinse the turkey and pat dry with paper towels. Sprinkle each cutlet with pepper. Coat a large nonstick skillet with cooking spray and warm over medium-high heat. Add the turkey and cook for 1 minute. Turn the cutlets and cook for 2 to 3 minutes, or until no longer pink.

Pour the reserved hoisin sauce mixture over the turkey and cook until the mixture comes to a boil. Sprinkle with the sesame seeds.

Makes 4 servings

Per serving: 142 calories, 28 g protein, 3 g carbohydrates, 0 g dietary fiber, 2 g total fat, 75 mg cholesterol, 148 mg sodium

Diet Exchanges: 3 meat

Note: To toast the sesame seeds, place them in a small nonstick skillet. Cook and stir over medium heat for 2 to 3 minutes, or until golden and fragrant.

STUFFED TURKEY TENDERLOINS

2 **turkey breast tenderloins (8–12 ounces each)**

¼ **cup fat-free ricotta cheese**

2 **tablespoons fat-free cream cheese**

2 **tablespoons diced red bell peppers**

1 **tablespoon grated Parmesan cheese**

1 **tablespoon chopped fresh oregano**

1 **tablespoon drained capers**

Salt and ground black pepper

1 **cup fat-free chicken broth**

2 **tablespoons fat-free sour cream**

2 **teaspoons lemon juice**

Cut a 3" horizontal slit into the center of each tenderloin. In a small bowl, mix together the ricotta, cream cheese, red peppers, Parmesan, oregano, and capers. Add salt and black pepper to taste. Stuff into the slit pockets.

In a large nonstick skillet over medium heat, brown the turkey for about 2 minutes per side. Add the broth. Cover, reduce the heat, and simmer for 15 minutes, or until the turkey is cooked through and no longer pink when cut with a knife.

Transfer the turkey to a plate and tent with foil to keep warm. Increase the heat and cook the broth for 3 minutes, or until reduced by half. Whisk in the sour cream and lemon juice. To serve, slice each tenderloin in half crosswise and drizzle with the sauce.

Makes 4 servings

Per serving: 164 calories, 30 g protein, 3 g carbohydrates, 0 g dietary fiber, 1 g total fat, 3 g saturated fat, 78 mg cholesterol, 285 mg sodium

Diet Exchanges: 4 meat

BEEF, PORK, AND LAMB MAIN DISHES

SPICY MEATBALLS WITH COCONUT MILK

1½ pounds extra-lean ground beef

3 scallions, finely chopped

1 large egg, lightly beaten

5 tablespoons + ½ cup coconut milk

2 tablespoons soy sauce

1½ teaspoons ground cumin

¾ teaspoon ground coriander seeds

½ teaspoon crushed red-pepper flakes

Place the broiler rack 3" to 4" from the heat source and preheat the broiler. Coat a large broiler-pan rack with cooking spray.

In a large bowl, combine the beef, scallions, egg, 5 tablespoons of the coconut milk, 1½ tablespoons of the soy sauce, and the cumin, coriander, and red-pepper flakes. Gently form into 1½"-diameter meatballs and arrange on the prepared pan, placing them at least ½" apart. Broil (without turning) just until browned on the top, no longer pink inside, and the juices run clear. Transfer to a serving dish and discard the fat drippings in the pan.

Pour the remaining ½ cup coconut milk into the pan and scrape up the browned bits, stirring until dissolved. Season with the remaining ½ tablespoon soy sauce and pour over the meatballs.

Makes 6 servings

Per serving: 213 calories, 24 g protein, 2 g carbohydrates, 12 g fat, 95 mg cholesterol, 389 mg sodium, 1 g dietary fiber

Diet Exchanges: 3 meat, 1 fat

Carb Choices: 0

NOT YOUR MOTHER'S MEAT LOAF

½ small onion, chopped

1 rib celery, chopped

⅓ cup finely chopped red or green bell pepper

1 clove garlic, minced

1 can (14½ or 15 ounces) chopped tomatoes, drained

⅓ cup chopped fresh parsley

⅓ cup fat-free milk

1 egg

2 teaspoons Worcestershire sauce

2 teaspoons Italian seasoning

1 pound extra-lean ground beef

1 pound ground turkey breast

1½ cups fresh bread crumbs

Preheat the oven to 350°F. Coat a 9" x 5" loaf pan with cooking spray.

Coat an 8" skillet with cooking spray. Add the onion, celery, pepper, and garlic. Coat with cooking spray and set over medium heat. Cook, stirring often, for 4 to 5 minutes, or until soft. Place in a large bowl. Add 1 cup of the tomatoes and the parsley, milk, egg, Worcestershire sauce, Italian seasoning, beef, turkey, and bread crumbs. Stir until well blended. Pat the mixture into the prepared loaf pan.

Bake for 1 hour, or until a thermometer inserted into the center registers 160°F and the meat is no longer pink. During the last 15 minutes of baking, spread the remaining tomatoes down the center of the meat loaf.

Remove from the oven and drain off any accumulated juices from the pan. Let stand for 5 minutes before slicing.

Note: When making meat loaf, you can double the recipe with little extra effort. Cook a loaf for dinner and wrap the uncooked loaf in plastic wrap and then in foil. Freeze for up to 1 month. Completely thaw in the refrigerator before cooking.

Makes 8 servings

Per serving: 287 calories, 33 g protein, 20 g carbohydrates, 8 g fat, 94 mg cholesterol, 368 mg sodium, 2 g dietary fiber
Diet Exchanges: 1 bread, 4 meat
Carb Choices: 1

SIZZLING BEEF KEBABS

- 8 ounces fresh orange juice
- 2 tablespoons reduced-sodium soy sauce
- 1 tablespoon rice wine or apple cider vinegar
- 2 large cloves garlic, minced, or 1 teaspoon garlic powder
- 1 tablespoon chopped fresh ginger or 1 teaspoon ground
- 2 teaspoons crushed red pepper
- 2 teaspoons ground black pepper
- 1 teaspoon orange peel
- 1 pound bottom round, trimmed and cut into 1½" cubes
- 1 large zucchini, sliced ½" thick
- 1 yellow bell pepper, cut into 2" chunks
- 1 red bell pepper, cut into 2" chunks

In a flat baking dish, whisk together the orange juice, soy sauce, vinegar, garlic, ginger, red pepper, black pepper, and orange peel. Place the beef, zucchini, and red and yellow bell peppers in the dish, coating well with the marinade. Cover the dish with plastic wrap. Marinate in the refrigerator for at least 2 hours.

Preheat the grill.

Alternate the beef and vegetables on eight 8" or four 10" to 12" skewers. Place the kebabs over heat and grill each side for 4 to 5 minutes, or until cooked through.

Makes 4 servings

Per serving: 237 calories, 27 g protein, 14 g carbohydrates, 8 g fat, 66 mg cholesterol, 348 mg sodium, 3 g dietary fiber
Diet Exchanges: 1 vegetable, ½ fruit, 3 meat
Carb Choices: 1

GRILLED FLANK STEAK WITH CHILE-TOMATO SALSA

2 tablespoons ground cumin

3 cloves garlic, minced

3 tablespoons lime juice

1 teaspoon coarsely ground black pepper

¼ teaspoon salt

1 beef flank steak or top round steak (1¼ pounds), trimmed of all visible fat

1 can (4½ ounces) chopped mild green chiles, drained

1 large tomato, finely chopped

3 scallions, thinly sliced

Lightly oil a grill rack or broiler-pan rack. Preheat the grill or broiler.

Place the cumin in a 6" skillet over medium heat and cook, stirring, for 3 minutes, or until fragrant and darker in color. Place in a small bowl and let cool.

Remove 1 teaspoon toasted cumin and place in a medium bowl. To the small bowl, add the garlic, 2 tablespoons of the lime juice, the black pepper, and ½ teaspoon of the salt. Mix well. Place the steak on the prepared rack and rub the cumin mixture over both sides of the steak. Let stand at room temperature.

Meanwhile, in the medium bowl with the reserved cumin, combine the chiles, tomato, scallions, and the remaining 1 tablespoon lime juice and ¼ teaspoon salt. Let stand at room temperature.

Grill or broil the steak for 4 minutes per side, or until a thermometer inserted into the center registers 145°F for medium-rare.

Place the steak on a cutting board and let stand for 5 minutes. Cut into thin slices and serve with the salsa.

Note: The steak may be rubbed with the spice mixture and refrigerated up to 1 day ahead.

Makes 4 servings

Per serving: 269 calories, 33 g protein, 7 g carbohydrates, 11 g fat, 58 mg cholesterol, 605 mg sodium, 2 g dietary fiber
Diet Exchanges: 1½ vegetable, 4 meat
Carb Choices: ½

ITALIAN-STYLE BEEF BURGERS

1½ **pounds extra-lean ground beef**

5 **tablespoons grated Romano cheese**

2 **tablespoons pine nuts, toasted and finely chopped**

½ **teaspoon salt**

1 **teaspoon dried oregano**

¾ **teaspoon garlic powder**

¼ **teaspoon ground black pepper**

Place the broiler rack 2" to 3" from the heat source and preheat the broiler.

Place the beef in a large bowl and break into pieces. Add the cheese, pine nuts, salt, oregano, garlic powder, and pepper. Using a fork, gently combine the beef and seasonings. Divide the meat into 4 even pieces and gently form into patties approximately 4" in diameter and 1" thick.

Place on a broiler-pan rack and broil until the top is browned, for 4 to 6 minutes. Turn and cook until a meat thermometer inserted into the center of a patty registers 160°F for medium, for 4 to 6 minutes.

Makes 4 servings

Per serving: 252 calories, 37 g protein, 2 g carbohydrates, 12 g fat, 98 mg cholesterol, 482 mg sodium, 0 g dietary fiber
Diet Exchanges: 4½ meat
Carb Choices: 0

SALSA BEEF PATTIES

- 1 **pound ground eye round**
- ¼ **teaspoon ground black pepper**
- 3 **plum tomatoes, finely chopped**
- 1 **jarred or freshly roasted red bell pepper, finely chopped (see note)**
- 2 **tablespoons finely chopped red onion**
- 1 **tablespoon finely chopped fresh cilantro**
- 1–2 **teaspoons finely chopped jalapeño pepper (wear plastic gloves when handling)**
- 4 **whole wheat buns, split**
  Romaine lettuce leaves

Preheat the oven to 450°F.

Form the meat into 4 patties ½" thick. Season with the black pepper. Place on a broiler-pan rack and bake for 8 minutes. Turn and bake for 8 to 10 minutes, or until no longer pink in the center.

In a small bowl, mix the tomatoes, bell pepper, onions, and cilantro. Stir in jalapeño pepper to taste.

Line the bun bottoms with lettuce leaves and spoon on half of the salsa. Place the patties on top of the salsa. Add the remaining salsa and the bun tops.

Makes 4

Per pattie: 356 calories, 26 g protein, 22 g carbohydrates, 3 g dietary fiber, 18 g total fat, 5 g saturated fat, 68 mg cholesterol, 323 mg sodium
Diet Exchanges: 1½ carb (1 bread/starch, 1 vegetable), 3 meat, 2 fat

Note: Blacken a red bell pepper on all sides under the broiler. Wrap it in foil and set aside until cool enough to handle. Remove and discard the charred skin, seeds, and inner membranes. Chop the flesh.

PORK CHOPS WITH APPLE CIDER, WALNUTS, AND PRUNES

4 pork chops (6–8 ounces each), each ¾" thick

½ teaspoon salt

½ teaspoon ground rubbed sage

¼ teaspoon ground black pepper

1 tablespoon walnut oil or olive oil

6 pitted prunes (2–3 ounces), chopped

½ cup apple cider

¼ cup dry white wine or apple cider

2 tablespoons chopped walnuts

Season the pork with the salt, sage, and pepper.

Heat the oil in a 12" skillet over medium-high heat. Add the pork and cook until browned on the first side, for 4 to 5 minutes. If desired, hold the chops on the edges and cook the edges until browned, for 1 to 2 minutes. Turn and cook until the second side is browned, about 1 minute. Reduce the heat to low and pour off any fat in the skillet. Add the prunes, cider, and wine or cider. Cook, turning once or twice, until the juices run clear and a meat thermometer inserted into the pork registers 155°F, for 12 to 15 minutes.

Transfer to plates and spoon the prunes on top. There should be about 2 tablespoons of juices left in the pan. If more, cook over low to medium heat until reduced. Spoon over the pork and sprinkle with the walnuts.

Makes 4 servings

Per serving: 296 calories, 22 g protein, 11 g carbohydrates, 17 g fat, 60 mg cholesterol, 342 mg sodium, 1 g dietary fiber
Diet Exchanges: 3 meat
Carb Choices: 1

BARBECUED COUNTRY SPARERIBS

2 cans (6 ounces each) tomato juice

⅓ cup apple cider or peach nectar

2 tablespoons Worcestershire sauce

1½ tablespoons apple cider vinegar

2 teaspoons Dijon mustard

¾ teaspoon ground black pepper

½ teaspoon chili powder

¼ teaspoon salt

¼ teaspoon garlic powder

8 boneless pork country spareribs (3½ ounces each), trimmed of all visible fat

Preheat the oven to 350°F.

In a roasting pan or baking dish, combine the tomato juice, cider or nectar, Worcestershire sauce, vinegar, mustard, pepper, chili powder, salt, and garlic powder. Add the pork and coat completely.

Cover with foil and bake, turning once, until very tender, 1¾ to 2 hours. If the sauce thickens too much, thin it with a little hot water.

Makes 6 servings

Per serving: 304 calories, 32 g protein, 5 g carbohydrates, 0 g dietary fiber, 16 g total fat, 6 g saturated fat, 102 mg cholesterol, 488 mg sodium

Diet Exchanges: 4½ meat, 1 fat

MEXICAN PORK STEW

- 2 tablespoons olive oil
- 1 pound pork tenderloin, cut into 1½" cubes
- 1 large onion, chopped
- 2 cloves garlic, minced
- ½ teaspoon ground cumin
- ¼ teaspoon ground cinnamon
- 2 cups low-sodium vegetable broth
- 1 can (15 ounces) diced tomatoes
- 1 can (4½ ounces) chopped green chiles, drained
- ¼ teaspoon ground black pepper
- 1 small butternut squash or pumpkin (2 pounds), peeled, halved, seeded, and cut into ¾"-thick chunks
- 1 medium zucchini, halved lengthwise and cut into ½"-thick slices
- 1 large red bell pepper, cut into thin strips
- ¼ cup whole blanched almonds, ground

Heat the oil in a large saucepan or Dutch oven over high heat. Add the pork, onion, garlic, cumin, and cinnamon. Cook, stirring, for 5 minutes, or until the pork is lightly browned.

Add the broth, tomatoes (with juice), chiles, and black pepper and bring to a boil. Reduce the heat to low, cover, and simmer, stirring occasionally, for 25 minutes.

Stir in the butternut squash or pumpkin, zucchini, and bell pepper. Cover and simmer, stirring occasionally, for 1 hour, or until the pork and squash are tender. Stir in the almonds. Cover and simmer for 5 minutes, or until slightly thickened.

Makes 4 servings

Per serving: 244 calories, 24 g protein, 18 g carbohydrates, 10 g fat, 45 mg cholesterol, 594 mg sodium, 4 g dietary fiber
Diet Exchanges: 1½ vegetable, ½ bread, 3 meat
Carb Choices: 1

SPICED PORK SCALLOPS WITH FRUIT CHUTNEY

1 teaspoon ground cumin

¾ teaspoon ground coriander

¼ teaspoon ground cinnamon

¼ teaspoon salt

¼ teaspoon freshly ground black pepper

4 well-trimmed boneless pork chops (1 pound)

2 tablespoons butter

1 small onion, coarsely chopped

2–3 small tart apples, cored and cut into ¾" chunks

⅓ cup dried apricots, halved

¼ cup pitted prunes, halved

¼ cup water

3 tablespoons frozen apple juice concentrate

In a cup, combine the cumin, coriander, and cinnamon. Reserve ½ teaspoon for the chutney. Stir the salt and pepper into the spice mixture in the cup. Rub over both sides of the chops. Place the chops on a plate, cover, and let stand at room temperature.

Meanwhile, melt 1 tablespoon of the butter in a medium saucepan over medium-high heat. Add the onion and cook, stirring frequently, for 3 minutes, or until soft.

Add the apples, apricots, prunes, water, apple juice concentrate, and the reserved ½ teaspoon spice mixture. Bring to a boil over high heat. Reduce the heat to low, cover, and simmer, stirring occasionally, for 20 minutes, or until the fruit is very tender and the juices have thickened into a glaze. Remove from the heat and cover to keep warm.

Melt the remaining 1 tablespoon butter in a large nonstick skillet over medium-high heat. Add the chops and cook for 6 minutes, turning once, or until a thermometer inserted in the center of a chop registers 160°F and the juices run clear. Serve the pork with the chutney.

Makes 4 servings

Per serving: 320 calories, 25 g protein, 33 g carbohydrates, 4 g dietary fiber, 11 g total fat, 5 g saturated fat, 90 mg cholesterol, 271 mg sodium
Diet Exchanges: 2 carbs (2 fruit), 3 meat

LAMB KEBABS

- 2 tablespoons lemon juice
- 1 tablespoon olive oil
- 2 tablespoons chopped fresh oregano
- 1 pound leg of lamb, trimmed of all visible fat and cut into 1" cubes
- 16 cherry tomatoes
- 2 yellow bell peppers, each cut into 8 pieces
- 2 zucchini, each cut into 8 pieces
- 1 large red onion, cut into 16 chunks
- ½ teaspoon salt
- ¼ teaspoon freshly ground black pepper

In a medium bowl, combine the lemon juice, oil, and oregano. Add the lamb and toss to coat well. Cover and refrigerate for at least 2 hours or up to 8 hours.

Coat a grill rack or broiler-pan rack with cooking spray. Preheat the grill or broiler.

Evenly divide the lamb among 4 metal skewers, leaving ¼" of space between the pieces. Discard the marinade.

Evenly divide the tomatoes, bell peppers, zucchini, and onion onto 8 metal skewers, alternating the vegetables. Sprinkle the meat and vegetables with the salt and black pepper.

Cook the kebabs 4 inches from the heat for 8 minutes, turning occasionally, or until the lamb is pink inside and the vegetables are tender.

Makes 4 servings

Per serving: 284 calories, 31 g protein, 15 g carbohydrates, 3 g dietary fiber, 11 g total fat, 3 g saturated fat, 90 mg cholesterol, 368 mg sodium
Diet Exchanges: 1 carb (3 vegetable), 4 meat

MINTED LAMB CHOPS WITH WHITE BEANS

3 anchovy fillets, rinsed and patted dry

1 teaspoon extra-virgin olive oil

3 tablespoons chopped fresh mint or 3 teaspoons dried, crushed

½ teaspoon freshly ground black pepper

4 lamb loin chops (about 1¼ pounds), well-trimmed

4 plum tomatoes, coarsely chopped

1 clove garlic, crushed

3 cups rinsed and drained canned cannellini beans

2 tablespoons beef broth

¼ teaspoon salt

Mint sprigs + additional chopped mint for garnish (optional)

Coat a broiler-pan rack with cooking spray. Preheat the broiler.

On a cutting board, finely chop the anchovies. Sprinkle with the oil, 1 tablespoon of the fresh mint or 1 teaspoon dried, and ¼ teaspoon of the pepper, then mash to a paste with the flat side of a chef's knife or a fork. Place the chops on the prepared rack and rub the anchovy paste over both sides. Let stand at room temperature

Meanwhile, in a medium nonstick skillet, combine the tomatoes and garlic and cook, stirring frequently, over medium-high heat for 2 minutes, or until the tomatoes begin to give up their juices. Reduce the heat to medium, cover, and cook for 3 minutes, or until very soft.

Stir in the beans, broth, salt, the remaining 2 tablespoons fresh mint or 2 teaspoons dried, and the remaining ¼ teaspoon pepper. Bring to a boil over high heat. Reduce the heat to low, cover, and simmer, stirring occasionally, for 10 minutes to blend the flavors.

Meanwhile, broil the chops 4" from the heat for 8 minutes per side, or until a meat thermometer registers 145°F for medium-rare.

To serve, evenly divide the bean mixture among 4 plates and top each with a lamb chop. Garnish with the mint, if using.

Makes 4 servings

Per serving: 515 calories, 47 g protein, 45 g carbohydrates, 12 g dietary fiber, 13 g total fat, 4 g saturated fat, 98 mg cholesterol, 667 mg sodium

Diet Exchanges: 3 carbs (3 bread/starch), 5 meat

FISH AND SHELLFISH MAIN DISHES

BREADED BAKED COD WITH TARTAR SAUCE

TARTAR SAUCE

½ cup reduced-fat mayonnaise

1½ tablespoons lemon juice

1 tablespoon finely chopped dill or sweet pickles

2 teaspoons mustard

2 teaspoons capers, drained and chopped

2 teaspoons chopped parsley (optional)

FISH

2 slices whole wheat bread, torn

2 eggs

1 tablespoon water

1¼ pounds cod or scrod fillet, cut into 1"–1½" pieces

½ teaspoon salt

¼ teaspoon ground black pepper

To make the tartar sauce: In a small bowl, combine the mayonnaise, lemon juice, pickles, mustard, capers, and parsley (if using). Cover and refrigerate.

To make the fish: Preheat the oven to 400°F. Coat a baking sheet with cooking spray.

Place the bread in a food processor and process into fine crumbs.

Place in a shallow bowl. In another bowl, beat the eggs with the water. Season the fish with the salt and pepper. Dip into the eggs, then into the bread crumbs. Place on the prepared baking sheet and generously coat the breaded fish with cooking spray. Bake until opaque inside, for 10 minutes. Serve with the tartar sauce.

Makes 4 servings

Per serving: 268 calories, 30 g protein, 14 g carbohydrates, 10 g fat, 174 mg cholesterol, 734 mg sodium, 1 g dietary fiber

Diet Exchanges: 1 bread, 3½ meat

Carb Choices: 1

SAUTÉED TUNA STEAKS WITH GARLIC SAUCE

2 large cloves garlic, minced

1 tablespoon + 1½ teaspoons olive oil

1 tablespoon balsamic vinegar

¼ teaspoon salt

⅛ teaspoon ground black pepper

4 tuna steaks (6 ounces each), each 1" thick

1½ teaspoons chopped fresh parsley or basil

In a 12" heavy nonstick skillet, cook the garlic in 1 tablespoon of the oil over very low heat, stirring until the garlic's aroma is apparent, 30 to 60 seconds. Immediately add the vinegar, ⅛ teaspoon of the salt, and half of the pepper. Transfer to a bowl and cover with foil to keep warm.

Season the fish with the remaining ⅛ teaspoon salt and the remaining pepper. Heat the remaining 1½ teaspoons oil in the same skillet over medium heat. Add the fish and cook until browned on the first side, for 4 to 5 minutes. Turn and cook until just opaque throughout, for 3 to 4 minutes. Cut each steak into two 3-ounce servings. Serve topped with the garlic sauce and parsley or basil.

Makes 8 servings

Per serving: 148 calories, 20 g protein, 0 g carbohydrates, 7 g fat, 33 mg cholesterol, 107 mg sodium, 0 g dietary fiber

Diet Exchanges: 3 meat

Carb Choices: 0

GRILLED SALMON WITH MINT-CILANTRO YOGURT

¼ cup + 2 tablespoons low-fat plain yogurt

2 tablespoons sour cream

1 tablespoon chopped fresh cilantro

2 teaspoons chopped fresh mint

¼ teaspoon salt

¼ teaspoon ground black pepper

Pinch of ground red pepper (optional)

4 salmon steaks or fillets (6 ounces each), each ¾"–1" thick

2 teaspoons vegetable oil

In a small bowl, combine the yogurt, sour cream, cilantro, mint, salt, ⅛ teaspoon of the black pepper, and the red pepper (if using).

Coat a grill rack with cooking spray. Preheat the grill.

Brush the fish with the oil and season with the remaining ⅛ teaspoon black pepper. Place on the prepared rack and cook until golden, for 5 to 6 minutes. Turn and cook until completely opaque but still juicy, for 3 to 4 minutes. Cut each fillet into two 3-ounce servings. Serve topped with the mint-cilantro yogurt.

Makes 8 servings

Per serving: 143 calories, 18 g protein, 0 g carbohydrates, 7 g fat, 49 mg cholesterol, 108 mg sodium, 0 g dietary fiber
Diet Exchanges: 3 meat
Carb Choices: 0

SOLE WITH STIR-FRIED VEGETABLES

3 tablespoons soy sauce

3 tablespoons dry sherry or fat-free reduced-sodium chicken broth

2 cloves garlic, minced

2 teaspoons grated fresh ginger or ½ teaspoon ground

2 teaspoons cornstarch

1½ teaspoons sugar

2 teaspoons vegetable oil

4 ounces snow peas

¼ pound shiitake or button mushrooms, sliced

1 small red bell pepper, cut into strips

1 cup mung bean sprouts

1 teaspoon toasted sesame oil

4 sole fillets (5 ounces each)

In a small bowl, combine the soy sauce, sherry or broth, garlic, ginger, cornstarch, and sugar. Stir to blend well and set aside.

In a 12" skillet or wok, heat the vegetable oil over high heat. Add the snow peas, mushrooms, and pepper. Cook, tossing, for 3 to 4 minutes, or until the pepper starts to soften. Add the bean sprouts and sesame oil. Toss to combine. Reduce the heat to medium. Add the reserved sauce and cook, stirring, for 2 to 3 minutes, or until thickened.

Place the fillets in a single layer over the vegetables. Cover tightly and cook for 10 to 12 minutes, or until the fish flakes easily.

Makes 4 servings

Per serving: 203 calories, 30 g protein, 10 g carbohydrates, 4 g fat, 68 mg cholesterol, 522 mg sodium, 0 g dietary fiber
Diet Exchanges: 1½ vegetable, 3 meat
Carb Choices: 1

SHRIMP AND CRAB CAKES

2 slices white bread

1 egg white

2 tablespoons low-fat mayonnaise

1 teaspoon Worcestershire sauce

1 teaspoon Dijon mustard

½ pound large shrimp, peeled, deveined, and finely chopped

½ pound lump crabmeat, picked over for shells and flaked

1 rib celery, finely chopped

3 scallions, white part only, chopped

2 tablespoons chopped parsley

Toast the bread and allow to cool. In a small bowl, crumble into fine crumbs. Set aside.

In a large bowl, combine the egg white, mayonnaise, Worcestershire sauce, and mustard. Whisk to blend. Add the shrimp, crabmeat, celery, scallions, parsley, and one-third of the reserved bread crumbs. Toss to mix.

Shape into 8 cakes, about ½" thick. Spread the remaining bread crumbs on a shallow plate. Dip the cakes into the crumbs, pressing lightly to adhere.

Coat a 12" nonstick skillet with cooking spray. Place the cakes in the skillet and cook over medium heat for 2 to 3 minutes, or until lightly browned on the bottom. Remove the pan from the heat and coat the cakes lightly with cooking spray. Return the pan to the heat and carefully turn the cakes. Cook for 2 minutes, or until lightly browned on the bottom. Turn the cakes two more times, coating with cooking spray each time. Cook for 2 minutes longer per side, or until cooked through.

Makes 4 servings

Per serving: 248 calories, 25 g protein, 24 g carbohydrates, 5 g fat, 121 mg cholesterol, 678 mg sodium, 1 g dietary fiber
Diet Exchanges: 1 bread, 3 meat
Carb Choices: 1½

ROAST SWORDFISH WITH HERBED CRUST

4 swordfish steaks (5 ounces each)	1 tablespoon minced fresh parsley
1 tablespoon lemon juice	½ teaspoon salt
⅓ cup fine unseasoned dry bread crumbs	¼ teaspoon ground black pepper
1½ teaspoons dried Italian herb seasoning	

Preheat the oven to 400°F. Coat a 9" x 13" nonstick baking dish with cooking spray.

Sprinkle the swordfish with the lemon juice and let stand for 10 minutes.

In a shallow bowl, combine the bread crumbs, Italian seasoning, parsley, salt, and pepper. Dip the swordfish into the bread crumbs and press gently to coat both sides.

Place the swordfish in a single layer in the prepared baking dish. Generously coat the fish with cooking spray. Bake for 20 to 25 minutes, or until the swordfish is opaque and flakes easily when tested with a fork.

Note: You can replace the swordfish with tuna, shark, or mahi mahi.

Makes 4 servings

Per serving: 220 calories, 29 g protein, 7 g carbohydrates, 6 g fat, 56 mg cholesterol, 474 mg sodium, 0 g dietary fiber
Diet Exchanges: 4 meat
Carb Choices: ½

FLOUNDER FLORENTINE

1 **package (10 ounces) frozen spinach, thawed and squeezed dry**

2 **shallots, minced**

1/3 **cup fish stock or fat-free chicken broth**

1/8 **teaspoon ground nutmeg**

1 **pound skinless flounder fillets**

1/2 **cup buttermilk**

1/2 **cup fat-free liquid egg substitute**

1/8 **teaspoon hot-pepper sauce**

2 **tablespoons grated Romano cheese**

In a medium saucepan over medium heat, combine the spinach, shallots, stock or broth, and nutmeg. Stir, then cover and cook for 5 minutes, stirring once more.

Coat an 8" ovenproof nonstick skillet or large pie plate with cooking spray. Spread the spinach mixture in an even layer in the skillet or pie plate. Place the flounder on top of the spinach in a single layer.

Preheat the broiler.

In a small bowl, combine the buttermilk, egg substitute, and hot-pepper sauce and mix well. Spoon evenly over the flounder. Sprinkle with the cheese. Broil 8" from the heat for 15 minutes, or until the sauce is evenly browned and the flounder is opaque and flakes easily when tested with a fork. Remove from the oven and let stand for 5 minutes. Cut into portions with a spatula and serve hot.

Note: You can replace the flounder with scrod, sole, or orange roughy.

Makes 4 servings

Per serving: 161 calories, 28 g protein, 6 g carbohydrates, 3 g fat, 65 mg cholesterol, 289 mg sodium, 0 g dietary fiber
Diet Exchanges: 1 vegetable, 3 meat
Carb Choices: 1/2

ORANGE ROUGHY VERACRUZ

4 orange roughy or red snapper fillets (5 ounces each)

1 tablespoon lime juice

1 teaspoon dried oregano, crushed

1 tablespoon olive oil

1 onion, chopped

1 clove garlic, minced

1 can (15 ounces) Mexican-style diced tomatoes

12 pimiento-stuffed green olives, coarsely chopped

2 tablespoons chopped parsley

Preheat the oven to 350°F. Coat a 9" x 13" baking dish with cooking spray.

Place the fillets in the prepared baking dish. Sprinkle with the lime juice and oregano.

Heat the oil in an 8" skillet over medium heat. Add the onion and garlic and cook, stirring occasionally, for 5 minutes, or until soft. Add the tomatoes (with juice), olives, and parsley. Cook, stirring occasionally, for 5 minutes, or until thickened. Spoon over the fillets and cover tightly with foil. Bake for 15 minutes, or until the fish flakes easily when tested with a fork.

Makes 4 servings

Per serving: 185 calories, 22 g protein, 11 g carbohydrates, 6 g fat, 28 mg cholesterol, 510 mg sodium, 2 g dietary fiber
Diet Exchanges: 1½ vegetable, 3 meat
Carb Choices: 1

CASSEROLES AND ONE-DISH DINNERS

BAKED POTATOES WITH MUSHROOM STROGANOFF

4 medium baking potatoes

1 small onion, finely chopped

1 tablespoon canola oil

8 ounces shiitake mushrooms, thinly sliced

¼ teaspoon dried thyme

¼ teaspoon salt

¼ teaspoon ground black pepper

2 tablespoons balsamic vinegar

1 cup low-fat plain yogurt

½ cup reduced-fat sour cream

Preheat the oven to 400°F.

Place the potatoes on a baking sheet and bake for 1 hour, or pierce several times with a fork and microwave on high for 15 minutes. When done, they will be easily pierced with a knife.

In a large nonstick skillet over medium heat, cook the onion in the oil for 3 minutes. Add the mushrooms, thyme, salt, and pepper. Cook for 5 minutes. Stir in the vinegar and cook for 1 minute, or until the liquid evaporates.

In a small saucepan, whisk together the yogurt and sour cream. Stir over low heat for 5 minutes, or until warm. (Do not allow the mixture to get too hot or it will separate.)

Split the baked potatoes. Top with the yogurt mixture and the mushrooms.

Makes 4 servings

Per serving: 250 calories, 9 g protein, 38 g carbohydrates, 4 g dietary fiber, 8 g total fat, 3 g saturated fat, 4 mg cholesterol, 209 mg sodium
Diet Exchanges: 2 carb (1½ bread/starch, ½ milk), 2 fat

EGGPLANT STUFFED WITH SAVORY BEEF

2 **eggplants (16 ounces each)**

3 **tablespoons olive oil**

1 **large onion, chopped**

1 **red bell pepper, chopped**

2 **cloves garlic, minced**

1 **pound extra-lean ground beef**

1½ **teaspoons dried oregano**

1 **tablespoon +1½ teaspoons tomato paste**

2 **anchovy fillets, finely chopped (optional)**

1 **tablespoon capers, drained and coarsely chopped (optional)**

½ **cup (2 ounces) shredded or grated Parmesan cheese**

¼ **teaspoon salt**

¼ **teaspoon ground black pepper**

Preheat the oven to 400°F. Pierce the eggplants in 2 or 3 places and place on a baking sheet. Roast, turning once or twice, just until tender when pierced with a fork, 20 to 25 minutes. Let cool enough to handle. Halve lengthwise and scoop out the pulp, leaving a ½" to ¾" shell. Chop the pulp and let drain in a colander.

Heat 2 tablespoons of the oil in a large skillet over medium heat. Add the onion and bell pepper and cook, stirring occasionally, until tender, 8 to 10 minutes. Add the garlic and beef. Cook, stirring to crumble the beef, until no longer pink, 5 to 6 minutes. Stir in the eggplant pulp, oregano, tomato paste, anchovies (if using), and capers (if using). Reduce the heat to low and cook, stirring occasionally, until thick, 15 to 20 minutes. Stir in ¼ cup of the cheese, the salt and black pepper.

Place the eggplant shells on a baking sheet and divide the beef mixture among them. Sprinkle with the remaining ¼ cup cheese and drizzle with the remaining 1 tablespoon oil. Roast until lightly browned on top, 15 to 20 minutes.

Makes 4 servings

Per serving: 372 calories, 31 g protein, 22 g carbohydrates, 8 g dietary fiber, 20 g total fat, 6 g saturated fat, 74 mg cholesterol, 380 mg sodium
Diet Exchanges: 1 carb (3 vegetable), 4 meat, 2 fat

CINCINNATI-STYLE TURKEY CHILI

1 tablespoon + 1½ teaspoons vegetable oil

1 large onion, chopped

1 large green bell pepper, chopped

2 cloves garlic, chopped

1⅓ pounds ground turkey

1¾ cups chicken broth

3 tablespoons tomato paste

2–3 tablespoons chili powder

1½ teaspoons dried oregano

1 teaspoon ground coriander

¼ teaspoon salt

½ teaspoon ground cumin

¼ teaspoon ground cinnamon

1 can (15 ounces) red kidney beans

6 ounces whole wheat spaghetti, broken into short pieces

½ cup (2 ounces) shredded Monterey Jack or Muenster cheese

Heat the oil in a large, heavy pot over medium heat. Add the onion, pepper, and garlic. Cook, stirring occasionally, until the onion starts to brown, 8 to 10 minutes. Add the turkey and cook, stirring to coarsely crumble, until no longer pink, 8 to 10 minutes. Stir in the broth, tomato paste, chili powder, oregano, coriander, salt, cumin, and cinnamon. Bring to a simmer. Partially cover and cook, stirring occasionally, until the meat is tender and the broth is slightly thickened, about 30 minutes.

Meanwhile, pour the beans (with juice) into a microwaveable bowl. Microwave on high for 1 to 2 minutes, or until heated through. Drain and cover to keep warm.

Cook the pasta according to the package directions. Drain and divide among 4 bowls. Ladle the chili over the pasta, top with the beans, and sprinkle with the cheese.

Makes 4 servings

Per serving: 306 calories, 22 g protein, 29 g carbohydrates, 7 g dietary fiber, 13 g total fat, 3 g saturated fat, 66 mg cholesterol, 519 mg sodium

Diet Exchanges: 2 carbs (1½ bread/starch), 2 meat, 1 fat

EGGPLANT PARMESAN

2 eggplants (32 ounces), peeled and sliced lengthwise into ¼"-thick slabs

3 tablespoons olive oil

½ teaspoon salt

1 can (15½ ounces) crushed or chopped tomatoes

1 tablespoon + 1½ teaspoons tomato paste

1 teaspoon dried basil or 3 large fresh leaves, chopped

½ teaspoon dried rosemary, crumbled

¼ teaspoon ground black pepper

1 cup (4 ounces) shredded mozzarella or Fontina cheese

½ cup (2 ounces) grated Parmesan cheese

Preheat the broiler.

Place the eggplants on a large baking sheet and brush both sides of each with the oil (work in batches if necessary). Sprinkle with ¼ teaspoon of the salt. Broil 5" from the heat, until just beginning to brown, for 2 to 3 minutes per side.

Set the oven temperature to 375°F.

In a medium saucepan, combine the tomatoes (with juice), tomato paste, basil, and rosemary. Cook over medium-low heat, stirring occasionally, until slightly thickened, for about 15 minutes. Season with the remaining ¼ teaspoon salt and the pepper.

Spread a layer of the tomato mixture over the bottom of a 1½-quart baking dish. Add a layer of eggplant and top with another layer of tomato mixture. Sprinkle with a thin layer of the mozzarella or Fontina and the Parmesan. Continue making 2 more layers with the remaining eggplant, tomato mixture, and cheeses, ending with a thick layer of cheeses. Bake until bubbling, for 25 to 30 minutes. Let stand for 10 minutes before cutting.

Makes 6 servings

Per serving: 224 calories, 11 g protein, 16 g carbohydrates, 14 g fat, 22 mg cholesterol, 628 mg sodium, 5 g dietary fiber
Diet Exchanges: 3 vegetable, 1 meat, 2 fat
Carb Choices: 1

SPICY CURRIED VEGETABLES

2 tablespoons vegetable oil

1 onion, chopped

2 cloves garlic, minced

1 tablespoon minced fresh ginger

¼–½ teaspoon red-pepper flakes

2 teaspoons curry powder

½ teaspoon ground cumin

½ teaspoon ground coriander seeds (optional)

1–1½ cups vegetable broth

1 small cauliflower (24 ounces), cut into 1½" florets

2 small red potatoes (3 ounces each), cut into 1" cubes

6 ounces string beans, halved

½ cup canned crushed tomatoes

1½ cup plain yogurt (optional)

Heat the oil in a large, deep skillet or saucepan over low to medium heat. Stir in the onion, garlic, ginger, and pepper flakes. Cook, stirring occasionally, until the onion is slightly softened, 2 to 3 minutes. Add the curry powder, cumin, and coriander (if using). Cook, stirring, for 30 seconds. Stir in 1 cup of the broth, the cauliflower, potatoes, beans, and tomatoes. Cover and cook, stirring occasionally and adding up to ½ cup broth as needed, over medium heat until the vegetables are tender, 20 to 25 minutes. There should be 2 to 3 tablespoons of thin sauce in the pan. Remove from the heat and gently stir in the yogurt (if using).

Makes 4 servings

Per serving: 180 calories, 7 g protein, 26 g carbohydrates, 8 g dietary fiber, 7 g total fat, 1 g saturated fat, 0 mg cholesterol, 448 mg sodium
Diet Exchanges: 1 carb (½ bread/starch, 1½ vegetable), 1 fat

MEXICAN LASAGNA

1 pound boneless, skinless chicken breasts, cut into strips

1 large onion, halved and cut into thin wedges

1 large clove garlic, minced

2 cups (16 ounces) fat-free ricotta cheese

1 cup (8 ounces) reduced-fat sour cream

1 jar (4½ ounces) chopped green chiles

½ cup chopped fresh cilantro (optional)

2 teaspoons ground cumin

⅛ teaspoon salt

6 plum tomatoes, chopped

8 corn tortillas (6" diameter), cut in half

1¼ cups (5 ounces) shredded low-fat Monterey Jack cheese

Preheat the oven to 350°F. Coat a 13" x 9" baking dish with cooking spray.

Coat a 12" nonstick skillet with cooking spray. Add the chicken. Cook over medium heat, turning several times, for 5 minutes, or until no longer pink. Transfer to a medium bowl. Wipe the skillet with a paper towel and coat with cooking spray. Add the onion and garlic. Cover and cook over medium heat, stirring occasionally, for 7 to 8 minutes, or until lightly browned. Add to the chicken in the bowl.

In another medium bowl, combine the ricotta, sour cream, chiles, cilantro (if using), cumin, and salt.

Spread 1 cup of the tomatoes in the prepared baking dish. Arrange half of the tortillas evenly on top. Spread half of the ricotta mixture over the tortillas. Top with half of the chicken mixture. Top with 1 cup of the remaining tomatoes and ½ cup of the Monterey Jack. Repeat with the remaining tortillas, ricotta mixture, and chicken mixture. Sprinkle with the remaining 1 cup tomatoes and ¾ cup Monterey Jack. Bake for 30 minutes, or until heated through. Loosely cover with foil if the cheese browns too quickly.

Makes 8 servings

Per serving: 259 calories, 28 g protein, 23 g carbohydrates, 5 g fat, 62 mg cholesterol, 333 mg sodium, 2 g dietary fiber
Diet Exchanges: 1 bread, 3 meat
Carb Choices: 1½

CHICKEN AND MUSHROOM PASTA CASSEROLE

½ pound boneless, skinless chicken breasts

1 large portobello mushroom cap, cut into strips

1 onion, halved and sliced

8 ounces small rigatoni pasta, cooked and drained

2 cans (10 ounces each) low-fat, reduced-sodium condensed cream of mushroom soup

2 cups water

2 roasted red peppers, coarsely chopped

¼ cup chopped parsley

¼ teaspoon salt

⅓ cup (1½ ounces) grated Parmesan cheese

Preheat the oven to 375°F. Coat a 13" x 9" baking dish with cooking spray.

Pat the chicken dry and coat both sides with cooking spray. Place in a 12" skillet over medium-high heat. Cook for 3 to 4 minutes per side, or until golden. Remove the chicken and set aside.

Add the mushroom to the skillet and coat with cooking spray. Cook, stirring, for 5 minutes, or until soft. Remove and set aside with the chicken.

Add the onion to the skillet and coat with cooking spray. Cook, stirring, for 5 minutes, or until lightly golden.

Cut the reserved chicken into strips and place in a large bowl. Add the reserved mushroom and the onion, pasta, soup, water, peppers, parsley, and salt. Stir to mix. Spoon into the prepared baking dish. Sprinkle with the cheese.

Cover loosely with foil and bake for 20 minutes, or until hot and bubbly.

Makes 6 servings

Per serving: 271 calories, 17 g protein, 39 g carbohydrates, 5 g fat, 29 mg cholesterol, 757 mg sodium, 3 g dietary fiber

Diet Exchanges: 2 bread, 2 meat

Carb Choices: 2½

ASPARAGUS QUICHE WITH BROWN RICE CRUST

CRUST

2½ cups cold cooked brown rice

⅓ cup grated Parmesan cheese

2 egg whites, lightly beaten, or ¼ cup liquid egg substitute

FILLING

12 ounces low-fat silken tofu

4 eggs, lightly beaten, or 1 cup liquid egg substitute

1 tablespoon cornstarch

½ teaspoon salt

⅛ teaspoon ground nutmeg

1 pound asparagus, trimmed, cut into 1" pieces, and steamed

3 ounces reduced-fat Swiss cheese, shredded

2 ounces ham-flavored soy deli slices, finely chopped

2 scallions, finely chopped

Preheat the oven to 350°F. Lightly coat a 10" deep-dish pie plate with cooking spray.

To make the crust: In a large bowl, mix the rice, cheese, and egg whites or egg substitute. Press evenly in the bottom and up the sides of the pie plate. Bake for 15 minutes.

To make the filling: In a food processor, combine the tofu, eggs or egg substitute, cornstarch, salt, and nutmeg. Process until smooth, scraping down the sides of the container as necessary.

Sprinkle the asparagus, cheese, soy slices, and scallions over the baked crust. Pour in the tofu mixture, stirring gently to blend slightly. Bake for 45 minutes, or until firm in the center. Let stand for 5 minutes before slicing.

Makes 6 servings

Per serving: 261 calories, 27 g protein, 25 g carbohydrates, 2 g dietary fiber, 8.3 g total fat, 3 g saturated fat, 151 mg cholesterol, 524 mg sodium

Diet Exchanges: 1 carb (½ bread/starch, 1½ vegetable), 3 meat

SPAGHETTI SQUASH CASSEROLE

1 spaghetti squash, halved lengthwise and seeded

1 tablespoon vegetable oil

2 cloves garlic, chopped

1 small onion, chopped

1 teaspoon dried basil, crushed

2 plum tomatoes, chopped

8 ounces low-fat cottage cheese

½ cup (2 ounces) shredded low-fat mozzarella cheese

¼ cup chopped parsley

¼ teaspoon salt

¼ cup (1 ounce) freshly grated Parmesan cheese

3 tablespoons seasoned dry bread crumbs

Preheat the oven to 400°F. Coat a 13" x 9" baking dish and a baking sheet with cooking spray.

Place the squash, cut side down, on the prepared baking sheet. Bake for 30 minutes, or until tender. With a fork, scrape the squash strands into a large bowl.

Meanwhile, heat the oil in a medium skillet over medium heat. Add the garlic, onion, and basil and cook for 4 minutes, or until soft. Add the tomatoes and cook for 3 minutes, or until the mixture is dry.

To the bowl with the squash, add the cottage cheese, mozzarella, parsley, salt, and the tomato mixture. Toss to coat. Place in the prepared baking dish. Sprinkle with the Parmesan and bread crumbs. Bake for 30 minutes, or until hot and bubbly.

Makes 6 servings

Per serving: 219 calories, 12 g protein, 28 g carbohydrates, 4 g dietary fiber, 7 g total fat, 3 g saturated fat, 10 mg cholesterol, 528 mg sodium
Diet Exchanges: 2 carbs (2 bread/starch), 1 meat

Note: Spaghetti squash can also be prepared in the microwave oven. Pierce the squash in several places with a knife. Place on a microwaveable plate and cover loosely with a piece of plastic wrap. Cook on high, turning twice, for 20 minutes, or until tender when pierced. Remove and let stand until cool enough to handle.

SIMPLY SUPER CHILE CASSEROLE

12	Anaheim chile peppers	2	cloves garlic, minced
6	egg whites	1	onion, finely chopped
1	egg	1	tomato, seeded and chopped
2½	cups reduced-fat ricotta cheese	1	cup well-drained canned corn kernels
½	teaspoon salt	½	cup shredded reduced-fat Cheddar cheese
2	teaspoons dried oregano		
½	teaspoon cumin		

Preheat the oven to 400°F.

Place the peppers on a baking sheet and bake for 15 minutes. Remove from the oven and let cool. Cut off the stems and slit each one lengthwise. Remove the seeds and set aside. Reduce the oven temperature to 350°F.

Whisk together the egg whites, egg, ricotta, salt, oregano, cumin, and garlic.

Coat a 9" x 9" baking pan with cooking spray. Lay half of the reserved peppers on the bottom of the pan. Evenly distribute the onion, tomato, and corn over the peppers. Spoon the cheese mixture over the vegetables. Lay the remaining peppers over the vegetables and sprinkle the Cheddar on top.

Cover the pan with foil and bake for 45 minutes. Remove the foil and bake for 10 minutes. Let cool for 10 minutes before serving.

Makes 8 servings

Per serving: 190 calories, 15 g protein, 18 g carbohydrates, 2 g dietary fiber, 8 g total fat, 5 g saturated fat, 50 mg cholesterol, 370 mg sodium
Diet Exchanges: 1 carb (3 vegetable), 2 meat

DESSERTS

PEANUT BUTTER COOKIES

6 tablespoons unsalted butter, softened

½ cup unsweetened smooth peanut butter, at room temperature

¼ cup packed light brown sugar

¼ cup Splenda

1 large egg, at room temperature, lightly beaten

1 teaspoon vanilla extract

1¼ cups sifted oat flour

¼ teaspoon baking powder

3 tablespoons salted peanuts, chopped

Place an oven rack in the middle position and preheat the oven to 350°F.

In a large bowl, beat together the butter and peanut butter until very smooth, about 1 minute. Add the sugar and Splenda and beat until well combined and light in color, for 1 to 2 minutes. Gradually beat in the egg and vanilla, beating until very smooth and a little fluffy, for 1 to 2 minutes. Mix in the flour and baking powder, beating until a moist but cohesive dough forms. Stir in the peanuts.

Drop the dough by rounded tablespoonfuls about 2" apart on nonstick baking sheets. Using the tines of a fork dampened in cold water, flatten each in a cross-hatch pattern until 2" in diameter. Bake until golden brown, for 22 to 25 minutes. Transfer to a rack to cool.

Makes 24

Per cookie: 94 calories, 3 g protein, 7 g carbohydrates, 7 g fat, 17 mg cholesterol, 56 mg sodium, 1 g dietary fiber
Diet Exchanges: 1 bread, ½ meat, ½ fat
Carb Choices: ½

CHOCOLATE HAZELNUT FLOURLESS CAKE

2 tablespoons unsalted butter

3 tablespoons unsweetened cocoa powder

½ cup blanched hazelnuts or almonds

8 tablespoons sugar

3 ounces bittersweet chocolate

½ cup (4 ounces) reduced-fat sour cream

2 egg yolks

1 tablespoon Frangelico or amaretto (optional)

1 teaspoon vanilla extract

½ teaspoon cinnamon

5 egg whites, at room temperature

¼ teaspoon salt

Fresh sliced strawberries (optional)

Preheat the oven to 350°F. Generously coat an 8" or 9" springform pan with 2 teaspoons of the butter and dust with 1 tablespoon of the cocoa powder (don't tap out the excess cocoa; leave it in the pan).

In a food processor, process the nuts with 1 tablespoon of the sugar until finely ground.

In the top of a double boiler over barely simmering water, melt the chocolate and the remaining 4 teaspoons butter, stirring occasionally, until smooth.

Remove from the heat. Place the chocolate mixture in a large bowl. Add the nut mixture, sour cream, egg yolks, Frangelico or amaretto (if using), vanilla, cinnamon, 5 tablespoons of the remaining sugar, and the remaining 2 table-spoons cocoa powder. Stir until well blended.

In another large bowl, with an electric mixer on high speed, beat the egg whites and salt until foamy. Gradually add the remaining 2 tablespoons sugar, beating until the whites hold stiff peaks when the beaters are lifted.

Stir one-quarter of the beaten whites into the chocolate mixture to lighten it. Gently fold in the remaining whites. Spoon into the prepared pan and gently smooth the top.

Bake for 30 minutes, or until the cake has risen, is dry on the top, and a wooden pick inserted into the center comes out with a few moist crumbs. Cool on a rack until warm. The cake will fall dramatically. Loosen the edges of the cake with a knife and remove the pan sides. Serve with the strawberries (if using).

Makes 12 servings

Per serving: 160 calories, 4 g protein, 15 g carbohydrates, 10 g fat, 46 mg cholesterol, 80 mg sodium, 1 g dietary fiber
Diet Exchanges: 1 bread, 2 fat
Carb Choices: 1

NUTTY BROWNIES

2 tablespoons melted butter	1 teaspoon vanilla extract
1/3 cup unsweetened applesauce	1/2 cup whole wheat flour
3/4 cup granulated sugar	1/3 cup finely chopped walnuts
1/2 cup unsweetened cocoa powder	Confectioners' sugar (optional)
1 egg or 1/4 cup fat-free liquid egg substitute	

Preheat the oven to 350°F. Coat an 8" × 8" glass baking dish with cooking spray.

In a large bowl, stir together the butter and applesauce. One at a time, stir in the granulated sugar, cocoa powder, egg or egg substitute, vanilla, flour, and walnuts until well mixed. Spread the batter in the prepared pan.

Bake for 25 minutes, or until the sides begin to pull away from the pan. Cool in the pan on a wire rack. Cut into squares and sprinkle with the confectioners' sugar (if using).

Makes 16

Per brownie: 88 calories, 2 g protein, 14 g carbohydrates, 4 g fat, 17 mg cholesterol, 21 mg sodium, 1 g dietary fiber
Diet Exchanges: 1 bread
Carb Choices: 1

ZUCCHINI–CHOCOLATE CHIP SNACK CAKE

1¾ cups whole grain pastry flour

1½ teaspoons baking powder

½ teaspoon baking soda

1½ teaspoons ground cinnamon

¼ teaspoon salt

2 eggs

⅓ cup packed brown sugar

½ cup (4 ounces) plain yogurt

⅓ cup canola oil

2 teaspoons vanilla extract

1½ cups shredded zucchini

¾ cup mini semisweet chocolate chips

Preheat the oven to 350°F. Line an 8" × 8" baking pan with aluminum foil, leaving extra foil over 2 opposite edges to use as handles after the cake is baked. Coat the foil with cooking spray.

In a large bowl, combine the flour, baking powder, baking soda, cinnamon, and salt.

In a medium bowl, with a wire whisk, beat the eggs, sugar, yogurt, oil, and vanilla until smooth. Stir in the zucchini and chocolate chips.

Add the zucchini mixture to the flour mixture and stir just until blended. Scrape into the prepared pan. Bake for 40 minutes, or until the cake is springy to the touch and a wooden pick inserted into the center comes out clean.

Let the cake cool in the pan on a rack for 30 minutes. Remove from the pan using foil handles. Discard foil and cool completely on the rack.

Makes 16 servings

Per serving: 146 calories, 3 g protein, 18 g carbohydrates, 8 g fat, 27 mg cholesterol, 127 mg sodium, 2 g dietary fiber
Diet Exchanges: 1 bread, 1½ fat
Carb Choices: 1

CHOCOLATE CHIPPERS

2¼ cups unbleached or all-purpose
  flour

¼ cup cornstarch

1 teaspoon baking soda

½ teaspoon salt

¼ cup butter or margarine, softened

2 ounces reduced-fat cream cheese,
  softened

¾ cup granulated sugar

¾ cup packed light brown sugar

1 egg

1 egg white

1 teaspoon vanilla extract

¾ cup chocolate chips

Preheat the oven to 375°F. Lightly coat a baking sheet with cooking spray.

In a medium bowl, combine the flour, cornstarch, baking soda, and salt.

In a large bowl, combine the butter or margarine and cream cheese. With an electric mixer on medium speed, beat for 1 minute, or until smooth. Add the granulated sugar and brown sugar. Beat until light and creamy. Add the egg, egg white, and vanilla. Beat until smooth. Reduce the mixer speed to low. Add the flour mixture in 2 additions, beating just until combined. With a spoon, stir in the chocolate chips. Drop the dough by rounded teaspoonfuls onto the prepared baking sheet. Bake for 9 to 12 minutes until golden. Transfer the cookies to a rack to cool. Repeat until all the cookies are baked.

Makes 40 cookies

Per cookie: 90 calories, 1 g protein, 16 g carbohydrates, 3 g fat, 6 g cholesterol, 72 mg sodium, 0 g dietary fiber
Diet Exchanges: 1 bread
Carb Choices: 1

RASPBERRY-ALMOND TART

CRUST

2/3 cup old-fashioned or quick-cooking rolled oats

1/2 cup whole grain pastry flour

1 tablespoon sugar

1 teaspoon ground cinnamon

1/4 teaspoon baking soda

2 tablespoons canola oil

2–3 tablespoons plain yogurt

1/3 cup mini semisweet chocolate chips (optional)

FILLING

1/4 cup raspberry all-fruit spread

3/4 teaspoon almond extract

2 1/2 cups raspberries

2 tablespoons sliced almonds

Preheat the oven to 375°F. Coat a baking sheet with cooking spray.

To make the crust: In a medium bowl, combine the oats, flour, sugar, cinnamon, and baking soda. Stir in the oil and 2 tablespoons of the yogurt to make a soft, slightly sticky dough. If the dough is too stiff, add the remaining 1 tablespoon yogurt.

Place the dough on the prepared baking sheet and, using lightly oiled hands, pat evenly into a 10" circle. Place a 9" cake pan right side up on the dough and trace around the bottom of the pan with a sharp knife, being careful to score only the surface of the dough. With your fingers, push up and pinch the dough around the outside of the pan to make a 9" crust with a rim 1/4" high. Remove the cake pan. Bake for 12 minutes on the baking sheet. Scatter the chocolate chips (if using) evenly over the surface of the crust and bake until the chocolate is melted and the crust is firm and golden, for 3 to 4 minutes. Remove from the oven and spread the chocolate over the crust to make an even layer. Set aside to cool.

To make the filling and assemble: In a small, microwaveable bowl, combine the fruit spread and almond extract. Microwave on high for 10 to 15 seconds, or until melted. Brush a generous tablespoon of the mixture evenly over the crust. Arrange the raspberries evenly over the crust. Brush the remaining spread evenly over the berries, making sure to get some of the spread between the berries to secure them. Sprinkle with the almonds.

Refrigerate for at least 30 minutes, or until the spread has jelled.

Makes 8 servings

Per serving: 138 calories, 3 g protein, 21 g carbohydrates, 5 g fat, 0 mg cholesterol, 43 mg sodium, 4 g dietary fiber
Diet Exchanges: ½ fruit, ½ bread, 1 fat
Carb Choices: 1½

RICH 'N' CREAMY BROWN RICE PUDDING

3 cups vanilla soy milk	¼ teaspoon freshly grated nutmeg
½ cup uncooked brown rice	2 eggs, lightly beaten
½ teaspoon salt	½ cup dried cherries

In a medium saucepan, combine the soy milk, rice, salt, and nutmeg. Bring to a boil over high heat. Reduce the heat to low, cover, and simmer for 45 minutes. Remove from the heat and let cool for 5 minutes.

Stir ½ cup of the rice mixture into the eggs, stirring constantly. Gradually stir the egg mixture into the saucepan. Stir in the cherries.

Place over medium-low heat and cook, stirring constantly, for 5 minutes, or until thickened. Serve warm or refrigerate to serve cold later.

Makes 4 servings

Per serving: 242 calories, 11 g protein, 38 g carbohydrates, 3 g dietary fiber, 7 g total fat, 1 g saturated fat, 106 mg cholesterol, 347 mg sodium
Diet Exchanges: 2 carbs (½ bread/starch, ½ fruit, 1 milk), 1 meat, ½ fat

SUMPTUOUS STRAWBERRIES IN SPICED PHYLLO

3 cups strawberries (if berries are large, slice into quarters)

¼ cup honey

2 teaspoons lemon juice

¾ teaspoon ground cinnamon

4 tablespoons confectioners' sugar

4 sheets phyllo dough

¼ cup fat-free milk

¼ cup finely chopped almonds

In a large bowl, combine the strawberries, honey, lemon juice, and half of the cinnamon. Fold gently with a spatula.

In a small bowl, combine the remaining cinnamon with the sugar.

Preheat the oven to 350°F. Coat a 6-cup nonstick muffin pan or 6 individual nonstick molds with cooking spray.

On a clean flat surface, lay out 1 sheet of the phyllo. Using a pastry brush, brush the sheet with milk and sprinkle with half of the cinnamon-sugar mixture. Lay the second sheet over the first and sprinkle with the almonds. Lay the third sheet on top, brush with the remaining milk, and sprinkle with the remaining cinnamon-sugar mixture. Lay the fourth sheet on top. Cut in half lengthwise, then crosswise twice to make 6 individual sections.

Using a 6"-round plate or upside-down custard cup, cut 6 disks from the phyllo stack and mold each disk to fit a cup of the muffin pan or molds. Bake for 10 minutes, or until the shells are crisp and golden brown on the sides and bottoms. Remove from the oven and cool completely in the pan.

Remove the phyllo cups and fill each with ½ cup of the berries. Serve at room temperature.

Makes 6 servings

Per serving: 160 calories, 3 g protein, 30 g carbohydrates, 5 g fat, 0 mg cholesterol, 65 mg sodium, 2 g dietary fiber
Diet Exchanges: 1 fruit, 1 bread
Carb Choices: 2

STRAWBERRY-WATERMELON SLUSH

4 ice cubes

6 frozen strawberries

2 cups frozen seedless watermelon
cubes

¾ cup calcium-fortified orange juice

1 tablespoon lime juice

In a blender, combine the ice cubes, strawberries, watermelon, orange juice,
and lime juice. Blend until smooth.

*Note: To freeze melon chunks, lay the chunks on a baking sheet and cover
with plastic wrap. Place in the freezer for about 1 hour. For best quality, store
the fruit in plastic freezer containers and use within 2 to 3 months.*

Makes 2 servings

Per serving: 112 calories, 2 g protein, 26 g carbohydrates, 0 g fat, 0 mg cholesterol, 6 mg sodium,
3 g dietary fiber
Diet Exchanges: 1½ fruit
Carb Choices: 1½

CHOCOLATE SOUFFLÉ CAKE

½ teaspoon + 1 tablespoon unbleached or all-purpose flour

2 ounces semisweet chocolate, chopped

1 cup granulated sugar

2 tablespoons butter or margarine, softened

5 tablespoons (2½ ounces) fat-free sour cream

1 egg yolk

¼ teaspoon vanilla extract

3 tablespoons cocoa powder

4 egg whites, at room temperature

⅛ teaspoon cream of tartar

2 tablespoons confectioners' sugar

Preheat the oven to 350°F. Coat an 8" springform pan with cooking spray. Dust with ½ teaspoon of the flour.

Place the chocolate in a microwaveable bowl. Microwave on high for 1 minute. Stir until smooth. Add ¾ cup of the granulated sugar, the butter or margarine, sour cream, egg yolk, and vanilla. Stir until well blended. Add the cocoa powder and the remaining 1 tablespoon flour. Stir until smooth.

In a large bowl, combine the egg whites and cream of tartar. With an electric mixer on medium speed, beat until soft peaks form. Beat on high speed, while gradually adding the remaining ¼ cup granulated sugar, until stiff peaks form. Fold about one-third of the egg whites into the chocolate. Gently fold in the remaining egg-white mixture in 2 additions. Spoon the batter into the prepared pan and smooth the top.

Bake for 30 to 35 minutes, or until a wooden pick inserted in the middle comes out nearly clean. Cool on a rack. The cake will fall as it cools, leaving a raised edge. Gently press down on the edges as it cools.

To serve, remove the pan sides and transfer the cake to a serving plate. Sift the confectioners' sugar over the top of the cake.

Makes 10 servings

Per serving: 160 calories, 3 g protein, 28 g carbohydrates, 5 g fat, 21 mg cholesterol, 29 mg sodium, 1 g dietary fiber
Diet Exchanges: 2 bread
Carb Choices: 2

INDEX

Boldface page references indicate photographs. Underscored page references indicate boxed text.

E

W

Waist measurement. *See also* Abdominal fat
    in metabolic syndrome, 256, <u>257</u>
Walking
    avoiding injuries from, 164–66
    for beginnners, 156–57
    benefits of, 155
    finding time for, 161–62
    increasing calorie burn from, 157
    interval training with, 150, 160–61
    motivational tips for, 214, <u>224–51</u>
    pace for, 157
    with pedometer, 158–59, <u>159</u>
    for reversing
        insulin resistance, 141–42
        prediabetes, 266, 267
    shoes for, <u>156</u>
    stretching after, 158
    in *Sugar Solution* fitness plan, 9, 144
    weather conditions and, 162, 164
    weekly plans for, <u>157</u>
Walking videos, 164
Wall push, <u>158</u>
Walnuts
    Adzuki Beans and Miso Dressing, 356
    Green Beans with Gingered Walnuts, 357
    Grilled Vegetable Melts, 344
    heart protection from, 67
    Nutty Brownies, 403
    Pork Chops with Apple Cider, Walnuts, and
        Prunes, 377
Water drinking, 121, 219
Watermelon
    Strawberry-Watermelon Slush, 409
Web site(s)
    with diet analysis tools, 94
    Sugar Solution, 23
Weight control, from stress management, 188
Weight gain, causes of, <u>39</u>, 187, <u>198</u>
Weight lifting. *See* Strength training
Weight loss
    breakfast for maintaining, 93
    diet analysis tools for, 94
    for metabolic syndrome, 259
    for polycystic ovary syndrome, 285, 287
    for prediabetes reversal, 266, 267
    promoters of
        attitude adjustments, 99
        blood sugar control, 6, 7
        calcium, 65
        fun fitness opportunities, 24–25
        low-GI diet, 19–20, 21–23, 59, 60, 63
        nuts, 67

protein, 64
        sleep, 25–26
        treats, 68–69
    saboteurs of, 98
Whole foods, <u>216</u>
Whole grains
    for blood sugar control, 16
    bread crumbs, 113
    breads, <u>216</u>
    for breakfast, 93
    cereals, 104
    flour, 105, 110, 113–14
    health benefits from, 57–60, 74
    menu choices of, 57
    pastas, 113, <u>217</u>
    for prediabetes reversal, 267
    preparation of, 74
    recommended servings of, 57
    uses for, 112–13
Wine
    heart protection from, 17
    as treat, 68
Work
    easing commute to, 200–201
    handling deadlines at, 202
Worrying, exercise reducing, 199

Y

Yamax SW-200 Digi-Walker pedometer, <u>159</u>
Yoga, 191–93
Yogurt
    Baked Potatoes with Mushroom Stroganoff,
        391
    Berry Good Smoothie, 317
    Blueberry-Yogurt Muffins, 320
    Grilled Salmon with Mint-Cilantro Yogurt, 385
    Spicy Curried Vegetables, 395
    Whole Grain Crepes with Banana and
        Kiwifruit, 315

Z

Zinc, 88, 138
Zucchini
    Grilled Vegetable Melts, 344
    Grilled Vegetables, 352
    Lamb Kebabs, 381
    Ratatouille Pizza, 330
    Sicilian Sausage Stew, 337
    Stuffed Chicken Breasts, 366–67
    Zucchini Bites, 325
    Zucchini-Chocolate Chip Snack Cake, 404